Available From the American Academy of Pediatrics

Achieving a Healthy Weight for Your Child: ^ ~ ^ ~

ADHD: What Every Parent

Autism Spectrum Disorder: What Eve:

Building Resilience in Children and Teens: (

Caring for Your Adopted Child: An Essential Guide for Parents

Caring for Your Baby and Young Child: Birth to Age 5*

Caring for Your School-Age Child: Ages 5–12

Co-parenting Through Separation and Divorce: Putting Your Children First

Family Fit Plan: A 30-Day Wellness Transformation

Food Fights: Winning the Nutritional Challenges of Parenthood Armed With Insight, Humor, and a Bottle of Ketchup

Guide to Toilet Training

My Child Is Sick! Expert Advice for Managing Common Illnesses and Injuries

Parenting Through Puberty: Mood Swings, Acne, and Growing Pains

The Picky Eater Project: 6 Weeks to Happier, Healthier Family Mealtimes

Raising an Organized Child: 5 Steps to Boost Independence, Ease Frustration, and Promote Confidence

Raising Kids to Thrive: Balancing Love With Expectations and Protection With Trust

Retro Baby: Cut Back on All the Gear and Boost Your Baby's Development With More Than 100 Time-tested Activities

Retro Toddler: More Than 100 Old-School Activities to Boost Development

Waking Up Dry: A Guide to Help Children Overcome Bedwetting

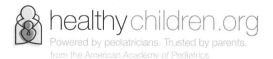

For additional parenting resources, visit the HealthyChildren bookstore at https://shop.aap.org/for-parents.

*This book is also available in Spanish.

Quirky Kids

Updated Edition

Understanding and Supporting Your Child With Developmental Differences

Perri Klass, MD, FAAP
Eileen Costello, MD, FAAP

American Academy of Pediatrics
DEDICATED TO THE HEALTH OF ALL CHILDREN®

American Academy of Pediatrics Publishing Staff

Mary Lou White, *Chief Product and Services Officer/SVP, Membership, Marketing, and Publishing*
Mark Grimes, *Vice President, Publishing*
Kathryn Sparks, *Senior Editor, Consumer Publishing*
Jason Crase, *Senior Manager, Production and Editorial Services*
Shannan Martin, *Production Manager, Consumer Publications*
Sara Hoerdeman, *Marketing Manager, Consumer Products*

Published by the American Academy of Pediatrics
345 Park Blvd
Itasca, IL 60143
Telephone: 630/626-6000
Facsimile: 847/434-8000
www.aap.org

The American Academy of Pediatrics is an organization of 67,000 primary care pediatricians, pediatric medical subspecialists, and pediatric surgical specialists dedicated to the health, safety, and well-being of all infants, children, adolescents, and young adults.

The information contained in this publication should not be used as a substitute for the medical care and advice of your pediatrician. There may be variations in treatment that your pediatrician may recommend based on individual facts and circumstances.

Statements and opinions expressed are those of the authors and not necessarily those of the American Academy of Pediatrics.

Any websites, brand names, products, or manufacturers are mentioned for informational and identification purposes only and do not imply an endorsement by the American Academy of Pediatrics (AAP). The AAP is not responsible for the content of external resources. Information was current at the time of publication.

The persons whose photographs are depicted in this publication are professional models. They have no relation to the issues discussed. Any characters they are portraying are fictional.

The publishers have made every effort to trace the copyright holders for borrowed materials. If they have inadvertently overlooked any, they will be pleased to make the necessary arrangements at the first opportunity.

This publication has been developed by the American Academy of Pediatrics. The contributors are expert authorities in the field of pediatrics. No commercial involvement of any kind has been solicited or accepted in development of the content of this publication. Disclosures: The authors report no conflicts of interest.

Every effort is made to keep *Quirky Kids* consistent with the most recent advice and information available from the American Academy of Pediatrics.

Special discounts are available for bulk purchases of this publication. Email Special Sales at nationalaccounts@aap.org for more information.

© 2021 Perri Klass, MD, FAAP, and Eileen Costello, MD, FAAP

All rights reserved. No part of this publication may be reproduced, stored in a retrieval system, or transmitted in any form or by any means—electronic, mechanical, photocopying, recording, or otherwise—without prior permission from the publisher (locate title at http://ebooks.aappublications.org and click on © Get permissions; you may also fax the permissions editor at 847/434-8780 or email permissions@aap.org). First edition © 2003 Ballantine Books as *Quirky Kids: Understanding and Helping Your Child Who Doesn't Fit In—When to Worry and When Not to Worry.*

The American Academy of Pediatrics would like to acknowledge the permission granted to reprint previously published material:

From A WRINKLE IN TIME © 1962 by Madeleine L'Engle. Reprinted by permission of Farrar, Straus and Giroux Books for Young Readers. All Rights Reserved.

From EASY WAY OUT by Stephen McCauley. Copyright © 1992 by Stephen McCauley. Reprinted with the permission of Simon & Schuster, Inc. All rights reserved.

From *To Kill a Mockingbird* by Harper Lee. Copyright © 1960, renewed 1988 by Harper Lee. Used by permission of HarperCollins Publishers.

Excerpt(s) from CELESTIAL NAVIGATION by Anne Tyler, copyright © 1974 by Anne Tyler Modarressi. Used by permission of Alfred A. Knopf, an imprint of the Knopf Doubleday Publishing Group, a division of Penguin Random House LLC. All rights reserved.

Excerpt(s) from BUDDENBROOKS: THE DECLINE OF A FAMILY by Thomas Mann, translated by John E. Woods, translation copyright © 1993 by Penguin Random House LLC. Used by permission of Alfred A. Knopf, an imprint of the Knopf Doubleday Publishing Group, a division of Penguin Random House LLC. All rights reserved.

From *Marjorie Morningstar* by Herman Wouk. Copyright © 1955 by Penguin/Random House. Used by permission of the Estate of Herman Wouk.

Printed in the United States of America
9-451/0221   1 2 3 4 5 6 7 8 9 10
CB0119
ISBN: 978-1-61002-419-8
eBook: 978-1-61002-420-4
EPUB: 978-1-61002-422-8
Kindle: 978-1-61002-423-5

Cover design by Rattray Design
Publication design by Peg Mulcahy

Library of Congress Control Number: 2020930664

What People Are Saying About *Quirky Kids*

"Every child is one of a kind, right from the start. But what about when the differences that make your child unique are uniquely challenging—at home, at the playground, at school, in life? With an empowering mix of accessible information, reasoned advice, realistic strategies, honesty, empathy, and perspective, *Quirky Kids* will guide you through the complex, sometimes frustrating, often draining, ultimately uniquely rewarding process of parenting and nurturing your uniquely quirky child."

–Heidi Murkoff, author of the *What to Expect* series of pregnancy and parenting books, creator of WhattoExpect.com, and founder of the What to Expect Project

"It's all too common for parents of developmentally different kids to feel isolated, ostracized, and confused. This book, written with uncommon clarity and compassion by Drs Klass and Costello, is an incredibly valuable resource for parents, family members, and friends of children who have their own special way of interacting with the world."

–Seth Mnookin, director of the Massachusetts Institute of Technology Graduate Program in Science Writing and author of *The Panic Virus*

"The ultimate comprehensive guidebook by 2 pediatricians whose comforting advice comes from years of professional experience. From early suspicion that something is different, to high school graduation, and into adulthood, this book covers all of the issues parents of quirky children face. It offers practical strategies and suggestions for getting a diagnosis, medication, disclosure, education, socialization, and managing life at home."

–Dania Jekel, MSW, executive director, Asperger/Autism Network (AANE)

Praise for the First Edition

"Highly recommended…Practical, compassionate, and thorough."

–Library Journal (starred review)

"Reassuring but frank, Klass and Costello walk parents through the steps of helping a quirky child, beginning with talking to the child's pediatrician, coping with the parents' sense of loss of a perfect child, getting a diagnosis and negotiating the maze of evaluations and evaluators….a good place for parents of quirky kids to start their research."

–Publishers Weekly

"Terrific…Thoroughly researched…An exceptional resource for anyone working to provide the best care for children with special needs."

–The Plain Dealer

"A wise and profoundly comforting book."

–Michael Thompson, PhD, coauthor of *Raising Cain*

"A superb, original, hugely needed book…The first and the definitive guide to understanding these marvelous kids. Free of jargon, full of facts and wisdom and practical advice."

–Edward M. Hallowell, MD, coauthor of *Driven to Distraction*

"As I read this wonderful and helpful book, I kept nodding in agreement: 'Yes, this is right, this is good, very true!' Parents and pediatricians need this book. A+."

–Carol Stock Kranowitz, MA, author of *The Out-of-Sync Child*

"Every parent of a 'quirky kid' needs this book."

–T. Berry Brazelton, MD

To our own families whose children we have taken care of,
with gratitude for all we've learned.

Contents

PART 1

A World of Quirky Kids

PART 2

Growing Up Quirky

PART 3

The Science, the Medical Science, and the Pseudoscience of Quirky Kids

PART 4

Looking Ahead

Acknowledgments

This book would not exist without the haven we were provided by the Ucross Foundation, in Ucross, WY, when we were writing the original edition. In the time we spent there, we found the opportunity to write, to think, and to talk, far from our clinical practices, our chaotic homes, and, of course, our 6 much-loved children.

To write this book, we interviewed a number of specialists and experts in fields ranging from special education to speech pathology. Many parents and grandparents generously agreed to be interviewed for this book and spent time and trouble detailing for us the complex and often very moving stories of the roads they had traveled with their children. Their accounts enriched our understanding of the subject, and we feel that their voices, as included in the text, enrich and illuminate everything we have written. They are the real experts, and the real champions. All of the names of the children have been changed, along with certain identifying details; we have taken some liberties in updating diagnoses and occasionally creating some composite accounts. We thank the children and their families.

Many professional colleagues took time from their busy schedules to talk with us about their experience and to read sections of the manuscript. This book draws on many specialized fields, and we are not experts in any of them. As practicing general pediatricians, we send our patients to the experts we most trust for further evaluation and advice, and we were incredibly fortunate that many of these same experts—those who actually evaluate and treat our patients and those whose writings and teachings have meant most to the parents we see and to us as well—were willing to help make this book more accurate, more representative, and more authoritative. We want to thank the many American Academy of Pediatrics experts who reviewed the content in this updated edition for technical and medical accuracy. We would also like to express our gratitude to colleagues who helped with the first edition of the book, some of whom may not even remember those conversations, and to the many friends and colleagues who have helped shape our thinking since 2003. The late Elsa Abele, professor of speech and language pathology at Boston University, was a tireless advocate for all quirky kids and a great inspiration. The staff at the Autism/Asperger Network (AANE) has been an enormous source of support and knowledge over the years since publication of the first edition. We are especially grateful to Dania Jekel, executive director of the AANE, for her review of and helpful comments about the chapters on disclosure and family life.

Marilyn Augustyn, MD, chief of developmental and behavioral pediatrics at Boston Medical Center and professor of pediatrics at Boston University School of Medicine, gave us the benefit of her expertise and experience pertaining to the issues of diagnosis, therapies, and school services. She is a powerful advocate for children from underserved communities in need of evaluation and services, and she reviewed the diagnosis chapter. We are extremely grateful for her input, which has made this edition better.

Andrea Spencer, MD, assistant professor of child and adolescent psychiatry at Boston University School of Medicine and director of the integrated behavioral health program at Boston Medical Center, reviewed Chapter 10, Medications and the Quirky Child: Drugs, Doses, and Daily Routines, and offered her expertise on the use of psychotropic medications to ease the burden on kids and families. Her insights have been invaluable to us.

We thank our colleagues in pediatric primary care at Boston Medical Center and Bellevue Hospital and our supportive chairs, Dr Bob Vinci, chairman of pediatrics at Boston University School of Medicine and Boston Medical Center, and Dr Catherine Manno, chair of pediatrics at New York University.

Our families, of course, have contributed to this book in a wide variety of ways. It's probably true, as we said earlier, that this book would not exist if we hadn't escaped them for a little while, but it is certainly true that it would not exist without their inspiration and support. They taught us much of what we know about the vagaries and realities of family life, and they put up with our often haphazard mothering styles. We would like to thank all 6 of our children—Nolan, Geoffrey, Isaac, Orlando, Josephine, and Anatol—for the many lessons on the limits of parental and pediatric wisdom and, of course, for the recurring joys that make everything else worthwhile. Larry Wolff cheered Perri on through all the stages of putting the book together and has been especially adept at identifying interestingly quirky adult specimens in the halls of higher academe. David Taylor supported Eileen with his life wisdom and culinary alacrity.

Last, with profound humility and gratitude, we thank the many children and families who have allowed us, as pediatricians, into their lives; we learn constantly from our patients and their parents, and we hope that with this book we may give back to families some of what we have learned in a way that will help them on their own journeys.

Introduction

You're worried about a child you love. There's something different, something off, something eccentric, something quirky. You want to understand what's going on, and most of all, you want to help. Your job as a parent is to help your child grow and develop and learn and thrive, and to do that job properly, you have to understand your child as an individual, quirks and all. The world is full of quirky kids. They live with us in our houses, but they live in slightly different zones, seeing the world around them through idiosyncratic lenses, walking just a little out of step, marching and even dancing to the beat of different drummers.

> As Aidan got older, I noticed more and more his inability to interact with other kids and his lack of interest in activities. I tried to take a music class with him. He had no interest whatsoever. He would not participate. He was more interested in the lights in the room, the stuff on the bulletin board, the numbers and letters. I felt so mad at him: "Why won't he do what the other kids do?"

The kids we are calling "quirky" are the ones who do things differently. Maybe you've noticed developmental variations—a child who doesn't talk on time or, alternatively, talks constantly but can't get a point across. Or maybe there's something about your child's temperament that makes daily life a challenge: a rigid need for absolute routine, a propensity for nuclear tantrums. Or perhaps you're uncomfortably aware of social difficulties because your toddler is always alone while the rest of the playgroup lives up to its name. These are the differences—skewed development, temperamental extremes, social complications—that define the group of quirky kids. As pediatricians and mothers, we are in contact with kids every day, and we have become interested in the quirky kids among us. Here are the voices of three parents telling us about three very different children:

> The weekend I decided our son, John, had autism—he was 3—we were on Cape Cod, and it was overwhelming for him. He put his arms around this little tiny tree and shook back and forth the entire weekend. He was wearing a sleeper with feet and sneakers, he was wearing a watch, and he was hanging on to this tree. And I said to my husband, "I think he's autistic—this is so far off the curve."

Caitlin is good at math, but she can get completely stuck if there is a typo in the word problem. She's idiosyncratic. She cannot stand to estimate; she must have a precise answer. If the graph paper doesn't have enough lines, she gets stuck.

Trevor is an anxious child who now, at the age of 9, very much wants to be like other kids and wants the other kids to like him. He's an avid baseball fan and player, and that has helped him out in the social area, but he still has some autistic-type behaviors, like running in circles when he is excited. He writes or draws in the air when he is bored or feels uncomfortable.

Forty or 50 years ago, these kids would have been thought of as odd or eccentric, but they would not have undergone medical or psychiatric assessments, and they would not have been given diagnoses. Nowadays, you may find that helping your quirky child grow up involves coping with a formal diagnosis or often multiple diagnoses or diagnoses that shift and change as the child grows. This book is not about the children diagnosed with severe developmental delay and intellectual disability or major mental illness. They are outside the scope of what we define as "quirky," and there is a great deal of specific expertise out there to help parents get them the help and support they need. We are talking about a group of children who inhabit a grayer zone, a zone of characteristics also found in typically developing children, a zone of overlapping diagnoses and evolving terminology. Some of them never need any special services or therapies, and they follow their own eccentric paths through school and through life, accomplishing all kinds of wonderful and unusual things. But others struggle, and nowadays, that usually means medical attention. You may find, for example, that concerns will be raised about whether your child has autism spectrum disorder, nonverbal learning disability, or social (pragmatic) communication disorder. Depending on their strengths and weaknesses, as well as on who does the diagnosing, children may also be diagnosed with sensory processing disorder, social phobia, or attention-deficit/hyperactivity disorder. It's important to note that these are all relatively recent diagnostic categories that may be used to describe children who, when we were young, might have just been called "eccentric"—or maybe harsher schoolyard names.

We're calling them *quirky kids*. We prefer this term for a reason. It's not pejorative. In fact, it's sometimes a compliment. But it does suggest the unusual features—challenging yet often charming—shared by an increasing number of children in our society. We don't mean to minimize the seriousness of your concerns or the pain that comes with worrying about a child, but it's also true that everyone gets only one childhood, one family, one set of parents. Look for ways to enjoy and appreciate the child you have, even as you look for answers and help.

The Purpose of This Book

This book is not an exhaustive resource and is not intended to enable you to diagnose your child. We don't recommend that. We do recommend arming yourself with as much knowledge as possible. You will find that it helps on this journey if you know more about the assessment process, the professionals who might help you and your child along the way, the therapies and medications that might be recommended, and what to expect as your child grows up. We'll try to be honest about our prejudices. We speak from a medical perspective, from within the pediatric profession. Still, we'll include plenty of quotes from parents who have felt ill-served by our professional colleagues, as well as from parents who have found help and support, and we'll help you get the best that medicine can offer.

Parents come to see us with stories and with patterns, habits, and behaviors that they've noticed in their babies and toddlers, preschoolers, and elementary school–aged children, and they ask for our opinion. Is this normal? Is something wrong? We hear stories about toddlers whose tantrums seem off the scale in comparison with their siblings, about young children with intense obsessive interests, about children who don't talk on schedule or who do talk but in peculiar ways, about children who don't enjoy the games that delight the other children in the playgroup. We hear about strong preferences and prejudices—children's habits and routines that can come to dominate an entire family. All of these parents look to us, the professionals who see hundreds and hundreds of children grow, for a little perspective and often a little help, if a child is struggling.

As we watch parents struggle with a multitude of assessments, diagnoses, therapies, and medications, we have come to appreciate that life with a quirky child can be complex and difficult. We wrote this book to help you navigate and do what you most want to do: know and recognize and appreciate these remarkable children and help them grow and thrive. Everything you do—looking for the right diagnosis, investigating possible therapies, looking for the best possible school, setting guidelines for life at home—is directed toward that end. It is by that standard that you should judge any advice you receive—including ours. Helping your quirky child become the person that child was meant to be will involve getting to know and understand a remarkable individual.

Why This Book Is Important

In practicing primary care pediatrics in Boston and New York, we see hundreds of families each year. That means that we are *generalists*, the regular pediatricians who are often the first people parents come to when they are worried. We send children to developmental-behavioral pediatricians and neurologists, psychiatrists and neuropsychologists, and physical and occupational therapists, and we assist parents in thinking about what is helpful. Between us, we have reared 6 children of our own. As mothers, we have had our share of visits to the pediatrician, referrals to specialists, teacher conferences, and childhood social snarls to untangle. We worked together for many years, starting as residents in training, and we have swapped many stories over the years about our own kids and the kids with whom we work. Like all pediatricians in this fortunate modern era of pediatrics, we see fewer serious infections than our colleagues did a few decades ago, and we find ourselves talking about child development much more than did those previous generations of pediatricians, who were busier with measles and meningitis.

In this book we tell you what we have learned from our practice, as well as from our colleagues in child development, child neurology, and psychiatry, about the spectrum of developmental differences and disorders, the patterns and problems and solutions that recur in the lives of quirky children. We offer help at every stage, from the early worries of virtually all parents who suspect they have children who tend toward the quirky to the successes and surprises and setbacks we have witnessed as these kids grow to adulthood.

We have tried not to make gender-based assumptions about children or adults, that is, not to assume that the sports-obsessed child is necessarily a boy or that the child who is obsessed with Barbies is a girl. We also did not assume that all children will grow up to have binary gender identities or, for that matter, that all children have a father and a mother or that all elementary schoolteachers are women. In fact, quirky kids have a higher rate of questioning their assigned gender, which we discuss later in the book. We sometimes alternate between the pronouns *he* and *she*, although we acknowledge that some kids will grow up to prefer a different pronoun.

We want to acknowledge that many children receive their primary care from family physicians and nurse practitioners, and we have tried to use terms such as *provider* and *clinician* to include everyone; however, we are both pediatricians, and some of what we write involves looking in the professional mirror, so we do occasionally use the term *pediatrician*, sometimes when we are talking about ourselves and also when we are talking about parents who feel their children's pediatricians may have dismissed their concerns.

We bring this up because we have spoken with many parents who feel they *knew* something was wrong yet had their concerns dismissed by pediatricians. We have also known many parents who worried desperately for awhile, only to see their children outgrow their problems. As pediatricians, we understand the dilemma well; when you have seen the full range of "typically developing" children, as well as the range of quirky kids, you often feel that the proverbial "tincture of time" is well worth a try. Many kids do outgrow so many things. Yet, there are situations in which an early assessment and early assistance can make a big difference.

This book follows children as they grow out of toddlerhood and into the pre-school years, when it's often easier to see which children are really off the scale and may not be able to manage well in their preschools and schools because of their developmental issues, social difficulties, or unusual learning styles.

We take you through the preschool and kindergarten years and into elementary school, looking at the kinds of evaluation that may help pinpoint your child's needs as well as the therapies and school settings that can improve relevant skills and offer a quirky child the most comfortable setting for growth and learning. We talk about finding the right teacher—and helping teachers do their jobs once you've found them. Although many quirky kids can function well in a regular education setting, others need additional supports, such as an aide in the classroom or a more specialized school environment. We discuss these situations in detail.

We talk about how things go at home—about your quirky child, your other children, your extended family—and even about what you as parents may experience. We talk about bedtime and mealtime and homework and birthday parties, the daily details of life that get shifted, a little or a lot, when living with a quirky child. We also talk about friends and come back to those social scenarios we mentioned; how do you help your child connect with other children and maneuver in the childhood social world?

We also help you anticipate the inevitable issues that child-rearing will present: how to talk about these sometimes prickly topics with relatives and friends; what and when and whether the child needs to know about what's going on; the effect on your other children, your marriage, and your other adult relationships as well as on you. We will remind you to take care of yourself so you can take care of your child. It's easy to get lost in the maze of appointments, therapies, expert recommendations, internet information, and bestselling books. But, in fact, as your child's parent and strongest advocate, as the one who knows and loves and appreciates this child best, you are fully capable of deciding what is and is not useful. Keep a healthy dose of skepticism and remember that this is *your* child. Don't listen to anyone—including us—who tells you something that doesn't jibe with what you know about your child. But do keep an open mind. Listen and learn, and at the same time trust your instincts and trust yourself to do the best by your own particular quirky kid.

As we worked on revising this book, the world was struggling with the coronavirus pandemic, with much disease, many deaths, and many schools closed. The long-term effects of this virus on our health and well-being are still unknown, and, of course, we cannot even predict what the situation will be by the time you are reading this, though we hope very much that the world will be in better shape. We do know, from talking with many families of quirky kids over recent months, that the pandemic brought disruptions in services and treatments, which worried parents concerned about their children's development, educational progress, emotional well-being, and quality of life. Life was hard enough before the pandemic for many families with quirky children, but it got even harder—as it did for families everywhere. Routines were disrupted, parents were under economic pressure, and kids—quirky and not—found themselves staying home from school and trying to video in for class.

Quirky kids need routines, and the routines of school, activities, and therapies were suddenly not there for so many children. Parents asked how to cope with the demands when they were suddenly thrust into the role of teacher, playmate, speech therapist, or occupational therapist, all while running a household, in many cases working from home, and worrying about the future. Many parents faced furloughs or loss of work and income, as well as multiple caregiving responsibilities, including for other children and elderly parents, and it was even harder—and in many cases impossible—to bring help into the home. There was, of course, no single answer; each family situation was different, and issues varied with children and their different developmental stages, needs, and areas of difficulty.

Many of the suggestions we offered were the general suggestions being offered to all families—to have a schedule, to build routines, including healthy sleep routines, to be careful about screen time, to build in physical exercise, and to look for strategies to deal with anxiety. Quirky children are particularly vulnerable because they tend to be even more dependent on routines, are often prone to anxiety, and face disruptions in many of their support systems so painstakingly created by their parents and teachers. We want to recognize the valiant efforts of so many parents and hope that there will be additional support for them and their children as the world recovers.

Last, and probably most important, we keep reminding you to treasure your child and your child's childhood. Quirky children can be incredibly endearing and often very creative. Many have unique views of the world to offer. This book is written in the spirit of embracing these kids and fostering their good health and growth, while recognizing and addressing the inevitable challenges that childhood, school, and family life hold for them. We don't minimize the real difficulties and heartaches of loving and living with a child who is different from other children, but we do urge you to not let those differences define your entire family, your feelings about your child, your sense of yourself. The frustrations and irritations you may feel at times are real, but so are the joys and the pride you will take in your child's victories and accomplishments. There also will be unexpected insights, the special quirky moments when you realize that your child's unusual perspective has enlarged and enriched the world.

PART

A World of Quirky Kids

What You Should Know

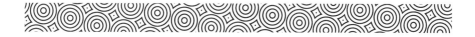

Let's start where most parents start: noticing that something is different, wondering what it means, and dealing with the emotional ramifications of that worry. There's no standard story here because quirky kids' behaviors are outside the common patterns. They have a hard time fitting in. What comes easily to other children is hard for them. In particular, their ability to socialize with other children is impaired—sometimes mildly, sometimes severely. They may have unusual interests bordering on obsessions and insist on restricting the conversation to these topics. They may have trouble fitting into the physical environment as well, finding themselves overwhelmed by sensations or sounds that the typical child wouldn't notice. They tend to be anxious, often unchildlike. Other kids don't always know how to deal with them, which is hardly surprising since their own families sometimes don't know either. In addition, their development is not by the book. Although eventually all of them walk and talk, they don't follow the expected time course, and they often have great difficulty with particular milestones. Developmentally and socially, these children are different.

Emma is 10 now, and she's obsessively interested in cats. If she did a self-portrait or portraits of her family, they would be of cats and cat families. She hates loud noises. Restaurants are too loud. Fireworks are overwhelming. She cannot stand the loudness of the toilet flushing or the bath being drawn. Someone has to do that for her. Then she is happy to take her bath.

George always had unusual obsessions, especially with the vacuum cleaner. We have photos of him hugging the vacuum cleaner at 6 months of age. When he was older, he drew pictures of the vacuum and talked about it all the time. He had phobias as well. One was a phobia of pinecones, not especially functional given that we live in a neighborhood with lots of towering pine trees.

3

We're going to start in early childhood, but as we all know, parenthood is for life, and we might as well say now that we plan to stick with you as your children grow. By the end of this book, we'll be talking about quirky teenagers. Be aware that almost all parents fear the complexities and turbulence of adolescence, but quirky kids can have an especially difficult time of it, given the often unforgiving culture of adolescence and the importance of fitting in. The more equipped the child and family are with knowledge and strategies for success, the better this time will be. Still, it will not be easy. To be fair, no one, quirky or not, is guaranteed an easy time of it in adolescence, and you have the opportunity to plan ahead and strategize with your child and with people who know your child so that supports are in place.

Adults are much more accepting than children and teenagers, and many quirky kids thrive in college or vocational schools where they can pursue their interests. Look around you. Quirky adults are everywhere: Think about the bonsai grower at the flower show who knows everything there is to know about bonsai and talks bonsai all day long and goes home to read about bonsai. Look at your family; is that math professor uncle of yours a quirky kid grown up?

The truth is, as every worried parent knows, that not every quirky child grows up to be a successful but quirky independent adult. However, the ability to succeed in life and to function independently depends on the whole package that is your developing child, not just the quirky aspects. The children we are discussing make up a varied group: from the mildly eccentric to those who will turn out to be more severely hampered in their daily lives. As we worked on this book, we tried to be mindful of this range. We know that to the parent of a child struggling desperately in school and at home and taking 3 different medications, it will seem patronizing and even callous to talk about quirkiness in a tone that suggests that eccentricity is charming and that quirky is a synonym for genius. As one mother said to us:

I'm so cynical about all the people who say that kids with special needs are "special," that there is some profound joy in taking care of them. If there is a beautiful side to this, I am still waiting for someone to point it out to me.

On the other hand, we don't want to make things sound too bleak or as if early differences mean that your life's destiny is set in stone. Many of these kids manage just fine. And many parents, especially when the children are doing well, do find much joy in their children and take pride in their achievements.

We see so many good things about Chrissie—her optimistic spirit, her warmth, her fun-loving personality, her offbeat sense of humor—that a lot of the time, we don't think about the stress that her problems have caused.

The more tools children have for understanding their differences, coping with their difficulties, and playing to their strengths, the greater the likelihood of having functional and sometimes quite wonderful adulthoods. There is a club—centered perhaps at Massachusetts Institute of Technology—of very successful nerds, and many of them went through hard times along the way. There are adults who make careers of their obsessions and those who find their way into the helping professions as nurses, counselors, or physicians precisely because they understand these struggles so personally. We have talked with a number of adults who, in retrospect, clearly fell into this group of distinctly quirky kids as they were growing up, before their parents or pediatricians had any way to evaluate their struggles or knew how to help. Many of their child-hood stories are heartbreaking, and, yes, some are struggling with adult issues of intimacy or with occupational difficulties, but there is much to be learned from them. Many needed extra help along the way—a little or a lot—and you have the opportunity, as a parent, to look for ways for your child to receive that help and encouragement. We want to help you do that, and to feel that you, and your child, are not alone.

1

My Kid Is Different: Wondering and Worrying

So what do you do when you're worried about your child? You wonder and worry, you scope out other children, you read books on child development and parenting magazines, and you go online looking for help. And you reach for your strengths as a family. You talk with your spouse or partner, your best friend, your own parents, or your child care teacher. Maybe you lock up all the worry inside and say nothing to anyone because you can't help feeling that by speaking the words, you will make them come true. Finally, you usually ask your child's doctor. Maybe you make a special appointment and come in to discuss your concerns, or maybe you just wait for your child's next checkup to mention it, more or less in passing, hoping to be reassured. Part of our job as pediatricians is to evaluate babies and young children and decide whether their development is proceeding normally and on schedule.

We see our patients for a brief amount of time, often at moments when they are feeling more than a little bit stressed out. No young child loves going to the pediatrician's office. Think of the 1-year-old, cranky after a long stint in the waiting room, less than eager to be handled by a stranger and maybe remembering all too well that this chilly room is where they sometimes stick you with needles. So, as pediatricians, we examine kids and watch how they behave, but we rely most of all on parents to tell us what's going on. We know that many behavioral and developmental problems are subtle and difficult to identify, and we worry that we may be missing something. On the other hand, part of our job is to reassure. If we sent every child who takes a little longer to walk for a full orthopedic, neurological, and developmental assessment, we would hardly be doing anyone any favors—not to mention what would happen if everyone who was a little slow to talk underwent a full oral-motor workup and brain scan. You want to partner with your child's primary care provider, you want to keep the conversation going, and you want to be able to come back with more questions.

Is Something Really Going On?

All children have bad hours, bad days, and even bad weeks. Many children experience difficult developmental stages or find particular developmental tasks frustrating and even miserable. Many parents who at some point consider requesting diagnostic workups and medical and developmental evaluations end up looking back on what turned out to be nothing more than a difficult episode in an otherwise relatively straightforward childhood. A persistent worry doesn't tell you what the end result is going to be, but it does signal a need to pay attention and ask the right questions.

Medical students famously diagnose themselves with every syndrome they study. And as pediatrician parents, reading about children and the various things that can go wrong in their health or development, we measure our own children against the most ominous medical syndromes.

But if you've picked up this book, your concern is more than the occasional reflexive anxiety that falls under the heading of parental love. You may be worried that your child is developmentally different in a significant way. You may be watching your child struggle in ways that other children don't seem to. You may already have started making your way through the maze of diagnoses and assessments, and a diagnosis—or a label or formulation—may have been assigned to your child. But wherever you and your child are in this journey, it probably began with worries that in some way this child was different; such worries didn't disappear with the morning sun or when teething ended or move to the back burner when you found a better child care center.

Early Signs

For many parents, this nagging worry that something is wrong begins early in the child's life. Maybe it's an unusually intense expression of a standard developmental stage: the infant whose colic doesn't end at 12 weeks or the toddler whose tantrums reflect an underlying frustration out of proportion to that of the average 2-year-old. Maybe it's an unusual pattern of behavior or interaction—the baby who won't make eye contact, the toddler who plays obsessively with only 1 or 2 toys and insists on lining them up. Or perhaps you're looking at developmental delays or differences that are just too numerous or intense to write off as a variant of normal.

We knew John was different from the beginning. He had a lot of trouble learning how to nurse. I remember this nurse at the hospital saying he's got a sucking disorder. I knew once I got him home, he would be fine. He was, but he nearly starved to death in the process. It was 3 or 4 days before he got the hang of it. Then, for the first 4 months, it went OK. I went back to work, started giving him some formula. But he couldn't make the transition to eating. His intake started dwindling. I remember thinking, "It's because I've gone back to work." He couldn't figure out what to do with baby food when it was in his mouth, and from 4 to 9 months of age, he had a totally flat growth curve—didn't gain any weight at all.

I first noticed differences between Abby and other kids as early as 2 months. We were in a playgroup, and I felt Abby wasn't with it to the extent the other babies were. Her fists remained clenched longer than theirs, she slept more, her motor milestones were slower even at that young age. Throughout her first year, I referred to all the usual books about milestones, and I couldn't relate to any of them.

These parents are looking back on the infancies of children who turned out to be genuinely quirky. For most of us, going forward, these early anxieties are more nebulous. You have this sense that your child just doesn't fit—doesn't fit the books, doesn't fit the group, doesn't fit your expectations. You listen to other parents, and you feel more and more certain that something in your own home is out of step.

So let's take a look at the kinds of concerns that often nag at parents and can send them looking for help and advice.

Developmental Milestones

Comprehensive lists of developmental milestones are available for parents who want to check out whether their children are keeping up with the normal trajectories (we recommend the milestones posted by the American Academy of Pediatrics on its website for parents: HealthyChildren.org). In this section, we take a somewhat more global look at the kinds of concerns that parents often have, which may be less about a particular age-related milestone than about a general sense that something is off, usually regarding the child's general behavior, language and communication skills, or social development—and often all 3 areas. We provide a few basic yardsticks for measuring general development and a website to visit for a more detailed tool. We also encourage you to follow up on your worries even if there is no specific missed milestone on which to pin them. And if your child has actually lost milestones—that is, has regressed in development so that speech or social skills are less advanced than they used to be—you should seek help immediately.

Temperament and Behavior

Parents may become concerned because their children's temperaments seem extreme: incredibly irritable, as if they are not quite comfortable in their own skin, desperately needy, or chronically frustrated. These are babies who arch, shriek as if in frequent pain, and never seem to settle down. They're the fitful, disorganized sleepers, or maybe the toddlers who don't seem to need any sleep at all.

> Andrew didn't sleep. We would walk him around. He was uneasy right from the beginning. He threw up all the time. He wouldn't eat. He had repetitive behaviors. The early intervention people would come with toys, and he would just open and close the doors but not play with the toys.
>
> I had planned to go back to work when George was 6 or 7 weeks old and put him in child care. I couldn't actually leave him there. He was just too delicate, and he actually had separation anxiety at 6 weeks. He always had a worried look on his face. He was an anxious, hyperaroused baby.

More rare are babies who are remarkably, even disturbingly, placid and don't seem to demand anything from the world. They're easier to care for, but their parents may become troubled—and rightly so—that they are somehow out of touch. Babies aren't supposed to be easy; it's a rare one who is truly undemanding, and this may indeed be a red flag.

With older children, parents may note unusual behaviors, repetitive movements such as spinning, hand-flapping, or rocking. They may run in circles and flap their hands whenever they become agitated. A child may constantly touch or spin or roll a particular object, ignoring all other toys.

Think about whether you're looking at repetitive behaviors, extraordinarily rigid routines, or any evidence, as children grow, of obsessional behaviors. One question to ask yourself is whether your family's daily routines are dictated by these aspects of your child's temperament. Do you truly live in fear of the meltdowns that occur if regular rituals are varied? Does the family's equilibrium depend on keeping this child calm?

As they grow out of the toddler stage, quirky kids may have difficulty transitioning from one activity to another. They may throw outrageous tantrums that last longer than routine toddler rages and that continue well after the child should have outgrown them. They also may exhibit extreme sensitivity to sensory stimuli and be unable to tolerate things that are routine for other kids, such as the noise of a movie sound track, the sensation of water on skin, or the motion of a swing at the playground.

What comes easily to most children can be terribly difficult for quirky kids. If you are watching your child struggle with some of the routine activities of daily life, and if your family life is being reshaped to accommodate a young child's needs and preferences because the child cannot accommodate others at all, it may be time to look more carefully at that child. Daily life shouldn't hurt.

Speech and Language

During the first 3 years, many parents become concerned about speech and language, noticing that the child is slow to develop speech or seems uninterested in the speech of others. All children with a true delay in speech should get tested for hearing loss, which is a rare and treatable cause of delays. Quirky kids may have normal speech and language development, but something is off. They may ignore human voices, for example, but respond to a certain tune played by a music box or on a favorite TV show. Some are slow to speak, but others speak early and precociously and, in fact, use their speech and language to manifest early obsessions.

> Aidan spoke early. He started talking at 9 months and knew the alphabet at 12 months; he could recognize some of the letters. By 18 months, he insisted on learning phonics. He read early and became interested in numbers, directions, things like that.

> Emma's language was slow to develop, and we used to say she spoke "Emmaese." She prattled on in her own language, which was incomprehensible to anyone else. By 2½, she babbled but did not talk at all. She did respond to speech. She always loved music and Disney movies. I just sensed that she was off the beam early on.

While some quirky kids are speech delayed and therefore use other forms of communication when they're young (eg, screaming, pointing, making grunting sounds, pulling on a parent's clothes), others develop speech that follows the standard trajectory. They learn and speak words more or less on schedule (refer to the following milestones) but find themselves with impaired *language*—that is, they may know words and say them clearly and form sentences, but they can't use those words and sentences for the types of communication that come naturally for most children. A child may be able to talk endlessly about an obsession but be unable to carry on a basic conversation. She may develop functional language that allows her to ask for what she wants but have no interactive language. In other words, she might be able to say, "I want juice," but be incapable of saying, "This juice is good!" Some children can only use and understand concrete words for concrete objects.

Patterns of speaking may also raise a red flag. Children with *echolalia* repeat the last few words of whatever is said to them. Children who perseverate may ask the same question or make the same statement over and over. Finally, some quirky kids have "robotic speech," and whatever they say comes out in a strange monotonous tone.

Some speech milestones to watch for include

- A baby should babble by 6 months of age, and the babbling should increase in complexity and in how close it sounds to spoken language. Most infants start with vowel sounds and begin using consonants by around 6 months of age.
- Even though there are no words, babble is very much about communication and usually involves the baby responding to adult overtures or comments or soliciting adult attention; it can seem very much like a conversation.
- By 9 months of age, a baby should respond to his or her own name.
- By 15 to 18 months of age, a child should be able to say a couple of words and understand simple spoken instructions.
- By 18 months, most children are putting two words together: "go out" or "want cookie."
- By 2½ to 3 years of age, a child should be speaking in sentences, with a certain amount of fluency and inflection—that is, a question should sound like a question.
- By age 4, speech should be completely intelligible to those outside the child's family.

Social Interactions

Some quirky children are uninterested in toys, or they play with their toys in unusual ways—lining them up or fixating on certain textures and stroking them over and over. Some fixate on one particular object to the exclusion of everything else. Many parents become concerned when their infants or toddlers don't seem to look at them or engage in early games of peekaboo. Then, of course, there's the social outlier, the child who can't or won't join in the sandbox games, the circle time at child care, or the birthday party mob.

Looking back, I think Abby's total disinterest in toys was a clue and also interfered with her language development, which remains her greatest challenge today. I went to a playgroup meeting with Abby and her "wiggle worm," which looked brand new. Another mom asked, "How did you keep that so clean?" While the other child's was tattered and well worn, Abby's was so clean from never being used!

Caitlin was always determined and knew what she liked. For example, she liked a certain color, a bluish-green color, and before she could walk or talk, she would crawl over to the laundry basket to let me know that she wanted to wear something that was that color. She has had severe temper tantrums from early on. And at her first playgroup, she had no interest in the other kids. She just clung to me.

With the increased publicity in recent years devoted to early child development and to autism spectrum disorder, many more parents are making careful observations about their children's social skills, understanding that social problems are a hallmark of autism. Some key behaviors that may raise concern in an infant include failing to make eye contact and failing to pay attention to nearby conversations. In a toddler, parents might notice that the child doesn't really seem to care whether the parent is present or not. But other children may be extremely clingy, as in the previous story, or too anxious to be able to explore any new situation without holding onto a parent. Sometimes, these children are uninterested in "joint attention"—in joining with you—whether by pointing or talking or looking at something and thinking about it together. They may also display a lack of reciprocal play; when they're babies, they may not respond to their names or play peekaboo; when they're toddlers, they may be unwilling to acknowledge another child's presence, let alone join in a group game.

As children grow up, there are usually more opportunities to see them with their peers. You may be concerned about a child who bonds tightly to some unlikely object, such as a certain DVD, as one of our patients does, or who is completely uninterested in being around other children. Generally, these kids have trouble with imaginative play. They just don't understand what the other kids are doing. Hardest to watch for most parents is the child who is deeply interested in other children and eager for social contacts but goes about it all wrong and ends up crying, making someone else cry, or feeling left out.

Some social milestones to watch for include

- Babies younger than 4 months should make eye contact and respond with a social smile when a parent smiles.
- By 1 year of age, a child should be pointing and waving bye-bye.
- Children younger than 2 years enjoy being around other children but don't necessarily engage them in play activities.
- From the age of 2 years on, children should have real interactions (not all of them positive!) with one another and be able to play games that involve some back-and-forth.

Will Saying It Out Loud Make It "Real"?

There are irritable babies and placid babies, children who talk early and children who talk late. Plenty of children, quirky or not, fixate on one particular toy or transitional object and melt down if it gets left behind. But when parents of young children become concerned about some combination of communication patterns, unusual behaviors, social interactions, and developmental irregularities, those concerns may indicate a child who needs extra attention.

Other parents experience the early years of their child's life without noticing anything particularly concerning but then see problems emerge once the child leaves the cocoon of the family and starts school. Looking back, these parents often can see patterns and behaviors in infancy and during the toddler stage that they now understand are part of a larger pattern.

> In the toddler room at child care, I remember them saying about him, "Brian seems to be fine just as long as he is allowed to use the certain trucks he wants, and the kids have learned that if they just leave a 6-foot radius around Brian and his trucks, everything is fine." And I said "OK," and I just accepted it. I think they were trying to say something to me and I didn't want to hear.

The Pivotal Moment

For many parents, there is a pivotal moment when they acknowledge that something is really distressing. Maybe it's some public fiasco, a child who can't enjoy what other children can, a child who falls apart at what ought to be a treat. It's not that this one episode is so decisive, but viewed against a backdrop of many concerning behaviors and parental worries, a particular episode may make a parent feel that it's time to take action.

By age 2, Abby started avoiding things that she couldn't control and was extremely fearful—afraid of noises like the vacuum cleaner, afraid of being touched, afraid of unknown people or anything unpredictable, like someone laughing when she was in a group of people. She was too scared to go anywhere. There was an episode at the zoo. She was so scared of all the strangers that she screamed and clutched me until I decided to put her back in the car and go home. We realized we needed help right away.

Virtually every parent has a story of a public meltdown, a disastrous tantrum in a public place. One disaster does not a quirky child make. But, on the other hand, one extreme performance may be what it takes to crystallize in a parent's mind all the floating anxieties and worries of many months. Other pivotal moments involve extreme behavior that is impossible to explain away and that reinforces the parent's long-considered and long-avoided fears.

The thing that really pushed us over the edge with Brian was that when he was in second grade he developed a phobia about going to the bathroom. He had to know where the bathroom was and how to get to it before he could be comfortable anywhere. It made it difficult to drive in the car, visit a zoo or anyplace. He got anxious. He was having trouble making sense of the world. In retrospect, it was clearly an anxiety disorder.

Acknowledging Your Concerns

Many parents find it difficult to put their worries into words. Sometimes parents feel that articulating this kind of observation about a child will make it real, will stamp their child with a disorder. Sometimes, as a parent lives with a growing suspicion that something is wrong, there is comfort in putting off the discussion, the moment when the anxiety is admitted to another adult, who may confirm the observation. While we understand this, we also have tremendous respect for those deep parental concerns and instincts; you know your child better than anyone else does, and if you are worried, you need to be heard.

When Jacob was about 18 months old, I started noticing some backsliding in terms of development and the onset of some unusual behaviors. He liked to watch the washing machine spin around. He played soccer obsessively, and he was fascinated by numbers

on elevators. Also, by 21 months, he had lost most of his language
skills and his social skills, and he became much less affectionate
and less "connected" to other people. He began making strange
shrieking sounds; having severe, prolonged temper tantrums with
lots of screaming; and banging his head. He became fearful of
new people.

So you start searching for information about child development and find some
scary symptoms that seem to match those of your child, as well as many more
that don't. How do you decide whether your worries are real enough to warrant
follow-up? And what would that entail? And maybe most important of all, how
can you keep doing the job you need to do with your child and your family
while watching and worrying? Where are you going to go for help and advice?

Your Partner

It is not uncommon for one parent to be worried, usually the one who spends
the most one-on-one time with the child and possibly sees the child around
other children and makes comparisons. The other parent may be untroubled,
absolutely sure that everything is going to be fine. These discrepancies can be
a major source of tension, with one parent feeling that the other is in denial or
one parent furious that the other keeps looking for problems when nothing's
really wrong. Some of these gaps and disagreements can persist for years, well
beyond those early suspicions and into the process of diagnosis and treatment.

My husband took a lot longer to accept that there was something
wrong with John, having come from a family where everyone was
high-achieving. When we were around his family, nobody knew what
to say about our son.

Talking It Over With Your Partner

- Think about your different personalities. Does one of you tend to be the
  worrier, whatever the subject? Do you naturally fall into roles, with one
  parent raising problems and the other dismissing them? Acknowledge these
  patterns and try to get past them to talk about your child.
- Discussing your concerns with your partner may make them seem more
  real and may carry significant emotional weight for you both. If you aren't
  both convinced that there really is a problem, you might agree to watch and
  wait for a short, well-defined period now that the issue has been brought out
  into the open.

- Even if one parent remains convinced that nothing is really wrong, when the watchful waiting is over, if the problem isn't clearly resolved (the child has in fact started talking, stopped throwing tantrums, or found good friends at child care), agree on some reasonable plan of action for getting your concerns addressed.
- Remember that you are in it together. Whatever worries you nurture, whatever judgments you make, you are both driven by love and concern. Even if you don't agree, you need to treat each other well, take each other seriously, and take care of each other. Your child needs you both and needs you to be working as a team.
- Having said all this, we need to acknowledge—and salute—the many parents who are raising children without partners. It's really difficult to hold these worries alone, and it's important to have good friends or family members you trust so that you can talk things over, ideally with someone who knows and loves your child.

Talking It Over With Friends and Family

Taking your worries outside of your immediate family may seem like a big step. Some parents consult friends, sisters, brothers, or cousins right from the beginning, but many hold back, and often for very good reason. Talking with family members can result in lots of unsolicited advice or, worse, judgmental comments that you as parents have created a problem in your own child. Later in this book, in the "What You Should Know" section at the beginning of Part 2, we discuss the disclosure issues that come up with quirky kids. But here at the beginning, when you aren't sure what you have to tell, it might be wise to confide in a few carefully chosen people as you start looking for expert help and advice.

- Talk with a few trusted friends, but be wary of sharing all your worries and the tale of every stressful moment to everyone you know or who knows your child. You run the risk that a year from now, when your child may have outgrown some of the worrying behaviors, other people will still remember your child as the one who used to throw those tantrums or didn't have any friends in the 3-year-old room.
- If, in fact, your child does receive a specific diagnosis and has ongoing challenges, think carefully about whom you want to tell and what you want to say. At these early undefined stages, you might want to hold off. If everyone in your child's world knows all your worst fears, it may be hard to dial them down later and have them see your child clearly. Give yourself time to absorb and acknowledge any diagnosis so you understand it well before you find yourself explaining it to others.

- If you cast this particular net too widely—that is, tell everyone you know about your worries—you may encounter certain parents whose own children have some particular problem and who therefore see the world from that very particular perspective. As one pediatrician told us:

> The mother of one of my patients had a sister with a severely disabled child who kept telling her, "This was just how my son started." And it was terribly upsetting for this mother, whose own child had mild learning problems, but who felt that what her sister was saying meant her daughter was going to end up inevitably with all the same problems her sister's child had, while being treated with these same medications.

Your Pediatrician/Pediatric Primary Care Provider

Most people begin with their child's health care provider, usually a pediatrician, family practitioner, or nurse practitioner. Parents come to us all the time with developmental worries—sometimes straightforward ("How come my sister's child is a month younger and she already knows how to go up and down stairs?") and sometimes complex and difficult to define. We also often find ourselves in the situation of having to bring up developmental concerns with parents who have not been at all worried. Some pediatricians have additional training in behavior and development, and many others have at least a special interest in the area. But every pediatric primary care provider spends many hours examining babies and young children and has some idea of the range of typical behavior and development, as well as of the variations that lie on the fringes of that range. That is not to say that your pediatrician knows everything about child development. Nobody knows everything about development.

You and Your Provider: Making It Work

In books about children with developmental issues, you may find bitter accounts of doctors who missed the boat. Parents were worried, they knew something was going on, and the pediatrician dismissed their concerns, saying, "He'll grow out of it." Then, of course, it turned out that the child really did have a problem, and valuable time had been lost. We know these stories, we know they happen, and we want to make sure you don't end up feeling that way. On the other hand, we know the other stories, too—the ones that don't end up in the books because the children really did grow out of it and the problems were resolved. In all honesty, many parents bring up developmental concerns with us, and many children deviate a little bit from the standard developmental charts, and most of these children turn out to be just fine.

Our job is to listen to your concerns, observe your child carefully, and make a reasonable judgment about whether it's time for further testing. We need to understand why you're worried and just how worried you really are. You may come to the conclusion that you're dealing with the wrong doctor and it's time to move on; however, we hope that most parents will find that their pediatricians are reasonably well informed and helpful during this complicated and sensitive process. Here are some important points about communicating with your child's primary care provider—and being heard:

- *If you feel you have an experienced pediatric clinician who listens carefully, has interacted with and examined your child, and is not worried, that means something.* Consider letting yourself be reassured. It's not a guarantee, of course (we're loyal to our profession, but not blindly so), but it may well mean that your child is indeed only going through a phase, that this too shall pass. Judging whether a 2-year-old is off the charts in oppositional behavior and tantrums can be difficult, especially with a first child (or a second child when the first was an easy kid). If you like and trust your doctor, you might consider letting it rest here, at least for a few months.
- *It's important to make these diagnoses early, but not on an emergency basis.* Obviously, we aren't talking about a child who's deaf or one with seizures. Children with medical disorders need to be diagnosed and treated as rapidly as possible. The more obviously and severely delayed your child is, the more quickly things should move. Most of the kids we're talking about—the quirky kids—can be watched a little more slowly or, most important, offered special help (eg, speech therapy, occupational therapy) with the developmental tasks that give them trouble while you're figuring out the big picture or waiting for an appointment with a specialist. It's also important to point out that sorting through the issues that affect these kids can be a long, ongoing process. Getting children help for the issues with which they're struggling and watching how they respond to that help can actually be part of the diagnostic process. Also keep in mind that the testing itself can be stressful and that even having diagnoses and labels under consideration may have an emotional effect on you. When warranted, testing is important, but when your child is not severely affected, the advice to give it a few months and watch closely is not going to harm your child, and children do grow and change.
- *If you are really worried about something, communicate that to your child's primary care provider.* It's sometimes hard for us to tell whether parents are making a casual comment or expressing a deep worry, rooted in days and weeks of careful observation. If you have any concerns, explain them to your provider in clear, distinct language. For example, "There's something I've been noticing for weeks now, and I'm really worried. I read an article and

it seemed to be describing my baby, so now I'm wondering if she has this syndrome. Could this be something really bad?" If the doctor doesn't seem to register your concern, repeat it. Parents may come away from a medical encounter believing they've told the doctor something, while the doctor leaves not understanding that it's a real worry. It's not at all uncommon for a parent to drop a casual question: "That birthmark—it's not going to turn into anything bad, is it?" "That funny sound he makes, does that mean he's going to have a stutter?" When the pediatrician is fully alert and understands that your question is not asked in passing, those concerns are properly explored. "What do you mean by anything bad?" or "Does stuttering run in your family?" But as we hustle through the day and try to remember all the items on the long checklist of any child's annual physical examination, we may not be paying proper attention. Stop us, look us in the eye, tell us you're worried, and tell us exactly why.

- *Schedule a visit specifically about your child's development.* Don't try to talk about it at the visit that's really about an ear infection. We all walk a fine line as parents between wanting to have our suspicions confirmed and wanting to have our worries set aside. However, when you come in, sit, and tell us what is worrying you, we listen—or we should. The fact that you were worried enough to make the appointment signals to us that we need to give this issue time and attention. If the visit is specifically scheduled to discuss your concerns, there should be time for your most pressing questions to be answered and for you and your child's primary care provider to agree on a next step.

- *Your concerns should prompt the pediatrician to perform some type of systematic developmental assessment, not just eyeball your child.* The pediatrician should take a more detailed history of your child's development and do an assessment of where your child stands, according to age-appropriate norms in gross and fine motor development, cognitive skills, language, and social interactions. Screening tools have been developed for use by general pediatricians, not specialists, and they can be done quickly and may give you a handle on whether a referral is indicated. While examining a child, a pediatrician might also make note of the child's response to the usual sensory stimulation in a doctor's office, such as an otoscope in the ear or a tongue depressor in the mouth. Children with sensory problems may find this sort of stimulation unbearable.

I had a friend who kept a developmental screening test on her refrigerator and checked off each developmental milestone her child reached. When I saw it, I realized I could never do it because John didn't have any of the check marks he should have had, and he didn't have most of the ones he should have had 6 months ago. It reminded me of how, when John was born, I wanted to keep baby books on each of my kids. At a certain point—he was maybe 1½ years old—I just stopped doing it. So much of our life was consumed with his delays—the fact that he couldn't talk—it was just too sad. I felt I would be fabricating his childhood, ignoring the major part of our life with him, which was early intervention, speech therapy, and occupational therapy.

- *If you really don't feel as if you're being listened to, obtain a second opinion.* Pediatricians are not all alike. Some are more attuned to these issues than others. Even those of us who consider ourselves to be interested in developmental differences and sensitive to parental concerns have gotten it wrong in certain cases.

Throughout Abby's first year, each time I talked to my pediatrician about it, he reassured me that everything was fine. I remember the lines people used to reassure me: "She's developing at her own pace." "She's on her own trajectory." "Don't compare her to others." "You're a first-time mom. Just relax." I felt that the doctors and our family and friends thought we were crazy. But I had a gnawing feeling something was up. In the pediatrician's office at age 2, something set Abby off and she started tantruming. She was fearful and overwhelmed, and she couldn't stop. The pediatrician said, "I would just ignore all this. This is just attention-seeking behavior," and told me he thought I was decompensating and referred my husband and me to counseling.

So why isn't your pediatrician concerned? First and foremost, your child's behaviors may not be as worrisome as you think. Range-of-normal infant colic can be pretty awful. Standard tantrums by a 2-year-old have driven many a parent over the edge. Second, your child may have some truly concerning quirks but come off overall as pleasant, appealing, and well connected to you and others. People may not worry as much about developmental problems in a happy and engaging child. Third, you may be observing certain extreme behaviors that are "saved" for you and just don't show up in the doctor's office. Last, you may be describing something that is beyond the knowledge and expertise of your clinician. In any of these situations, you need a second opinion, either to confirm your own suspicions or to dial down your anxiety.

Aidan's pediatrician felt he was within the norm. He became oppositional as soon as he could talk, and he talked very early. His tantrums simply couldn't be ignored. He would scream and hang on to me, save his worst behavior for me. Again, the pediatrician felt these were the usual oppositional/control issues with a toddler, and his recommendations didn't help. It was impossible to do a time-out with Aidan. You would have to hold him down the whole time, which defeats the purpose of the time-out.

- *Where do you go for further evaluation?* Ideally, the next step is a referral to a specialist in child development and behavior, so your child can be more fully evaluated. (Every major academic medical center and children's hospital has such a clinic.) Your health insurance may require a referral from your primary care provider. Be aware that the waits for some of these clinics can be very long. In the next chapter, we discuss some of the other types of specialists who might be able to help, sometimes depending on your paramount concerns.

The Big Picture

As you observe your child, be sure not to focus on only one developmental milestone. Every child reaches some milestones early and others late. Ask yourself whether there's a pattern. Does my child have trouble with many motor skills? Does my child seem weaker or clumsier than other children? Does my child have trouble with words or with communication in general?

Our son just wouldn't eat. It was mind-boggling. People would say, "Oh, he's not going to starve to death. People don't starve to death," but he certainly did not have a normal drive to eat. We used to count those little rotini pastas. Oh, he ate 6 of those for dinner! We were so excited. Plus, his head was small, his motor skills were so weak, and he wouldn't talk. By 1 year, he wasn't doing most of what a normal 1-year-old would do.

Different Trajectories

Children develop in many directions at once. Some kids are motor machines who roll, sit, crawl, and walk early, yet their language skills lag. Other babies happily sit in one place and babble away. It's as if some of them can't do both at the same time. When you observe your child, look not just at gross and fine motor skills but also at cognitive skills, communication, talking, and understanding. Look at social skills and personality. Does your child cry and act up around strangers but talk and laugh with familiar people? A child who is doing fine in most respects but has one particular area of difficulty is not as worrisome as a child who seems to struggle on several fronts. Even if you have a specific concern you want addressed, it's important to keep all these developmental trajectories in mind and recognize the many kinds of progress, wherever they occur.

In our clinic, we discussed a 9-month-old girl who wasn't crawling. Her mother had come in very concerned because she thought her daughter should crawl. We asked her, "What *is* your daughter doing?" It turned out she was doing a lot. We asked all the questions about gross motor and fine motor skills. Does she pull to stand? Does she sit upright in her high chair? Does she pick up a raisin? Does she know her name? And yes, this infant wasn't crawling, but she was doing every other thing. She was babbling, she was communicating her wants, she was beginning to say "Mama," and sometimes it even seemed to mean Mama. We concluded that this infant was, on some basic level, completely on target developmentally. And sure enough, on physical examination, she was strong and vigorous, and her muscle tone was normal. Under those circumstances, as doctors, we take a deep breath and tell the mother not to worry. When this little girl came back for her next visit, at 1 year of age, she was walking. She skipped crawling and went right to walking. While we were happy to see this progress, we were also relieved that our reassurances had turned out to be on target. Every time we make the decision to reassure parents, we think of the occasional child who *doesn't* go on to crawl or walk, the child who is truly signaling a developmental delay.

Even as you pursue diagnosis and testing, don't reduce your child to a symptom, a problem, a set of missed milestones. Look at your child, with strengths and weaknesses, preferences and quirks, and find as many ways as possible to cherish the days of childhood.

As parents, we move from vague worries to special appointments to talk about a concern that won't go away to evaluations at specialty clinics, where we find ourselves surrounded by children with the full spectrum of developmental difficulties. As pediatricians, we move from observing and examining the patient a little more closely—checking and rechecking the child's muscle tone perhaps or asking additional questions about speech development and social skills—to articulating our concerns to the worried parents and to involving our specialist colleagues and waiting for their multipage assessments. As you make your way across these borders, consider how the journey fits into the lifelong story of you and your child.

Hindsight Is 20/20

- *Everything looks different in retrospect.* If you end up with a diagnosis, with a child whose life is truly shaped and affected by a developmental disorder, you will look back at your early anxieties as loud warning signals and at everyone who did not take them seriously as dangerous and incompetent. On the other hand, if there is no specific diagnosis and your child outgrows most or all of the worrying behaviors, you may forget all those moments when you thought something might be wrong. In judging the people from whom you sought help along the way—and most of all, in judging yourself—remember that these are all complex, individual stories. Predicting the future is impossible. Don't be too hard on yourself if you feel you missed various warning signals. Don't kick yourself for not understanding right away that your child needed speech therapy or would never be one to enjoy crowds or loud noises or parties. You weren't blind or obtuse or cruel. You were just figuring things out as you went along. All kids are works in progress, and developmental trajectories and family dynamics shift with time. Your job with a quirky kid is a more challenging and complex version of any parent's job: to find what works; to help, protect, and teach; and to shape the world to fit your child even as you help your child learn how to handle the world.

- *Last, and maybe most important, do not let your worries or anxieties overshadow your relationship with your baby or child.* You need memories of your child's early years that are more than anxieties, diagnoses, testing, problems, and therapy. While you pursue diagnoses and workups, make sure you build in time for whatever comes most easily and gives most pleasure—to you, your child, and your family.

Despite all these difficulties, we carried on our life. We traveled with him, we took him to visit relatives. These things that bothered us didn't bother him at all. He was a happy kid. He liked to do a lot of things. There was a lot of pleasure in him. We had to try very hard, being who we were, not to let these things color our whole lives, but he was a fun little baby. He liked being around people. He had a nice disposition. And now that we know that he's basically doing pretty well, it's easy to look back and remember the things we had fun with.

2

Specialists, Labels, and Alphabet Soup: Diagnosis or Difference?

Once upon a time, most quirky children did not get assigned to formal diagnostic categories. They were called eccentric or odd and were humored as oddballs or tortured as weirdos, coddled as infant geniuses or ostracized as misfits, and sometimes even immortalized as geeks. Chances are, they received no special therapies, took no special medications, and carried no medical or psychological terminology on their journeys through childhood, unless they had what we would now call an intellectual disability. In such cases, they were lumped together into separate classrooms, sometimes in different parts of the school building.

Times have changed. Look around those same classrooms and schoolyards now, and, depending on your point of view as a parent or an educator, you will see these children in a different light. Certainly, they are not all the same and we've learned that it is not appropriate to lump all children with differences into one classroom and assume they will thrive. A child who doesn't quite fit the mold is likely to receive an evaluation, often leading to a diagnosis and sometimes more than one diagnosis over time, which, in turn, leads to an individualized program of therapies, home-based interventions, and possibly medications. This, we believe, is on the whole a good thing. We no longer accept that certain children, the ones who have a harder time, ought to be left to struggle alone. They can benefit from careful attention to their strengths and weaknesses, from extra help at an early age, and from a more understanding attitude on the part of the important adults in their lives.

As clinicians, we sometimes tend to speak of "having a diagnosis" as if it were a special distinction. "Well, does he have a diagnosis?" "So after all that, did the kid get a diagnosis?" As medical students, we were rewarded for coming up with long lists of possible diagnoses—the *differential diagnosis*, as it is called in medicine—and then, even more, for coming up with the one true diagnosis. In fact, later in this chapter, we provide a sense of what we look for in the pediatric examination room. Many parents do start with the child's primary care provider, and we can play important roles, but the diagnostic journey often doesn't end with us.

Some physicians, because of their training, have a generally positive reaction to the idea of a diagnosis, or of making the right diagnosis. We tend to see it as a step forward. But parents experience a different set of emotions when they find themselves considering the possibility of this kind of identity for a quirky child. To parents, a diagnosis may seem like a label, a limitation, or a confirmation of their inner fears. You ask a variety of specialists to quantify your child's strengths, weaknesses, oddities, and quirks, and then perhaps they offer you a name, a syndrome, or a single formulation. As we've said earlier, we know this is not where any parent starts out, and sometimes it's a painful step. We need to discuss a couple of important matters regarding quirky children and diagnoses:

1. *What does a diagnosis mean?* What does it mean to the parent and child or adolescent? Some parents see their children's quirks as wrinkles in development, personality variations rather than problems. Others, although grateful for help with whatever their children find most difficult, don't want any specific label applied to the child to explain those difficulties. Many fear that a label may become a self-fulfilling prophecy, marking a child in the eyes of teachers and classmates and even family members. On the other hand, many parents feel a strong desire to give their child's quirks a name, so that they can educate themselves, help their child as much as possible, maybe link up with other parents facing the same situation, and perhaps anticipate the problems that may lie ahead.

I'm one of those people who wants to give things labels. This way, I can know the worst-case scenario. I thought if [there was] a label, there was a body of knowledge out there and I could learn what I needed to know and see where he was on the spectrum. Also, I wanted to know about recurrence and the risk to other kids we might go on to have. I thought it would be useful to know the likelihood we would have to deal with it again.

As a little kid, Abby was one of those kids who was just bothered by everything. When we got her first diagnosis—sensory processing disorder—we felt that the weight of the world was off our

> shoulders. She was very tough to take care of. And when we got that
> first label, we felt as if everything made sense.

We find ourselves saying the following over and over to families in the examining room: *Many children will receive more than one diagnosis over time, as they grow and change and face different challenges and expectations.*

For many quirky kids, a single diagnosis does not fit. Depending on the child's age and developmental stage, as well as the orientation and training of the person doing the assessment, these children can receive many diagnoses as they grow. Some diagnoses fit for a while and then are outgrown, whereas others continue to be relevant as the child grows and changes. You may find yourself holding on to a particular diagnosis, not because it fits so well but because it helps you with the school system.

The nomenclature to describe children with autism spectrum disorder (ASD) has changed in recent years, and many quirky kids will receive an ASD diagnosis that specifies the level of support they will need: mild, moderate, or extensive. We discuss this in more detail later in the book. And some children will receive no diagnosis at all because they function just fine in the world, even with some mild characteristics consistent with ASD. It may be more helpful to look at an individual child in terms of strengths and weaknesses, rather than using diagnoses, and this is increasingly common in the field.

> Ben has a diagnosis of autism, made when he was 7, although along
> the way he has had a huge number of diagnoses or formulations
> of what his particular brand of quirkiness is. Included in the list:
> prolonged colic, attention-deficit/hyperactivity disorder, general-
> ized anxiety disorder, bipolar disorder, learning disorder, and so
> on. He's also been described as having sensory issues and as being
> impulsive and reactive. Sometimes I still wonder whether they've
> got it right, but he's getting what he needs, so the label isn't that
> important.

2. *Many of these conditions overlap or occur in tandem.* This is known as *co-morbidity*. Depending on children's ages and what is expected of them at those ages, different skills become more or less important and different problems seem major or minor. In kindergarten, for example, whether or not a child plays easily with other children may determine how happy she is in the classroom. By third grade, learning issues may have become paramount. As we get better at recognizing kids with differences, older

children are being diagnosed as well. Often, after years of persistent, but not devastating, school problems or social issues, they are given "official" diagnoses during adolescence. This is especially true for highly intelligent kids who breeze through the early grades and struggle later on.

Before getting into the nitty-gritty of diagnosis, we want to stress that the purpose of the workup, testing, and careful consideration of your child by multiple experts is *not* to come up with the right label, the right name, or the right answer on some cosmic medical student examination. The reason to have your child tested is to help your child—and to help you help your child. Diagnoses are helpful only insofar as they point the way to reasonable and realistic expectations, useful therapies, and greater understanding.

Looking More Closely at Your Child

So let's say you and your child's primary care provider have decided that your child needs testing by experts. Maybe you raised concerns during a visit, or your responses on a developmental screening form indicated the need for further evaluation. You need answers, advice, and explanations. Where to turn?

In a perfect world, you would turn to an erudite but sensitive team of experts who would view your child without preconceptions and take the time and trouble necessary to get to know her or him. Their recommendations would be realistic and practical, and the evaluation, along with any necessary follow-up appointments, would be fully covered by your insurance. Unfortunately, we don't live in that world, and the reality is that it can be a real challenge to find the experts you need without waiting a long time. Our goal is to help you get all or most of what you need, even in this imperfect world. Where you live may determine what is available, and we know that insurance coverage issues may matter a lot. Further, it can be frustratingly difficult to make appointments with some specialists in a timely way. We lay out several possibilities and encourage you to think strategically, ideally together with the primary care provider who knows your child and knows the local landscape.

Autism Spectrum Disorder

In today's world, a child with clear developmental differences or quirks early in life should raise concerns about ASD, because early diagnosis and intense intervention improve the outcome over time for the child and family. So it's worth talking this over with your pediatrician if your child's development or your responses on screening questionnaires suggest that further evaluation for ASD is indicated. General pediatricians are increasingly well-versed in early ASD detection. Some may have specialized training that allows them to take on some of the roles traditionally played by specialists, while others will at least be able to expedite the referral process and support families while they wait for complete evaluations. Most families will end up wanting to have ongoing partnerships with their child's primary care provider and a specialist. Unfortunately, the wait times in communities across the country for formal medical and developmental evaluation can be painfully long. One way we usually try to help sort things out and offer support in the interim is by connecting the child and family with early intervention (EI). It's an excellent place to start.

Early Intervention Programs

Early intervention programs are available in every state as federally funded services for children with developmental needs and medical problems in the first 3 years. Children younger than 3 with developmental or behavioral concerns can—and should—be referred to EI. Your child's primary care provider can do this, but you can also do it yourself. (The following link has information on each state: https://www.cdc.gov/ncbddd/actearly/parents/states.html.) Early intervention programs offer developmental testing, and if your child qualifies—that is, if delays or concerns of a certain magnitude are identified—therapeutic services are provided while you wait for further diagnostic evaluation. The EI programs are not in the business of making official diagnoses; rather, they look for delays or problems in the developmental domains, such as speech and language and communication, gross motor and fine motor skills, and social-emotional, and provide targeted therapies when a child's delays are significant enough to qualify.

Pediatric Specialists

Because of the importance of determining whether a child fits somewhere along the autism spectrum, it's worth reviewing that process, which varies depending on access to the specialists who are credentialed to make this diagnosis. Four types of pediatric specialists are highly trained in the evaluation process: developmental-behavioral pediatricians, child neurologists, child psychiatrists, and child psychologists. Some states require that a diagnosis be made by a medical doctor for a child to qualify for services. Your primary care provider should be familiar with those regulations and know which specialists are available in your geographical area.

In the following section, we look at the array of specialists to whom parents turn as they try to sort out their children's behavior and development and help them over some of the hurdles encountered in the early years at home and out in the world. We look at different specialists—with different training, orientation, and assessment tools—and the various types of information they offer, with some more oriented toward helping the child's practical everyday function and others more attuned to recognizing syndromes and making diagnoses.

Developmental-Behavioral Pediatrician

Often, the person directing the workup will be a pediatrician with additional specialty training in behavior and development. Although these are often the most overbooked physicians in town, you'll want to look for a developmentalist who specializes in kids on the quirky spectrum (as opposed to someone who specializes in kids with intellectual disability and cerebral palsy, for example). Check out the Society for Developmental & Behavioral Pediatrics (http://sdbp.org) for links to clinicians in your area. This evaluation may take more than one visit; it will involve going through your child's medical and developmental history in detail and reviewing any other evaluations that may have taken place, as well as testing, including a variety of carefully calibrated screening tools to assess a child's strengths, weaknesses, play skills, interests, ability to transition, and verbal and social communication skills. Finally, the pediatrician will review the results with you and offer support and referrals to agencies that can help. In some cases, you may complete vast amounts of paperwork instead of having that first visit and then skip right to the testing appointment. Expect to be asked a lot of repetitive questions about your child's development: how old he was when he first rolled over, sat, stood, walked, talked. Also, expect to be asked about problems that run in your family, including any pregnancy losses or miscarriages and kids with ASD, learning disabilities, attention-deficit/hyperactivity disorder (ADHD), or mental health problems. The developmental-behavioral pediatrician will perform a careful examination of your child, looking for anything unusual physically and paying particular attention to the child's nervous system. The pediatrician will note physical strength and coordination as well as behavior and will pay close attention to social responsiveness. For example, a developmentalist will want to see whether the patient makes eye contact and responds to her name, and will check speech and nonverbal communication. As part of the assessment, the pediatrician also should review your child's experience in preschool or school and consider ability to focus and social functioning, both at home and in any group setting.

Child Neurologist

A child neurologist is a physician with specialty training in the brain and nervous system of children and adolescents. Within the field, there are subspecialists with particular interests in kids with atypical behavior or development. Many child neurologists also have an interest and additional training in specific areas, such as ASD or ADHD. A child whose overall picture includes a neurological disorder, such as seizures, persistent tics, or possible Tourette syndrome, will most likely be seen by a neurologist, who may stay involved as the diagnostic questions expand past that particular disorder. A neurologist will examine your child in great detail, paying attention to the strength of each group of muscles and the ability of the nerves to register sensation, as well as to reflexes, coordination, and mental skills—regardless of whether the child is 9 months old or 9 years old. Most important, a neurologist will be strongly oriented toward sorting out the possibility of medical problems that are not just developmental differences. For example, if the child's weakness or clumsiness has raised the possibility of cerebral palsy or one of the muscular dystrophies, a neurologist's examination will be essential. A neurologist may order an imaging study of the brain, such as a CT scan or an MRI scan if a child seems to have intellectual disability or any physical features that suggest a disorder of the brain. The likelihood of a significant finding on a brain scan is extremely low (this is why insurance companies often will not cover the cost of brain imaging without a good reason upfront); most often, it serves to reassure parents that the overall appearance of the brain is normal.

Because children with ASD have an increased risk of seizures, a neurologist may also order an electroencephalogram (EEG), a test used to find problems related to electrical activity of the brain. This test can usually be performed on an outpatient basis.

Child and Adolescent Psychiatrist

At some point in the assessment, your child may see a child and adolescent psychiatrist, a physician who has done subspecialty training in psychiatric disorders of children. For many kids, evaluation by a psychiatrist occurs later in the process, perhaps because the child develops obsessive interests or because depression or anxiety has become an issue or because the psychiatrist may be able to help where there's diagnostic uncertainty. Some children receive diagnoses such as anxiety or depression for which they see child psychiatrists, then later concerns about ASD may be raised. Some child psychiatrists have additional training in the evaluation of a child with possible ASD, and in those cases the child psychiatrist may direct the entire workup.

> We have two kids on the spectrum and have really enjoyed and
> appreciated our relationship with the child psychiatrist over the
> years. They both look forward to seeing him, and we need his
> counsel and experience from time to time. He, more than the other
> professionals we have seen, seems to really enjoy the kids and sees
> them as interesting rather than as problems that need to be fixed.
> The kids sense this and appreciate it as well.

Child Psychologist

A child psychologist has an advanced degree, usually a doctorate in psychology, but is not a medical doctor. Psychologists conduct evaluations of a child's behavior, intelligence, and cognition. A school-based psychologist is often called upon to perform a psychoeducational evaluation to determine the child's educational potential and achievement and to spell out which accommodations on the part of the school may be helpful. Community or hospital-based psychologists have undergone training in the evaluation of a child with developmental differences, and they are equipped to make a diagnosis, although in some states, the child may need to be evaluated by a physician to obtain services for ASD.

Neuropsychologist

A neuropsychologist has special training in the biological and neurological bases of learning and thought. This evaluation includes a battery of tests that most kids describe as "like being in school." The purpose of a "neuropsych eval" is to assess the child's level of cognitive and behavioral functioning and to use the findings to make recommendations about school placement and overall care of the child. This is the tool that is most likely to be used to diagnose a learning difference, such as dyslexia or a language-based learning disability. Children whose achievement in school is below what their intelligence test results would suggest should come out of this testing with a better understanding of their learning difficulties and the strategies that may help. A neuropsychological evaluation may indicate attentional problems that interfere with learning. The neuropsychologist uses these tests to look at the child's ability to sit still, focus, process visual and auditory information, and organize thoughts and plans—the skill set we call *executive function*. The particular learning difference most common in quirky kids—the nonverbal learning disability—is characterized by a specific pattern on intelligence tests administered during this exam. Most neuropsychological evaluations include an interview with parents in which they review the history of the child's birth and growth and development, focusing on areas of special concern. Neuropsychologists are experienced with quirky kids, including those on the autism spectrum, and will be alert for this as a possible diagnosis. Neuropsychological testing is likely to be the most lengthy evaluation, and therefore the most stressful for your child and for you. Check with the evaluation team in advance to understand the schedule and what you and your child should expect over the course of the evaluation, which in some cases may involve more than one visit.

If you're concerned about ASD, it's important for your child to undergo a thorough evaluation as early as possible. But some children whose behavior and development have not been particularly worrisome to their parents start to struggle as they grow up and find themselves facing new educational and social challenges.

Evaluations and Experts

The following are experts and evaluations that parents may encounter as they try to understand what's going on with children who are having a hard time meeting expectations as they grow.

School-Based Evaluations

If a child older than 3 is struggling in preschool or elementary school for any reason, even if the parents and the primary care provider have not been worried in the past, a school-based evaluation can be a great place to start, and it may be required before more specialized medical evaluations can take place. Parents can write letters requesting a school-based evaluation, and you may well find yourself beginning this way because you think it will provide some answers, your insurance company requires it, or the school usually covers the expense. Most important, services to help the child in school will not be provided without a school evaluation that determines such services are indicated, as is mandated by the Individuals with Disabilities Education Act (https://sites.ed.gov/idea).

The school-based perspective is oriented toward problems that prevent a child from functioning well in the school setting, and therefore the evaluation tends to focus on learning issues. When a child receives a diagnosis that requires extra educational support, the school is required by law to supply that support, so parents sometimes wonder if schools may be reluctant to recognize edu-cational needs or recommend strategies that require expensive school-based services in the early elementary years, even though such help may make a huge difference over time. All of this is to say that, although you may need or want to start with a school evaluation, and it may provide you with helpful information, you may decide to go further in your diagnostic quest. Kids will still need an outside diagnosis in most instances, because like EI programs, schools do not assign a diagnosis. But to qualify for federally mandated special education support (an individualized education plan [IEP], which spells out the particular services the child needs), a child must have one of the following 13 educational classifications:

1. Autism spectrum disorder
2. Developmental delay
3. Deaf or hearing impairment
4. Emotional disturbance
5. Hearing impairment
6. Specific learning disability
7. Intellectual disability
8. Orthopedic impairment
9. Other health impairment
10. Speech and/or language impairment
11. Traumatic brain injury
12. Visual impairment including blindness
13. Multiple disabilities

Children with ASD most often qualify for services under the diagnosis of ASD, but in some cases it may be their communication difficulties or emotional disturbance that qualifies them for assistance.

Parents who do not live near any center that conducts a full developmental evaluation or who are more interested in functional help than in diagnosis may find themselves taking their children to several specialists individually. Thus, quirky kids may be assessed, in turn, by developmental pediatricians, speech and language pathologists, neurologists, physical therapists (PTs), occupational therapists (OTs), psychologists, psychiatrists, early childhood educators, EI specialists, and/or social workers—and that's not even counting those who are taken to nutritionists, allergists, homeopaths, and toxicologists!

Before we look at the different perspectives these specialists can offer, we have a few last words of advice on choosing your direction.

Trust your instincts. Go into this process with an open mind but also with a healthy degree of skepticism. If someone tells you something that absolutely does not fit with your sense of your own child, consider it objectively. Look at it to see whether it's going to help you help your child. Don't pursue a long-term therapeutic relationship with someone who can't answer your questions adequately or who makes you uncomfortable.

Be patient. If one specialist is not right, you may need to check out other specialists. If you know right away it's not a good fit, it's okay to respectfully decline working with the specialist. Keep in mind that sometimes it takes time to build a relationship with a specialist, so do your homework, ask lots of questions, take notes, and trust your instincts.

> **We have taken Abby to so many specialists over the years, I have antennae for those who don't really "get it," and I don't have a lot of patience with them. My task is to cut it short as soon as possible without being too rude, but there have been times when a specialist has shown such a lack of understanding that I've had to say, "I don't really care what you think." Life is too short to waste time with people who do not understand my child.**

Early Intervention Program

Parents with infants and toddlers who seem to be having developmental delays often begin with EI programs. This evaluation usually includes the following:

- A home visit to evaluate the child's social environment
- An assessment by a developmental educator, focusing on play skills, such as the use of toys and the ability to engage in pretend or symbolic play, as well as social interactions with familiar people and strangers. A child's attachment to her caregivers is evaluated as well. Does a toddler snuggle up with Dad out of fear of the strangers in the living room, or does he avert his eyes and seem to be in a world of his own? Does the child make good eye contact, respond when her name is called, point with a finger and follow with her eyes when someone else points? How does she make her wishes known to others? Does she use gestures and words?
- Assessments by OTs, speech and language therapists, and PTs. These specialists form teams within many EI programs and are skilled at evaluating infants and toddlers.

Early intervention programs conduct evaluations of needs and provide services, but they do not make formal diagnoses. Their job is to assess where the child is within the various developmental domains and provide whatever help is appropriate in areas in which catch-up is needed.

> **Many of the kids in our therapeutic playgroup shared the same basic difficulties, though they were coming from many different places. There was one who'd had a stroke after birth, there was one**

> with Down syndrome, one who was born very prematurely.
> Early intervention does a great service, but it doesn't give you a
> diagnosis. That's not what they are about. I wish I had known that
> at the beginning.

The combination of directed therapeutic help and no diagnosis may be exactly what some parents want and all that a child really needs, especially in the early years. More EI programs are now identifying young children who have delays or behaviors that suggest they may be along the autism spectrum. Once identified, these children will require a medical diagnosis and are then referred for more intensive behavioral programs with outside agencies. Given the data that suggest that intensive EI can improve long-term outcomes and the rising rates of ASD, EI has become a higher priority.

As children grow older, they show us the kinds of therapies that help them most. For example, we've heard OTs describe "a real OT kind of kid," that is, a kid who derives the most benefit from the work that OTs do. For those children, an early experience in EI may point the way to particular therapies that need to continue as the child grows. However, no matter what your child's issues are, EI services are provided only up to age 3. Clearly, many of these problems may last longer. Occupational therapists, PTs, and speech and language therapists are part of all EI teams, and most schools also retain these specialists to help kids as they "age out" of EI at age 3.

Assessments by Therapists

And so you set out, armed with a notebook, questions, reasonable expectations, and a certain amount of skepticism. The following are descriptions of professionals who may be involved in an assessment that will inform you and the medical specialists charged with making a diagnosis, if there is one to be made. It's important to remember that different professions mean different kinds of training and different professional experiences. Distinct perspectives will be brought to bear on your child, depending on who is doing the evaluating. Each specialist will view your child against the backdrop of the other children regularly seen in that specialty. Each specialist will ask different questions and use a different set of diagnostic tools to obtain answers. These are the people who will help you figure out your child, and it's worth understanding a little bit about who they are, what they are likely to do by way of evaluation, and what they bring to the story.

Occupational Therapist

Occupational therapy and PT overlap, but OTs are generally more interested in the smaller muscle groups such as the hand muscles or the facial muscles used in eating. *Dysgraphia* (terrible handwriting), for example, is a problem for many of these kids and falls within the OT's expertise. An oral-motor assessment is often performed by an OT for kids with difficulties such as excessive drooling, speech problems, or restrictive eating due to textures or tastes, a common problem among quirky kids. A subgroup of OTs have special certification in sensory processing disorder for those quirky children who seem uneasy in their skin, not confident moving through space, and uncomfortable with the usual sensations of daily life. As they assess your child, they look for problems such as gravitational insecurity and rotational insecurity, referring to the child who cannot tolerate having her feet off the ground (on a swing, for example) or rotating or spinning around. They also observe your child's sensitivity to sensory stimulation (for example, the child who can't tolerate the tag on the neck of his shirt rubbing against his skin).

With slightly older children, the OT focuses on whether the child can write, be taught to type, tie her shoes, eat with a fork, and follow multistep directions, as well as on larger questions. Can she organize her body in space? How about her thoughts on a page?

Speech and Language Pathologist

Many people know that speech therapists help children learn to talk and they address specific problems such as stuttering or speech impediments. They can also help assess a number of additional concerns in the realm of speech, language, and communication. Many quirky kids are not terribly language delayed. They can make words and talk, but they may not be able to carry on a conversation in an age-appropriate way.

A speech and language assessment includes not only your child's ability to make words but also her *ability to communicate* using words as well as her *prosody*—the character of her voice as she speaks. The assessment takes into account the child's frustration tolerance and the nature and quality of her tantrums. And, like the OT, the speech pathologist looks at oral-motor function. A child who uses speech or language lifted from movies or books, called "scripted speech," or one who repeats what others are saying but doesn't spontaneously use her own language to communicate, a pattern called *echolalia*, benefits from the support of a speech and language pathologist. Any child with language regression, that is, the loss of words previously used, should also be evaluated.

Physical Therapist

Physical therapy evaluation and treatment focuses on muscle strength and weakness and on coordination. The therapist looks at whether the child's muscles are weak, at whether she can throw and catch a ball, sit in a chair adequately enough to eat, and walk up and down stairs. Many quirky kids are physically awkward, either from clumsiness or weakness. They may have instability of the trunk in which their muscles are not quite strong enough to control their upper bodies. Such a child might do better sitting in a chair with back support, whereas a peer can sit on a picnic bench quite comfortably. Evaluation by a PT may include playing games and carrying out the activities of daily living.

Applied Behavior Analyst

Applied behavior analysis (ABA) requires special mention here and is discussed in more detail on pages 242 and 243. Children who are given a diagnosis along the autism spectrum qualify for ABA therapy, which is intensive and time-consuming, but also has the strongest evidence base for helping. A behavioral analyst, often a board-certified behavioral analyst, evaluates a child's concerning behaviors in great detail and develops a program for a therapist or technician who works directly with the child. Applied behavior analysis is based on the science of behavior and learning and is effective at decreasing undesirable behaviors such as tantrums and outbursts or meltdowns and increasing desirable behaviors such as language and communication. Many quirky kids benefit from ABA if their behaviors are challenging for those living with or teaching them, but it represents a serious time commitment for a child and family. Also, some people with ASD take issue with ABA because they feel that it is an attempt to extinguish the quirkiness and make a child more typical; they believe parents should be striving to understand and accept these children as they are.

Evaluating the Evaluators

As you move with your child through this maze of experts (the physicians, psychologists, therapists), your job is to track and evaluate the information offered and to make important decisions about when to look further and when to pause.

- *Make sure you understand the team. Look up your specialists online, and when you meet them ask about their qualifications, experience, and particular fields of expertise.* It's important to know whether you're dealing with a neurologist or a neuropsychologist or with a neophyte speech pathologist versus a master's-level expert with a special interest in ASD. Even if you aren't sure how to integrate the specialist's background with the assessment and advice, your child's primary care provider and the other specialists you see may better understand the information you've already collected if you can let them know who was doing the evaluating.

- *Talk to the evaluators, ask questions, write down what they say.* Some parents come away feeling they didn't—or couldn't—get their questions answered in any kind of detail by the people doing the evaluating. Sometimes this happens because there are still tests to be scored or conversations that need to take place among members of the team doing the evaluation. But even so, at the very least, you should leave knowing *when* you will hear and *how* you will hear what the assessment has yielded. For the most part, someone who has just spent some time with your child should be able to give you at least a few reactions or observations, but if you have an appointment scheduled in a week specifically to go over the results, it may make the most sense to wait so formulations can be more clearly discussed. The evaluating team may need to talk through their different observations and put the pieces together. It is completely reasonable to let evaluators know that you'd like a few minutes at the end of the session to get a sense of what they think. Bring your partner, if you have one, or a good friend or family member to listen and help you remember. Take notes. You may be more tense than you realize, and it may be difficult to remember exactly what you heard. Ask to have unfamiliar terms spelled out and explained. Ask whether there's anything you can read for more information. If a full multispecialty evaluation has been conducted, you might consider making an appointment to review and discuss the results, even if evaluators don't routinely do this.
- *Keep a notebook. Write everything down.* As time goes by, you will think of questions you want to ask, observations about your child that seem significant, ideas for further assessment or therapy. Write them down. Keep a record of the specialists you see, the tests they perform, the information they provide. Jot down phone numbers of programs or specialists you learn about from other parents, as well as contact data for someone who isn't that helpful now but may be in a few years. A notebook helps you track your child and your own understanding. It also helps you use your time wisely with the specialists by asking the questions you've been wanting to bring up.
- *Don't expect a single eureka moment.* We'll say it again because it's so important. **Many quirky kids don't fit neatly into diagnostic categories.** Parents may wonder, if he doesn't have ASD, what *does* he have? Having your child assessed and asking different experts to consider different diagnoses is an ongoing process that is valuable if it points the way to

helping your child. Still, it may not yield a single all-explanatory answer when you finally find out what's really going on.

- *Remember that some specialists—and some clinics—will give almost anyone a diagnosis.* If you look hard enough and long enough, eventually you will come across someone who pins on a label—maybe because it's the same label everybody gets at that particular clinic. Be especially wary of labels that carry immediate recommendations for expensive therapies. Don't let anyone prey on your desire to help your child. If you're uncomfortable with what's going on, or if you feel you're being pressured to sign up for treatments, it's probably worth getting a second opinion or discussing the recommendations with your child's pediatrician.

Most of the people you encounter with your child as you look into assessment and diagnosis will be honorable and professional. It must be said, however, that there is something of an industry out there in providing diagnoses and therapies to kids with developmental variations. This underscores our preference for academically affiliated specialists and the thorough unbiased evaluation.

Finally, it's worth saying that no matter how skilled and experienced the evaluator, no one can actually predict your child's trajectory, and it isn't fair to expect that. Medicine in general is not an exact science, and quirky kids grow up to do all sorts of unexpected things that no one can predict. We don't—any of us—know how any individual child will do, and just like typically developing children, quirky children will follow their own paths, and we don't—any of us—know exactly what those paths will be.

Diagnoses and Labels

You've now been to a specialist—or specialists. You've asked your questions and jotted down the answers, kept copies of all the assessments, and sat with your child's primary care provider to discuss the results. Bear in mind that each of these experts looks at your child through a different professional lens. Thus, a diagnosis of ASD is more likely to come from a developmental-behavioral pediatrician, a child neurologist, a psychiatrist, or a psychologist; an OT might describe the same child as having sensory processing disorder. And both are probably true. A child with ASD is likely to struggle with sensory difficulties. A speech and language pathologist might call the problem a social communication disorder, meaning the child may need support regarding the nuances of social conversation—as many quirky kids do. A neuropsychologist may call it a *nonverbal learning disability*, the most common learning profile of the quirky child. While any of these problems may exist in a child's life, it's worth noting that any one of these diagnoses does not preclude another. Your child is your child—not the sum of any number of these diagnoses. And the child you brought in at the start of the evaluation is the same child you will go home with that day. You may have a different lens through which to understand and support that child, but the evaluation process does not change the child you love. The objective of the diagnosis is to point the way toward something you can do to help. Different ways of understanding what's wrong may actually point you toward different ways of helping.

Some diagnostic labels are new, and some labels from 10 years ago are no longer in use. Although the new diagnoses may be relevant and useful, and they may represent our current best guess as to what is going on, we have to face the fact that many of these diagnoses will probably evolve in the years to come. Some may even disappear as our understanding changes. It's OK to feel a little wary if you sense that your child is being bent and twisted in order to fit the hot diagnosis of the moment.

The terms that follow may be spoken to you about your child by any of the specialists. Some are nothing more than descriptions. Some are more global terms that can describe difficulties in many areas. For any of these problems, entire books have been written to address the details, and we try to point you toward some good ones.

All of these words can be scary. Depending on your experience, your reading, and your background, some can be downright terrifying in their implications. We won't promise that what we say will reassure you, but we would argue as strongly as we can that none of these diagnostic terms should be viewed as the end of the world or as a distinct and final pronouncement on your child's potential. They are clues and constructs, approximations, best guesses, and often works in progress. And speaking of best guesses, because quirky kids are, in fact, quirky, you may find yourself being told that your child has some features of a certain diagnosis, or perhaps of more than one, but doesn't really fit neatly into any particular category. While that can be frustrating to hear, try to understand it as evidence that the people doing the evaluating have really looked closely at your particular child.

That said, what are some of the words you may hear or read or lie awake worrying about? The following diagnoses help sort out kids according to the symptoms and behaviors that are most prominent and problematic. Even if your child does not fit the descriptions exactly, careful testing and thoughtful diagnosis ought to give you a boost toward a relevant body of knowledge and experience and, most important, toward therapies and techniques that may be helpful.

We've tried to present these diagnoses roughly in the order in which they are most likely to come up in children's lives, starting with the ones that are more likely to be applied in early life.

Speech and Language Delay

A speech and language evaluation is often the first a quirky child will undergo, as parents are attuned to typical language development and will notice when a child is not talking like the other children his age. The description of speech and language delay reflects your child's progress in speech norms for age. In fact, a full speech and language evaluation provides detailed information about what your child can and cannot do with language. Older kids with communication difficulties probably should undergo an assessment of *pragmatic language skills* (the ability to understand the give-and-take of conversation, to pick up cues about when the other person is bored or no longer interested). Speech and language therapy can be helpful for both verbal and nonverbal aspects of communication. Not all quirky kids are speech and language delayed. Some actually develop language early. Some, quite dramatically, learn to read as they learn to talk—called *hyperlexia*. Thus, not all quirky children will be evaluated early in childhood for speech and language delay, but even some of the precocious talkers may need to be seen later in childhood when their communication difficulties emerge. For some children, initial concerns about speech and language delay lead to other questions about communication, social relations, and patterns of thought.

Trevor was developmentally delayed and had no language at age 2. Then, almost before he learned to talk, he started reading, and my husband saw an article about hyperlexia. So his first evaluation was with a hyperlexia specialist, who said yes, he does have this syndrome. When he did start to develop language, it was slow and echolalic. He had other unusual mannerisms, like waving backward, his palm facing himself, and mixing up pronouns.

George talked a lot but used "scripted language" from movies or books. He had an incredible memory and would remember a line appropriate to a situation, but it would be directly from a book or movie. When he was 3½, we had a storm and lost our power. We took out the flashlights, and his grandfather told him not to play with the flashlight because it wasn't a toy. George responded by saying, "I know, Grandpa. It's a big responsibility, but I'll take good care of it." His grandfather looked at me and said, "And you are worried about his language?" But it was a line directly out of a book we had read about taking care of puppies. At about this time, he had his first full evaluation, and the speech therapist said he had no "functional language."

Motor Delay and Motor-Planning Difficulties

Children with motor delay have fallen behind with respect to the motor skills you would expect them to be developing at their ages. Motor delay can refer to a specific skill or milestone that a child has not mastered, or it can refer to the quality of a child's movements, to clumsiness or unsteadiness or muscle weakness. A great number of quirky kids have difficulties with motor coordination and weakness, which can show up early as delayed motor milestones such as sitting up or walking, or you may notice it later if, for example, a child cannot hop or kick a ball or seems to lose her balance easily. Motor clumsiness may persist throughout life, but many children make tremendous gains in this area with a combination of OT and PT. Some kids may be diagnosed with developmental coordination disorder, which describes a child who does not have motor delay, but is persistently, well, clumsy. These children may have delays in their gross and fine motor development, visual-perceptual difficulties, and other problems holding them back.

The term *motor-planning difficulties* refers to the inability to plan an action with your brain and carry it out with your body. Many quirky kids have motor-planning difficulties. In medical terms, this is similar to what you see in an adult who has had a stroke in a particular area of the brain. She may know exactly what she wants to do but cannot get her body to do it. One part of the brain is not working right, and, therefore, despite her intelligence, memory, and understanding, a simple task such as buttoning her shirt is a difficult, if not impossible, assignment. In kids, motor-planning difficulties manifest as the inability to carry out tasks, perhaps simple tasks such as chewing and swallowing or more complex tasks such as getting dressed and tying shoes.

We noticed early that John had trouble getting things done. He was never motivated to get dressed on his own, and we coaxed him to try when we got busy with the younger children. We would watch him lay his pants over his legs. He knew how they were supposed to look once they were on, but he couldn't figure out how to get his legs inside.

Autism Spectrum Disorder

Autism spectrum disorder (ASD) is now the widely used term for a diagnostic category that captures a good number of quirky kids. Although already in wide use among parents and professionals, it first appeared in the fifth edition of the *Diagnostic and Statistical Manual of Mental Disorders (DSM-5)* in 2013. The term is applied to kids with social communication problems as well as repetitive behaviors and fixed interests, hallmarks of this diagnostic group. A child who receives a diagnosis of ASD is assigned a level of severity in social communication difficulties and another in repetitive behaviors; each realm is noted as 1 (requiring support), 2 (requiring substantial support), or 3 (requiring very substantial support).

Certain terms are no longer used when children undergo a diagnostic evaluation today, and for some kids that means a previous diagnosis now has a new name. For example, children who had a diagnosis of pervasive developmental disorder or Asperger syndrome are now considered part of the autism spectrum. Researchers argue that this streamlined category makes it easier to follow kids over time.

Severe classic autism—outside the province of this book—has shadowed this terminology so that many parents are terrified to hear that their child may have ASD, assuming that it means an intellectual disability. In fact, autism is a spectrum, with a wide range across both of the core features—social communication and restricted and repetitive behaviors. What children on the autism spectrum have in common are problems with communication and social interactions, as well as the tendency toward repetitive interests or activity.

> I miss the Asperger diagnosis because I felt it really helped me to understand myself, and I have a community of people like me who understand and feel they are "aspies." We don't like to call ourselves autistic.

Less severe ASD in children is more difficult to detect early. With the increasing incidence of these diagnoses, it is important not to rush to conclusions. On the other hand, an early diagnosis, even if it turns out to change over time, might help your child qualify for services and therapies that will really make a difference. So, take a deep breath and ride the wave. Get the help for your child, and take some time to consider whether a given label really fits.

> One time in a playgroup video, my husband and I saw our 2½-year-old Caitlin sitting in a corner by herself while the other two girls played ring-around-the-rosy. We were worried. Thus began a series

of evaluations and therapies. I called the pediatrician's office looking for the name of a child psychologist and was sent to someone who said that Caitlin's main problem is that she is just so smart! This was not helpful. After a couple of other visits to psychologists, we went to a child psychiatrist who saw her when she was about 5 and said, "This is Asperger's." What characteristics of Caitlin's behavior made it so easy for him to make this diagnosis? She was always very rigid and insisted that things had to be the same. As a toddler, she would only wear clothes that had frogs or clocks sewn on them. She had terrible eating habits and horrendous temper tantrums. She could not engage with other kids. She loved swings, but to an extreme degree.

Global Developmental Delay

For children with delays in two or more domains (speech/language, gross or fine motor, cognition, social/personal, activities of daily living) but who do not meet the criteria for ASD, a diagnosis of global developmental delay (GDD) might apply, and this diagnosis is usually given in the first 5 years. As your child ages, and intelligence testing becomes more reliable, the diagnosis may change. A child with GDD should be evaluated and monitored by a child neurologist or developmental-behavioral pediatrician over time. The more severely affected the child, the more likely an underlying etiology (cause) can be discovered, and genetic testing or imaging of the brain may be recommended. Some children subsequently may be diagnosed with an intellectual disability or a specific learning disability.

Social (Pragmatic) Communication Disorder

The term *social (pragmatic) communication disorder* (SCD) is used to describe the idiosyncratic social impairments of quirky kids who struggle with difficulties in verbal communication, although they do not meet criteria for ASD. Although some kids may be able to wax eloquent about their area of special interest, they may *not* be able to figure out when it is time to stop. This is *pragmatic language*—using words and the nonverbal behaviors that go along with them to understand another person. Much of interpersonal communication is actually nonverbal, such as body language and facial expressions. Quirky kids often miss the boat in this regard. They keep on talking. They talk in monotonous voices. They change the subject midstream. Or they do not understand the facial expressions of the person with whom they are speaking. They interrupt with no regard for the person being interrupted; the concept of turn-taking in a conversation is foreign to them. This is a major handicap, even for a comparatively young child in the first few grades of school. Pragmatic language therapy, or social skills training (discussed in more detail on pages 245–247 in Chapter 9), is directed at teaching children these skills. Given the rules of the game, many quirky kids can learn what comes naturally to most of us.

> There was one boy in my second-grade class who just didn't seem to understand that when I stood silently at the front of the room with my hands on my hips, they needed to settle down and get to work. He would just keep going about his business. It took a while for me to understand that this behavior was part of his disorder, not that he was being intentionally oppositional.

This diagnosis was introduced in 2013 when the medical literature began officially referring to the term ASD. Social communication disorder includes the social communication challenges of ASD without the restricted and repetitive behaviors. It is sometimes difficult for families to find appropriate treatment, precisely because the diagnosis does not include the word autism and, thus, children in some school systems may not qualify for the same level of support.

Sensory Processing Disorder

Most likely to be used by OTs, the term *sensory processing disorder* describes a child who seems out of sync with her environment. We have worked with a number of kids who fit this description and have benefited from treatments directed toward this problem. Sensory integration refers to the capacity to take in information from the senses—visual, tactile, auditory, taste, and smell—and process it. This capacity is hardwired in the central nervous system in the right hemisphere of the brain. The ability to integrate this sensory information enables us to understand the big picture. When this system is faulty, it is nearly impossible to make it through the day smoothly.

> Ben doesn't like loud noises but has no trouble with movies or loud performances. He has sensory abilities most of us don't have or screen out without thinking about it. He suffers from recurrent ear infections, and at age 6, he told his pediatrician, "I can feel fluid moving around inside my ear."

A child with sensory processing disorder may be oversensitive or undersensitive to sensory input. Some children are extremely sensitive to touch or textures, loud noises, or visual stimulation, and because of this sensitivity may try to minimize the stimulation. Alternatively, if children are much less sensitive than usual to such input, they may seek more of it than most people can tolerate. When you think about the oversensitive child, think of the kid who cannot stand the wind or the sand at the beach, not to mention the water. Or the boy who covers his ears at movies. Or the girl who cannot stand the seams on her socks or the tags on her sweater. However, the child who *seeks* stimulation of her senses may need the volume up high, may put everything in her mouth, or may enjoy spinning or twirling around as a way of sensing the world. In retrospect, parents often describe these oversensitive kids as fussy, prone to screaming or arching, and difficult to console. The undersensitive child may be remembered as excessively placid or so easy that the parents were worried—but probably didn't get much sympathy from anyone! Sensory integration treatment is designed to help kids with these issues.

> I was at the beach with my two children, Sam and John. I knew it was going to be hard for John, but I love the beach myself so I decided to just give it one more try. One breezy afternoon, Sam was so happy he just couldn't get enough of it. He jumped in and out of the water, rolled around in the sand, squealed and shrieked with joy in the brisk breeze. At one point, we decided to take a walk along the beach. Sam was completely naked except for his sunglasses and was thoroughly enjoying himself. John, on the other hand, was fully clothed with socks and shoes, a terry-cloth bathrobe, a bicycle helmet, and goggles so as not to feel the wind or get any sand in his eyes. I knew other moms were noticing us. We must have been quite a sight.

Nonverbal Learning Disability

The term *nonverbal learning disability* (NVLD) describes the learning profile often seen in quirky kids, with particular findings on neuropsychological testing—for example, a stronger verbal score than the performance score. It is a *nonverbal* learning disability because the child's verbal scores are fine; she runs into trouble with her nonverbal skills of integration and abstract reasoning. Children with NVLD tend to be bright, have a great vocabulary, are terrific at rote learning, and they reliably notice details, but they cannot integrate them into a unifying concept. Although these kids may be strong in math in the sense that they have excellent computation skills, a word problem can really throw them off. Anything that requires abstract reasoning is a challenge to a child with NVLD, and academic performance may falter as they move into higher grades where this kind of reasoning is required. Problems with visual perception can manifest as physical awkwardness or clumsiness. Many of these children also have sensory processing disorder, usually manifested as sensitivity to certain kinds of touch or textures, loud noises, and so on. Nonverbal learning disability is a global disability that makes processing of new information challenging. These kids are quite literal in their interpretation of language and cannot appreciate metaphors or "read between the lines." This can be of great concern to parents, as it puts the child with NVLD at risk for abuse or other dangerous situations. These kids need help from special education services, pragmatic language therapy, and sometimes OT.

Executive Function Difficulties

The executive function skills are the higher-order thinking skills required to organize a plan and carry it out. Many quirky kids, despite high intelligence, have great difficulty in day-to-day activities because of executive function difficulties. These problems can impede their progress academically, socially, and in the working world. They might answer any individual academic question perfectly well—maybe even brilliantly—but can't put it all together, can't actually outline the project and see it through, or can't complete the assignment. Teachers with special education skills can be helpful, and some OTs can work on organizational skills.

> Despite his high intelligence and encyclopedic knowledge of facts, Gabriel can't put it all together in a decent report for school. He's much better off with short answer questions or multiple choice—anything that doesn't require organization.

Anxiety

Anxiety is probably the single most common comorbid mental health condition for quirky kids, and sometimes it's the anxiety that brings them to medical attention. Familiar to all of us, anxiety is more familiar to quirky kids and their families. Children can manifest their anxiety in any number of ways, but it is almost always part of the quirky-kid package. That is not to say that all quirky kids qualify for the diagnosis of an anxiety disorder. Some manage anxiety much better than others. Some are truly debilitated by their anxiety, whereas for others, it's a smaller piece of the puzzle. Still, most quirky kids tend to be anxious. Perhaps your child needs someone in his bedroom until he has fallen asleep. Perhaps he does not separate and explore the world at the expected time because he just can't let go of you, or perhaps his fear of strangers is all-consuming and debilitating. As children get older, anxiety can show up in many ways in particular situations—around animals or about having to perform in class—or with anxiety-driven behaviors. Anxiety disorders are broken down into 3 subtypes:

- *Generalized anxiety disorder* describes a person whose worry is pervasive and difficult to control and is out of proportion to any real threat. The worry is associated with physical symptoms—trouble sleeping or palpitations—and causes enough distress to interfere with everyday life.
- *Social phobia* means the anxiety is focused on social situations or situations in which the child must "perform" in public. In young children, this may manifest as excessive shyness or fear of strangers.

Abby was so afraid in social situations, we stayed home most of the time. In her toddler years, she was terrified in groups, and anything unexpected could set her off—like a sudden laugh or someone coughing. We avoided family gatherings, or one of us would go and the other would stay home with her.

- *Separation anxiety disorder* describes a level of distress and worry about leaving home or separating from a parent that is unexpected for the child's age. Some of these kids are unwilling to go to school because it means separating from the parent, or they may even be unwilling to go to sleep for fear of something happening to the parent.

Obsessive-Compulsive Disorder

Obsessive-compulsive disorder (OCD) is a syndrome in which the compulsion to do something over and over is an attempt to ward off anxiety. Previously, it was classified under the anxiety disorders but recent research has shown that it seems to have differing manifestations as well as a distinct natural history. Hoarding and skin picking (newly recognized in *DSM-5*) fall within this category, along with hair pulling and body dysmorphic disorder, which is manifested by a negative preoccupation with body image that is focused on a minor or perceived flaw. For some families, this is the first symptom that brought them in for evaluation.

Eventually, Brian developed an hour and a half of going-to-bed rituals. I used to read to the kids every night, and he would have to go to the bathroom after I finished—and he would do it again and again.

When John was about 3, he learned to tell time, which was a great surprise to all of us. By 4 or 5, he had a collection of watches and clocks—some analog, some digital, some on military time. He often wore 3 or 4 watches at the same time. By age 5, he started lining up his clocks along the side of his bed and synchronizing them before he fell asleep. If they weren't synchronized when he woke up, he'd become very anxious. This prompted our first visit to a child psychiatrist.

The OCD-like symptoms can be a major source of stress and disability for quirky kids. Although this is not a primary quirky-kid diagnosis, a good proportion of quirky kids deal with these issues along the way, though comparatively few of these children actually meet the criteria for an OCD diagnosis.

Many quirky kids have a special interest in certain subjects, such as the Civil War, movie technologies, tax codes, or the weather. Intense special interests can be obsessive, and it can be challenging to determine when an obsession becomes a disorder. The *DSM-5* definition of obsession has also changed, with "urge" replacing "impulse." Sometimes what looks like OCD is better understood as a manifestation of the repetitive behaviors or interests that are part of ASD. Many kids will have obsessions and compulsions, but not to the degree that leads to an OCD diagnosis; even so, these issues may loom large for them as they grow up.

Adults are allowed to have special interests and become experts in obscure areas. For kids it's much more difficult to function socially if you are hyperfocused on trains, plumbing supplies, or sports statistics. If you're trying to figure out whether a child really is struggling with OCD, a child psychiatrist may be able to help sort all this out.

Attention-Deficit/Hyperactivity Disorder

Attention-deficit/hyperactivity disorder is a common diagnosis applied to quirky kids. Although it often fits the bill, this diagnosis is *so* common that parents need to be sure the evaluation is thorough. Identifying an attentional problem does not tell you whether or not ADHD is the whole story.

More common in boys, ADHD is found in as many as 11% of all children in the United States. Kids with ADHD can't maintain their focus, and this manifests itself in two major ways: inattention and hyperactivity-impulsivity. Children with inattention are easily distracted and disorganized; they have a lot of trouble following through, and, of course, they have a hard time paying attention. Hyperactivity means constant motion—from squirming and fidgeting at rest to nonstop running and climbing. And, as you would expect, impulsivity suggests a tendency to act without thinking. A child may have only inattention (often how ADHD shows up in girls) or only hyperactivity with impulsivity, but most commonly, children have both sets of symptoms.

To meet the *DSM-5* definition of ADHD, a child must manifest these behaviors in different settings (not just act up in school, for example, while behaving well at home) over the course of at least 6 months, and they must interfere with the child's functioning, which should become evident before 12 years of age. The ability to concentrate for long periods on television or video games does not mean that a child does not have ADHD, as those activities offer a kind of repeated stimulation that actually works well for children with this problem. Therefore, a child who can't pay attention in school or to activities with friends and siblings at home may have ADHD, even if he spends long periods watching TV or videos or playing games on a screen.

This diagnosis can be made by some general pediatricians, although others prefer to send kids to neurologists, developmental-behavioral pediatricians, or psychiatrists for a full assessment. The diagnosis should involve asking parents to fill out questionnaires describing the child's behavior at home while the teacher is asked for a description of school behavior.

Children with ADHD can be quite isolated from their peers because of their difficulties, which require a disproportionate amount of attention from adults. Teachers, coaches, camp counselors, and even parents may think of these kids as particularly troublesome and labor intensive. Other kids may resent them for taking up so much attention or for disrupting activities and making trouble in school. The children themselves end up lonely and depressed and sometimes act out even more wildly.

There are 3 components to the treatment of ADHD: behavioral supports such as counseling or parental training, educational supports such as a classroom accommodation, and medication. Medication is standard therapy for children whose ADHD is interfering with school function, and 85% of kids will respond well to medications.

Kids with ADHD have a higher-than-normal risk of developing many comorbid conditions, including other behavioral disorders, Tourette syndrome and other tic disorders, anxiety, depression, learning disabilities, and speech and language problems. Up to 15% to 20% of these kids will have some kind of learning disability, compounding their attentional problems with other academic struggles.

Oppositional Defiant Disorder

Although all kids are oppositional at times, the term *oppositional defiant disorder* is reserved for the child who is constantly disobedient and uncooperative. It is commonly seen along with ADHD, and we hear quite a lot about otherworldly tantrums in quirky kids who have difficulty modulating their reactions to fit the situation. This is a *DSM-5* diagnosis, which means it is a category of mental health disorder—children who lose their tempers easily, argue with adults, often defy or refuse to comply with adult requests, provoke people on purpose, blame others for their own misbehavior, are easily annoyed, and come off as angry, resentful, and spiteful. These are challenging qualities in a child and sometimes these are the reasons that parents look for some type of help.

> I told my pediatrician that I thought my son must have ADHD because he is always in motion, can't seem to sit still, and has tantrums that frighten me and my 8-year-old daughter. He's only 21 months old.

Although the diagnostic criteria are descriptive, they do nothing to explain the cause of this behavior. Our experience suggests that many quirky kids are overwhelmed by the world around them, aren't flexible enough to go with the flow, miss all kinds of cues that might avert a meltdown in the average child, and pop a gasket when they can't manage any other way. Sometimes called "explosive," these kids are not well liked by their peers or their teachers. By and large, they are not happy—and neither are their parents. Many end up on medications, and they often find it useful to see counselors and learn to discuss their feelings and impulses.

Tourette Syndrome and Other Tic Disorders

Many people have heard of Tourette syndrome, although some expect this neurological disorder to involve outbursts of profanity as its most prominent feature. In fact, the hallmark of Tourette syndrome is the presence of both vocal and motor tics, which are sudden involuntary movements or sudden involuntary sounds. Tics can range from brief jerks or twitches to head shaking or gyrating, as well as unexpected vocalizations, sniffing, or throat clearing. Very rarely, they can include obscene gestures or bad language.

Tic disorders are, in fact, quite common in all kids, quirky or not. Pediatricians see a lot of kids with tics, which are more common in boys than girls, and they often appear in kindergarten or first grade. A provisional tic lasts less than

12 months. We sometimes see a tic that disappears, only to see a new one appear later. All first- and second-grade teachers are familiar with tics because they are quite common. Kids often are not bothered by them, and other kids don't notice them, at least in elementary school, nearly as much as parents and other adults do.

> Kai had a cold for a week or two, but never stopped sniffing. He'd do
> it all the time except in his sleep. The pediatrician thought it was
> a tic, not an allergy symptom. Eventually it went away but then he
> started his eye blinking, which he has been doing for a few months.
> He doesn't seem to be aware of it. It's more intense when he is
> anxious or in a new situation, and it goes away when he is sleeping.

For a child to have Tourette syndrome, his symptoms must meet a set of criteria: multiple motor tics as well as at least one phonic (sound-related) tic and tics that occur multiple times during the day or continue to recur at least occasionally for more than a year. Tics in general, and Tourette's, are much more common in people with ADHD and OCD, and, as with many of these syndromes, they tend to run in families. Tourette syndrome typically shows up between the ages of 3 and 8 years, and it is most severe around the age of 10. Tics disappear by the age of 18 for more than half of the kids with Tourette's. Medication helps many children with tic disorders.

Processing What You've Learned

These diagnoses may seem like an overwhelming number of things to worry about, but they are meant to include the problems faced by a diverse group of children, and no two quirky kids are the same. The trajectory for most of them, especially with support and therapies over time, is positive; most of the diagnoses we've just described allow for a great deal of progress. As parents, you need to understand the landscape so you know the range of problems that might come up over time, but you should go into this expecting growth and improvement. Most important, remember that regardless of the diagnosis (or the new diagnosis, or the changing diagnosis), your child needs your love and support. And, as we said earlier, your child is the same child he or she was before any diagnostic label was applied, and you love that child like crazy.

3

Understanding the Diagnosis: Grief and Loss and Moving Forward

Your child now has a diagnosis, which is a way of understanding the things that have worried you. You've been given a name—a label—and told that it belongs to your child. Maybe it's a familiar name, or maybe it's a term you've never heard before. Perhaps it feels strange, unexpected, unrelated to your perception of your child and what's really going on. Or maybe it seems so right that it has a kind of inevitability. Maybe it's even the diagnosis you've been expecting all along. Or perhaps—and this can feel worse—you've been told that your child doesn't fit neatly into *any* particular category, and you're left wondering what to do next.

As pediatricians, we've seen parents in the days after they received these diagnoses. Sometimes we've even been the ones to deliver the news, explaining evaluation results or interpreting an overly technical letter. However well-educated and well-prepared parents may be, the experience of dealing with a diagnosis of this kind is intense, emotional, and highly charged.

Nothing hits as hard or hurts as much as finding out that your child has a problem. When you think something might be wrong, you lie awake and agonize. When those worries are confirmed, you're often devastated, no matter how well prepared you thought you were.

Despite me expecting the opposite, I was hoping our doctor would say, "Well, your child is definitely a little different and he's got this, this, and this, but he isn't on the spectrum." But I was still sad when he said, "Yes, he's pretty classic." Afterward, I wept and my husband said, "I don't see why you're so upset. You were expecting this." I think it was because a person in a position of authority and expertise had said this. I wasn't just a neurotic parent. We were going to be dealing with this his whole life. It was really mammoth.

A Sense of Loss

As parents, we start out with a mixture of hopes, expectations, and fantasies. It's the great adventure of our adult lives, this remarkable experience of starting out with an infant and looking ahead to helping shape a new life. It's a complicated blend of falling madly in love, working harder than you've ever worked before, and redefining your family and your sense of self. These fantasies typically do not involve thoughts about when the first early intervention evaluation will take place. Thus, your child's diagnosis will probably evoke a certain sense of loss and sadness.

Every year at the school where I taught, parents would come to see me to talk about their kids. I could see that they didn't know what to do and were in between denial and grieving. "This is not the child I was expecting. This is not the way I expected my child's upbringing to go." There's a grieving process that goes along with getting this kind of diagnosis.

We enter parenthood with lots of expectations and complications—in fact, lots of baggage. We're going to do it right even if our own parents didn't. We're going to protect our precious children from every danger; make their childhoods as happy as possible; control, as far as possible, the environments in which they live and the schools in which they learn. This isn't wrong or evil or arrogant—only impossible, as we come to learn. But in addition to our unrealistic fantasies of child-rearing, we bring fantasies of how our children will perform, how they will follow in our footsteps—or surpass us—and how they will do us proud. These fantasies are part of the anticipation and enjoyment of parenthood.

Your quirky child has served you notice that all will not go as planned. The reality is that it never goes as planned for any parents. However, this feels different, because it is. The diagnosis, when it comes, may seem to be the epitaph for all your fondest hopes and dreams. Many parents hear that first diagnosis as the end of fantasies. *No, my child will not [fill in the blank.] Won't be at the head of the class. Won't go further than I did in tournament tennis. Won't have the successful, untroubled, socially confident adolescence I never had. Won't grow up to take over the family bike shop. Or simply, won't grow up to be a happy, normal, independent, well-adjusted adult with a strong central relationship and a family.*

Understanding the ramifications of the diagnosis may mean coming to terms with some scary realities about what you will have to contend with as your child grows, as well as some of the difficulties your child may face physically, emotionally, or socially. There may be real limitations in the immediate and distant future. In our pediatric and personal experience, we've learned that parenthood is never what you expected it to be. Still, we also acknowledge that, right now, this generalization may be cold comfort.

No matter how much you thought you wanted it and needed it, you may experience your child's diagnosis as a blow and a loss. That's perfectly fair. Your job is to adjust and find ways to use this new information, to become informed as a caregiver, a supporter, and an advocate. But before you do that, you may need time to mourn and adjust to the new normal.

> I am not the support-group type but have met many parents in various waiting rooms over the years, and that became a support group of sorts. We'd share anecdotes, laugh about how weird the kids were, and reassure one another that we were not alone. When my son was really young, it helped me to see the older kids who had made great progress and to hear their parents say, "You wouldn't believe it if you saw him a few years ago!" It gave me hope, a sense of perspective, and someone to call when the going got rough.

After you acknowledge your grief at the loss of some of your hopes and fantasies, you must then build and maintain new hopes for your child's future, even as you adjust your expectations. Your parental job of helping your child grow and thrive as an individual is going to require that you believe in that individual.

That doesn't mean we're telling you to doubt or question the diagnosis. If it makes sense to you and is being offered by experts you trust, we urge you, at this difficult and emotional moment, to keep the diagnosis in perspective, to use it as a tool toward understanding and helping your child, and to keep an open mind about what the future may hold.

Moving Forward

- Remind yourself that the purpose of the diagnosis is to direct you toward information, resources, and therapies that can help your child function as well as possible, at home, in school, and in life. So much progress has been made in the past 20 years that the outlook is much brighter for the majority of quirky kids.
- Take the diagnosis seriously, but remember that many kids may accumulate several diagnoses as they grow, and the first one given may or may not have long-term relevance or predictive value.
- Consider joining a support group or another network of parents.
- Whatever diagnostic term you're dealing with, remember that it necessarily reflects a range of children—from those who struggle more to highly functional kids—so don't let your expectations be colored by examples from the more severe end.
- Most of these diagnoses are works in progress. The diagnoses themselves are likely to evolve over time, as they have done since the first edition of this book was published.
- Above all, don't let the diagnosis cast a heavy shadow on your own picture of your child and your sense of future potential.

Parental Reaction

Parents' reaction to a new diagnosis will depend on how they handle stress in general. We've watched parents in two-parent households divide up the intellectual and emotional work, with one parent insisting on obtaining more information, while the other cries or looks stunned. Some parents, given a clue, turn into desperate detectives, spending hours on the internet, accumulating shelves of books and scientific reprints, and trying to out-expert the experts. Although this can be admirable, watch out if you've completely split the duties and one of you is in charge of information while the other confronts the emotional implications. Chances are, you really need each other right now. You both need to acknowledge head and heart. For single parents, don't try to manage all the work and emotion alone. Call in the troops—family and friends—for support, meet with other parents through school or early intervention, and create a community for yourself for the long haul. It really makes a difference.

You also need to acknowledge the mourning process. Is there a person in your family or someone you remember from your own childhood who comes to mind when you worry about the future? Are there specific fantasy images of parenthood to which you feel you are bidding goodbye forever? There are certain parental experiences that perhaps only the other parent can truly understand, and we urge you to give each other some help and comfort. Also, be ready to seek outside help and support if either or both of you need something more. There are moments in life with a quirky child when you may need to talk with someone—a therapist, counselor, member of the clergy, or psychiatrist.

> **Yes, I am in therapy and on meds myself now—both things I thought would never happen. But my life as a mom is not at all what I expected and has been so deeply affected by having a child like David that I needed something to help me stay the course.**

Many people respond to a child's diagnosis by demanding a cause, an etiology, a reason for what has gone wrong. We have had parents ask us whether the problem was caused by an illness in infancy, a medication the mother took during pregnancy, or, of course, environmental toxins, childhood immunizations, or any of the other theories people read and hear about as possible causes of developmental differences. As we discuss in Chapter 5, there are many parents for whom the quest for a cause becomes a mission, even an obsession.

Even more commonly, though, what we hear in the office is a parent assigning familial responsibility:

- "It's from my family, I know. My brother's oldest child is hyperactive."
- "My husband's really upset because he knows where this is coming from. He has this brother who has seizures and tics, and he's scared our son is going to be the same way."
- "My mother told me about a cousin who was described as slow. Does that mean this is in my genes?"

Not so rarely, this takes on a tone of accusation, whether bitter self-accusation or even more bitter accusation of someone else. "I should never have had children." "You should have told me about your cousin before we got married." While genetic explanations are only established in a small proportion of kids, it's quite clear that there are as-yet unidentified genes involved, and many people can point to family members who seem to have related problems. Part of the reason for this is the high frequency of quirks and quirky kids in the general population, which was evident even before most of these diagnoses existed, but part of the explanation is that these diagnoses do indeed run in families. We discuss the genetic components in greater detail in Chapter 11.

> Chrissie's dad has a history of ADHD and learning disabilities, and he was held back in the fifth grade. He used to get locked in the closet because of his high activity level. I wonder whether I myself am on the spectrum. As a child, I listened to music obsessively, all day long. I wanted to be a disc jockey, and I read all the disc jockey magazines. In fact, I still want to be a disc jockey.

> Where did this come from? I feel that I am the most likely culprit. I've always been excessively shy. In school, I was the quiet smart one in the class. And I'm still shy. I have several very close friends I've had for years but not a lot of acquaintances.

Thinking in terms of blame and guilt when it comes to heritable conditions is a slippery slope for parents already facing a situation that requires them to summon all their strength and to support each other through difficult times and tough questions. So although you may want at some point to consider the genetics of whatever is going on with your child—seeing a geneticist, tracing out a family pedigree, and looking at the odds that a future child may be affected—this should not be your top priority in the days and weeks after receiving a diagnosis.

Try to be understanding and sympathetic. Any illness or major life stressor puts an enormous strain on a couple's relationship. Take time now to confront this new challenge and come together for the sake of your child, yourselves, and your family. You need to be able to discuss what's going on without assigning blame. No one deliberately passes on a problem to a child. You want to understand and help, and you want to do it together. Build on what you have in common—your commitment to each other and to your child—and don't rip yourselves apart.

> I always felt that my husband and I were in it for the long haul,
> whether we drove each other crazy or not, but once we had our
> son's diagnosis, I felt it much more acutely. John really needs us
> both, and he's doing as well as he is because he has two loving
> parents.

Make sure you look around and see how your other children are doing too. We've seen parents become so preoccupied with the new diagnosis and its implications that a sibling feels neglected.

> Brian started having problems and getting these diagnoses when
> his sister Jennifer was about 14, and she just withdrew. At the time,
> she felt she needed to become more self-sufficient because her
> parents had this problem that they needed to deal with. She orches-
> trated her applications to middle school all by herself. I was amused
> and thought this was sweet and cute at the time, but now I under-
> stand that she felt she had to do it because if she didn't, I wouldn't,
> because of what was going on with her brother. I think she's wrong. I
> hope she's wrong.

Who Needs to Know?

You're handling the diagnosis, you've allowed yourselves to grieve a little, you've helped each other and refrained from casting blame, you've started to put together a community of other parents and kids with similar issues, and you're feeling ready for the complex parental task of finding ways to use this new information to help your child. That's all really important work. Here are a couple of things to consider.

Who needs to know and who probably should know? We're not talking here about how you discuss this with the child, since we're focused for the moment on fairly young children, and on the question of discussing what may be an evolving picture with family members, caregivers, preschool teachers, friends, and even the wider community. There are no easy answers, but there are a few guidelines to consider as you make your decisions. In the years since our first edition was published, ASD has become a part of the lexicon of common speech. People often describe friends, relatives, or colleagues as "probably being on the spectrum somewhere." Many people are familiar with the terminology and what it means, and it engenders less fear and dread than it used to. The quirky child has found a way into popular culture as well, from

The Curious Incident of the Dog in the Night-Time to *The Big Bang Theory* to *Parenthood* and *Atypical*. So, while it's worth considering whether—and how—to share a diagnosis with members of your circle, you may find that the diagnosis does not come as a surprise.

If you have close friends, family members, or others who care about your child and who have been involved every step of the way in your child's evaluation, obviously, you're going to tell them about the diagnosis. Anyone who knows your child well will understand the importance of figuring out what's going on, and these are the people who will become part of your child's "team" as you all move forward together. The world is certainly more accepting of neurodiversity than it used to be, even since the first edition of this book.

On the other hand, the world is full of busybodies and self-appointed experts, and you do not owe lengthy explanations to people who are not part of that team. Telling folks may mean you have to talk about it more than you'd like. You need to take care of your child and yourselves and you have a right to protect yourself and your family from unwanted attention around a difficult topic.

> **I told one friend who is a little too hovering. Every time she reads an article about autism, she sends it to me. She means well, but she's more neurotic about this than I am.**

Tell people whatever they need to understand and help your child. That doesn't mean that if he acts up in public, you have to stand there saying over and over, "I'm so sorry. He's on the spectrum." All children act up in public. The correct thing to do is to set things to rights as much as possible, remove the child when that isn't possible, and apologize to anyone who has been bothered or inconvenienced. (In extreme situations, such as when you're trapped on a delayed flight on the tarmac with 300 total strangers, you may find yourself explaining, and you may be pleasantly surprised by the understanding and sympathy you encounter.) However, close relatives will need to be given some information to help them understand a child they love who may behave strangely at times. You can explain the behavior, offer your best strategies for dealing with it, and present and explain the diagnosis, but you might want to do this by degrees. Chances are, close relatives and friends also have been concerned but may have been reluctant to say something to you, so they may be relieved to know the behavior has been evaluated and has a name, and there are things that can be done to help. They will be your allies in the years ahead.

You may also have family members you find harder to talk to. There is no right answer. Our advice is to give yourselves a break; have the helpful and necessary conversations and wait on the ones that seem more problematic.

> My advice is to lie low for a while and not go blabbing it to the whole neighborhood or the schools—unless you have to. Also, don't talk about it with your child (unless he asks you directly or is disturbed by his differences) until he's old enough to understand.

> We have been very careful about who we said what to. One of our relatives is a child psychiatrist, and he had a lot of opinions. He made us feel as if this was all our fault.

> I have told my mother, but it doesn't mean anything to her. She loves her grandson; she knows he's different; she knows he needs a little extra help. The name doesn't mean anything to her. For his teachers, it's been very helpful. They've read about it; they've talked to his psychiatrist and his therapists. They've taken him on as a project.

One reason to think about this carefully is your immediate family. If you have other children, and they are old enough to understand, the way you present your quirky child to grandparents, aunts, and uncles quickly transfers to siblings. There are situations in which a child's behavior is so extreme that siblings need special explanations, but it cannot be denied that there are also many situations in which the best thing for a quirky child is to be treated normally by his less quirky siblings.

> We don't talk about Gabriel in our family as if he has a diagnosis. I think we can address the fact that he doesn't know his nose is running without saying, "Oh, it's your sensory processing." If my other kids ask, I say, "He doesn't like loud noises, and we're his family and we have to make sure he doesn't have to hear too many of them." And then I point out ways we accommodate to their quirks, too. He just has about 20 times more!

In other words, the decision about what you say within your immediate family is affected by the ages and personalities of your other children and, possibly most of all, by how extreme the behaviors are with which you need to deal.

It's possible that siblings may need to understand that one child has a special problem and mustn't be teased about it, but you may be better off casting this—at least at first—as standard household politeness; you are not allowed to tease your brother about his obsessions (eg, trains, clocks), and he is not allowed to tease you about yours (eg, Taylor Swift).

Informing the school makes good sense for the school-aged child. She may require special services to succeed academically, occupational or speech therapy, or applied behavior analysis at school, and the diagnosis will help you receive those services. Also, a diagnosis that school personnel understand may help when a child's behavior becomes difficult to manage. Because schools can be quick to ascribe a child's classroom difficulties to willful behavior problems, diagnoses may help schools and teachers understand that the children are actually doing the best they can. And that is an important message to get across. Kids with ASD are often misunderstood, and their behaviors can be misinterpreted as mischief, when in fact they are just trying to figure out the world around them.

Perhaps the most complex decision of all is what you are going to say to the quirky child himself. Some people and some organizations feel that disclosure is almost always right, and the sooner the better. Certainly, it is better for your child to learn about the diagnosis from you—with understanding, love, and information—than to have it thrown at him in school or by an angry sibling. The main issue is your child's developmental and intellectual stage; children need to be given information as they are ready to understand it. Some quirky kids, in particular, can be very young for their ages. We're going to come back to this issue and approach it as an evolving understanding in which the child may need new language, new information, and new definitions as time goes on.

Your own understanding of what may lie behind some of your child's unusual behaviors does not mean that anything goes. It is perfectly legitimate to look for new strategies and, of course, to forgive what the child cannot help, but the quirks and the diagnoses don't excuse you from your job as a parent. You still must help your child learn to behave and get along as well as possible.

Here are the most important take-home messages of this chapter and, possibly, of this book:

- *Keep loving your child, and do not confuse the child with the diagnosis.* See her for who she is—strengths and weaknesses, quirks and quibbles—and love her for it. Don't let your vision of her be affected too strongly by new terminology. You already knew she was different in certain ways. She's the same child she was before she received a diagnosis. Make sure she knows how much you love her.

- *Take a deep breath.* A diagnosis is not the end of anything—not the end of your fantasies, not the end of your child's potential and possibilities, and not even the end of your quest to understand and help your quirky child. We don't want to minimize the complexities that may be implied by the diagnosis or the special challenges your child may face as she grows, but a diagnosis is not the end.

- *Keep an open mind about what the future holds.* Remember that these diagnoses encompass a wide range of behaviors, problems, and complications. Also keep in mind that children grow and change, and any given child may evolve from one diagnosis to another. You need to find a blend of realism, good sense, and hope. All parents do, in fact, but in your case, that blend has to take into account the diagnosis and its implications without letting them define your child's entire future. Life with quirky kids is full of surprises; we've had the long view on lots of them over many years, and we often find ourselves just delighted by unexpected developments.

- *Don't fixate on blame, and don't fixate on a cure. Focus on your child and what she needs and how you can help.* It's completely normal to fantasize about a cure and to search for magic bullets, but none of these diagnoses is amenable to easy answers or overnight cures.

- *Don't forget to take care of yourself, your other children, and your spouse or partner.* Living with a quirky son or daughter or sister or brother can be a challenge, and there's a danger of forgetting that everyone else in the family has needs and emotions too. Your quirky child will profit immeasurably from growing up in a caring family. Take care of everyone, and keep the family on course.

- *The diagnosis is a tool. Now it's time to learn how to use it to help your quirky child.*

2

Growing Up Quirky

Literary Glimpses

Bradford...their genius five-year-old son...was sitting on the living room floor, pulling books off the bottom shelf of the bookcase that took all of one of the few existing walls. Without looking up at us, he started to mumble some barely coherent comments about how we'd interrupted him in the middle of what he was doing.

"He's arranging all of the books in the house according to height."

"According to color!" Bradford cried, "I'm arranging them all by color."

"Would you be willing to reveal your system for arranging the colors?" Arthur asked.

"Yes; it's a very simple alphabetical arrangement. If you'll look on that bookshelf behind you, you'll see that the black ones are first, then the blue, then the green, the orange, the red, and the yellow. Those are the basic categories."

"Hey, Brad," I said, "what about the browns?"

"I'm putting the browns together on a bookshelf in the other room, off by themselves."

—Stephen McCauley, *The Easy Way Out*, 1992

Was it because people were a little afraid of him that they whispered about the Murrays' youngest child, who was rumored to be not quite bright? "I've heard that clever people often have subnormal children," Meg had once overheard. "The two boys seem to be nice, regular children, but that unattractive girl and the baby boy certainly aren't all there."

It was true that Charles Wallace seldom spoke when anybody was around, so that many people thought he'd never learned to talk. And it was true that he hadn't talked at all until he was almost four. Meg would turn white with fury when people looked at him and clucked, shaking their heads sadly.

"Don't worry about Charles Wallace," her father had once told her. Meg remembered it very clearly because it was shortly before he went away. "There's nothing the matter with his mind. He just does things in his own way and in his own time."

—Madeleine L'Engle, *A Wrinkle in Time*, 1962

"He's five, just turned five," Morris Sapersteen said. … He set down the suitcase with a sigh. "Gosh, you'd never believe how heavy those things can be."

"What have you got there?" Marjorie said.

"Airplanes."

"Airplanes?"

"Forty-seven airplanes. Neville won't go anywhere without them. …"

Neville left his chair and catapulted into the dining room, yelling, "Daddy, I want my airplanes! Give me my airplanes!"

Morris jumped up, forgetting that the suitcase was open on his lap; the suitcase slipped, he clutched at it and upset it, and the forty-seven airplanes went clanking and tinkling all over the floor under the table.

"No, no," screeched Neville. "I don't want them picked up. I've got to make a parade!" He dived under the table and could be heard crawling, and sliding airplanes along the floor.

"What's he going to make?" Mrs. Morgenstern said nervously. "Get him out from under the table, please."

"A parade," [his mother] said. "He won't harm anything. He just lines them up three abreast. In perfect formation."

—Herman Wouk, *Marjorie Morningstar*, 1955
(Note that this is happening at a large
family Passover seder.)

What You Should Know

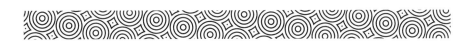

Entire parenting books have been written about children and school, about family life, and about children and their peers, but parents tell us that the advice in most books does not really apply to quirky kids. Having a quirky child can shift your perspective, causing all the usual worries and concerns to become more complex or slightly turned around or maybe arranged in a different order. Or it can mean a whole new set of problems to solve while getting through activities that are routine for most children.

There are many shades of quirky, and many children, over the course of their childhoods, move in and out of different phases. All children, quirky and not, wrestle at some points with school issues, social life issues, and family issues, and parents need to be a little wary of attributing every problem that comes up in a child's life to that child's quirks. It's also true that navigating all of this can be harder, more complicated, and sometimes more painful when you're grow-ing up on a different path.

In Part 2, we take a closer look at the 3 most important domains in which your child has to function on a daily basis: family, school, and peer group. It is probably safe to predict that how children feel about themselves as they grow up reflects their sense of how well they are doing in these arenas.

Not everything in Part 2 will be relevant to every quirky child because no two quirky kids are exactly alike. Navigating school will pose a different set of issues for the eccentric math genius whose town supports a math and science honors school than for the child who struggles with letters, numbers, and attention. And how chil-dren do in school affects other areas of their lives; that math genius, by virtue of being at a school with others like her, may find many aspects of her adolescent social life much more straightforward than she would have if she'd been in the big general high school.

We look at the educational choices—and issues—from preschool through high school. We take the same through-the-years approach to discussing a quirky child's social life and try to offer some philosophy and helpful strategies for navigating each stage. And we talk about the quirky child in the context of home and family, from the small everyday challenges and logistics to the larger emotional ramifications of being part of a quirky child's family.

Before we take on these big issues of the external domains in which your child must function, we want to address the most basic domain of all: your child's sense of self.

Children's sense of themselves and how different they are from other children varies tremendously, according to intelligence, self-awareness, social awareness, and perceptiveness. Some children, especially when they are younger, may hardly notice their own quirks, or may assume that the rest of the world is like them. Some kids remain blissfully clueless and go about their business without being afraid of social isolation. Other children are painfully aware from the very beginning of even minor differences. Some of this awareness—or lack of awareness—reflects the family, school, and social milieu.

Disclosing the Diagnosis to Your Child

How do children understand why they need to attend social skills training and occupational therapy once a week? How do they think about it if they can't ride a bike or swim when everyone else can do it? How would they explain the reason they get pulled out of class 3 times a week for extra help or why nobody else in the second grade is interested in train schedules or what those pills every morning are all about? For toddlers and preschoolers, their daily routines are just their daily routines. It usually doesn't occur to young children to think that their *experience is different from that of other kids their age.* However, as your child grows up, you will need to give some thought to self-consciousness, self-image, and self-knowledge. Many experts recommend explicit disclosure to a child with a specific diagnosis. This means telling your child, for example, "*You have what is called autism spectrum disorder and this explains many of the ways in which you think and function. There are many other people with autism spectrum disorder and you will have things in common with those people that will make you in some ways different from other kids. Your brain is special and a little different than a lot of other people's brains. You have skills that most people don't have, and you are more sensitive than others might be."*

In talking with their kids, parents should lead with their child's strengths and explain that because their brains are different, they will have challenges too, like everyone else. Many of the organizations and parental support groups that work with individuals with autism spectrum disorder feel that full disclosure is essential. There are plenty of published examples in which children—and adults—describe the relief that came with knowing that their differences had a name and that there were other people with similar differences.

In third grade, Caitlin found the article about Asperger syndrome [a former diagnostic category] that I had saved from the newspaper to share with my husband. Caitlin read it, brought it to me, and said, "I think I have this!"

But what about the child who doesn't fit a diagnostic category, who is thought to have social communication disorder or hard-to-categorize learning difficulty, or motor planning problems and sensory issues? Or what about the child who has already received several serial diagnoses and seems to be outgrowing the most recent? For these children, the question of disclosure can be more complicated. What if a child does not seem to sense herself as different from others? How do you know whether your child is ready or what she needs to hear?

Kids realize early on that they are different from other kids, and you need to find a positive way to have an open conversation about that in your family. We hear from adolescents and adults that when families think they are shielding their children, they are in fact hurting them. Not disclosing to children that they have diagnoses suggests that something is wrong, and that in itself is harmful. Think about children who were not told they were adopted until they were much older. This used to be common, but there is general consensus that the earlier this sort of information is shared, the better kids do. If it's too much information, though, it will go right over their heads until the next conversation.

Some general points on talking with children about their quirky and unusual behaviors:

- **Developmental stage.** The single most important determinant of what you say and how you say it is where the child is developmentally. You may need to explain to a 3-year-old why he is getting occupational therapy ("because your hands don't always do what you tell them to"), to an 8-year-old why she is taking a stimulant for attention-deficit/hyperactivity disorder ("because it makes it easier for you to focus at school and get your work done the way you want to"), or to a 10-year-old why he has to be in a different class from the kid next door ("because you learn things in a different way, and this teacher has some special ways of teaching that we hope will fit better with the way your brain learns"). Whatever the case, you need to adapt your language and images not just to your child's chronological age but to your child's developmental stage.

We were fortunate that the discussion about his differences came up while Brian was in elementary school when it was easier for him to accept. His self-image wasn't formed yet. I talked to a woman who had an older son whose problems were more clearly social, and he wouldn't accept the autism diagnosis at all. He refused to have anything to do with it and felt as if it was saying there was something wrong with him. With Brian being 10 or 11, it was easier to get the concept across that we need to think about doing things with him a little bit differently.

- **Ongoing conversation.** This conversation is not something you have once, and then it's done. It is an ongoing conversation, involving you, your spouse, your child, friends and family, teachers and therapists. As children grow, they refine their understanding of their quirks as their general cognitive levels and understanding deepen and change. Your goal in the earliest discussions could well be just to open the door and to emphasize that all questions are welcome and that you are happy to have these conversations whenever the child wants. As your child grows, this discussion should continue. You

want to avoid leaving a child with the sense that something important is being kept secret. Your child should hear all the most relevant
words from you in a positive and affectionate context.

- **Positive mindset.** You want this to be a positive experience, and, as
  much as possible, you want to present the information in a positive
  light. With a young child, that might mean saying something like,
  "Your brain learns in its own way, and that's part of what makes you
  who you are." It means reminding the child of her skills and talents
  any time that you are discussing her deficits and limitations and
  emphasizing that people vary, that everyone finds some things easy
  and other things difficult.

- **Know your timing.** Disclosure should never happen in the midst of
  a bad moment—a school failure, a disciplinary meltdown, a major
  social frustration. If a child asks why he is different in such a setting, deal with the immediate problem first and promise to sit down
  together and have a talk about all the other issues soon. Keep the
  promise. Similarly, if a child brings the subject up on line at the
  supermarket or while you are driving madly across town to pick up
  his brother, answer whatever short question is closest to the sur-
  face and then acknowledge that this is an important subject and
  deserves a serious talk. Promise that the talk will happen soon and
  keep that promise.

- **Listen and respond.** Listen to the question your child is asking and
  make sure that you answer it. There are lots of stories about 3-year-
  olds who ask an innocent question like, "Where did baby Lulu come
  from?" and get the whole fallopian-tubes-and-seminal-vesicles she-
  bang from an anxious but thorough parent, when all the child really
  meant was, "Is it true babies come from their mommies' tummies?"

- **Be straightforward and honest.** If a young child asks why she has to
  get some kind of special help or therapy, the best answer is concrete
  and practical (eg, "to help you do this, to make it easier for you to
  do that"). Having given that specific and functional answer, listen
  to whether your child wants to take it a step further. Why is it so
  hard for me to do that when it isn't hard for most kids? How come
  I always need special help with stuff? If those bigger questions
  are being asked, they need to be answered. And yes, there are 6- or
  7-year-olds out there who want the formal diagnoses. There are also
  11-year-olds who don't want to take it any further than,

"My hands don't always do what I want them to, and I worry more than other kids." Either way is fine. Tell your child what your child wants to know.

- **Direct the discussion accordingly.** Older children need more complex and complete answers, sometimes more complex and complete than you can give. If you know that it's time to sit down and talk with your 10- or 11-year-old, you might read up on the questions you'll need to discuss or have a book ready that your child can read herself.

However, by the time a child is 10 or 11 years old, you probably have a pretty good idea of that child's makeup, strengths and weaknesses, and the relevant diagnoses. You will be able to direct the discussion accordingly. Our experience as pediatricians is that children of this age will ask about what makes them different. (Our patients with chronic illnesses, for example, ask why they are always at the doctor, are always having their blood drawn or x-rays done, or are taking medications that their friends do not take.)

Chrissie is 10, and she's very relieved to know that her difference has a name and that there are other kids like her.

- **Preparation is key.** Be prepared for how you want to handle these questions. If you have a good working relationship with your pediatrician or another clinician or therapist, consider doing it together. We have had many such conversations with families over the years and have found them useful and moving for all concerned. Kids feel cared for and attended to, and the parent and pediatrician benefit from having this discussion in a supportive environment where questions can be answered and the future discussed.

Adolescence presents its own challenges, even for kids who previously seemed comfortable with having a diagnosis. Dania Jekel, MSW, executive director of the Asperger/Autism Network, reports that adolescents will sometimes outright reject a diagnosis and want nothing to do with it. This typically happens at around age 14 years and can be a real challenge for parents and professionals.

Moving Forward

We wish we could offer you hard and fast guidelines for helping children understand and appreciate their own unique perspectives as they grow. You need to be aware of your child's level of under-standing at any given point, his level of self-consciousness, and her feelings about herself and how she is doing. The only way for you to be aware of these things—especially as your child grows into a middle schooler and then an adolescent—is to keep the conversa-tional door open. Ask questions and listen carefully to the answers. Be sure that you are answering the questions asked of you, whether asked directly or indirectly. Your goal is not to protect your child from the knowledge that she is different but to help her integrate that knowledge into a reasonably happy picture of who she is. Just as you have learned to cherish her for all her different attributes, including her quirks, eccentricities, outsized talents, and struggles, you have to help her learn to understand herself, appreciate herself, and cherish herself. There is no more important single thread to growing up quirky, no more important responsibility for parents, and no more important developmental task for the child.

The disclosure process with George (now 14) has gone on over a few years. His older sister, who is a junior in college, has been very helpful in the process. She has attention-deficit/hyperactivity disorder herself, so she used this to explain to him that he, too, had learning differences. Since he adores her, it didn't seem so bad that he had something she also had, because he thinks of her as so smart and competent.

Logistics of Everyday Life:
The Home and the World

The single most famous line ever written about family life is probably Tolstoy's opening sentence in *Anna Karenina*: "Happy families are all alike; every unhappy family is unhappy in its own way." As pediatricians who have spent countless hours sitting with families, we humbly suggest that all happy families are sometimes unhappy and that no two families are actually alike for more than a few minutes at a time. In this chapter, we talk about family life with a quirky child.

Family life is intense, highly charged, and for most of us, extremely concentrated in terms of time and space. It's hard. It is colored for all of us by our own childhood experiences, our fantasies of what marriage and child-rearing would be like, and the images and messages sent to us by the culture in which we live, including television, YouTube, Facebook, and Instagram.

Finally, we measure ourselves constantly, and often rather harshly, against the parents and children we know: the other families at child care, our siblings and cousins and their families, our friends, and our colleagues. Parents play all kinds of subtle and not so subtle competitive games. There's the mother who casually drops into conversation that, of course, her 6-year-old is rereading the Harry Potter books now, and she's just desperate to find him something else that will really *challenge* him (often said after some other parent has just bemoaned the fact that her own 6-year-old refuses even to attempt *The Cat in the Hat*). Or how about the father who agrees that your daughter will have a wonderful time playing casual intramural soccer this year but happens to mention that his own daughter, the same age, has been recruited for the all-state team, and what a schlep that's going to be for everyone. Child-rearing turns out to be an oddly public activity, and we seem to be quick to judge one another's parenting, whether on an airplane, the playground, or more generally, the internet.

For parents of quirky children, these realities are particularly intense and charged. Life at home can sometimes feel like an hour-by-hour struggle. It doesn't help much to have well-meaning friends assure you that they understand—young children are always messy or siblings are always fighting; it's just the way of the world. In fact, for many parents whose children are outside the usual developmental parameters or manifest consistently eccentric habits, it can be particularly frustrating to be assured that their off-the-scale family stresses are just what everyone goes through. This chapter covers some of the common life experiences of families with quirky children and offers practical help for getting over the humps.

Family life with a quirky child is more fraught, more difficult, and subject to all types of stresses, or to more intense versions of the usual stresses. The daily routines of family life can be complicated by your child's eccentricities. Your relations with your spouse, your other children, your own parents, and your entire extended family will all be colored by this brush. You will find that you need to keep relearning to focus on the positive, to go easy on yourself, and to find occasions of joy. Although we don't mean to make light of the stresses and strains that families encounter, we do encourage you to hold on as tightly as possible to your sense of humor. Every parent needs one, and the parent of a quirky child needs a sense of humor that is downright, well, quirky. It may be hard to believe, but you will probably get to the point at which all your worst family disaster stories become familiar jokes. When you tell them, don't be surprised if you find at least a few other parents groaning in recognition.

Temperament and Goodness of Fit

Let's begin with a couple of concepts dear to pediatricians and early childhood professionals: temperament and goodness of fit. The child's temperament and the goodness of fit between that temperament and your family environment, not to mention your own temperament, will shape and color the tenor of your life together. By temperament, we mean the behavioral and psychological characteristics and personality of the child, which many experts believe are inborn or hardwired and that certainly appear to be established quite early in life. Parents will notice certain traits in their infants and young children and often connect them to similar traits in themselves. We describe temperament by looking at where a child lies along a continuum for each of several qualities, including:

- *Distractibility.* How hard does the child concentrate? How easy is it to draw her attention away to something else?

- *Irritability.* Everyone knows that some babies are easier than others. Many parents, looking at two siblings, are astonished by the contrast between the easy one, who is readily comforted, and the screamer, who arches and cries at any stimulation.
- *Ability to manage transitions.* Can he move from the car seat to the crib without waking up and screaming? Is child care pickup a fun reunion or a nightmare?
- *Ability to self-soothe.* Can the child calm himself when he gets upset? Infants and toddlers who suck their thumbs or twirl their blankets when they become overwhelmed will be easier to live with than the ones who howl, scratch themselves, or withdraw completely.
- *Mood or outlook.* Does the infant or child have a generally positive outlook or is he wary and unhappy?

A young child's temperament, skills, and problems don't exist in a vacuum. The concept of goodness of fit refers to the way a child is or is not in sync with the family environment, family expectations, the physical setting, and the temperaments of other family members. There are all kinds of classic examples of bad fits, children who might be just fine in a different family setting, but who pose all sorts of difficulties in the family to whom they were dealt. The high-energy child in the calm, serene home with 2 older contemplative parents—she might have had an easier time as the third of 4 in a busier, crazier, noisier household where her demands would have had to compete with those of the other children. Or the quirky math genius living in a highly active sports-oriented household—wouldn't it be nice if we could give *him* to those two older contemplative parents who are going out of their minds chasing that little girl! Or the fussy, difficult-to-transition child with the parents who are anxiously determined to do everything right and interpret every cry as an accusation—let's give him to that happy-go-lucky, take-it-as-it-comes family over there in exchange for their obsessive little girl, who will fare much better with these equally anxious parents. She'll show them how to do everything right, and they'll do it.

It doesn't work that way. You love your child and your child loves you, and you are bound together for life. But there are easier fits and harder fits, and it's important to look at your quirky child and see clearly that the puzzle piece has more than one side. Don't let yourself think of him as a square peg without carefully looking at what makes the hole so round. Be aware of your own temperament, expectations, and habits. Although we don't mean to suggest that you are the one who has to do all the adjusting, you *are* the grown-up and therefore the one who is supposed to figure out how to make this work. Over time, you and your child will both grow and change, and you will find ways to accommodate one another.

> My son has never had much ability to entertain himself. I remember
> when he was a toddler, there was none of that exploring indepen-
> dence and then checking back with us to be sure we were still there.
> One of us was always right beside him, holding his hand, exploring
> the environment. Now I understand that this was his anxiety getting
> the best of him. And now, many years later, it takes a different form,
> yet one of us still has to be right near him in order for him to do
> anything he needs to do—such as reading for school and doing
> homework. I find myself craving the child who sits down and does
> something, anything, alone. And I know this isn't fair. I try to keep
> these feelings in check, and when I can't, I know it's time for a break.

Nuclear Tantrums and the Nuclear Family

Life is harder when a child is miserable all or most of the time or subject to tantrums and uncontrollable rages. Some parents remember that their quirky children cried all the time as infants or toddlers, and this behavior may become more intense in children who are deeply sensitive to sensory stimuli or who are language delayed and crying in frustration at not being able to make themselves understood. If you have such a child, it may be worth asking your primary care clinician to refer you to a behavioral psychologist or developmental-behavioral pediatrician. We know too well that many pediatricians feel that the excessive crying of a baby or toddler who otherwise seems to be healthy and who is growing and developing well is something that the parents have to live with and wait out. The standard pediatric response is to offer strategies: set limits, try time-outs, consider behavior modification, reward him when he's good, or try a sticker chart. These strategies work for some typical kids. But a child who is off the scale, or a parent who is truly worried that something else is going on, warrants a second look.

> My daughter had a tantrum right there in her pediatrician's office on
> the exam table. I hoped that the doctor would finally see what I was
> talking about and offer some suggestions or advice, or at the very
> least a little compassion. Instead, I felt that he, like our family and
> friends, thought I was crazy.

Many quirky children go through periods in their lives when they are subject to intense rages or tantrums. Again, many children, quirky or not, have tantrums, but the quirky kids tend to have tantrums that are more extreme—the tantrums that can't be touched by any of the wise strategies advised by the pediatrician, magazine article, or well-meaning passersby.

Quirky children have tantrums that don't go away if you ignore them, and that don't lend themselves to limit-setting and time-outs. It's not our intention here to provide you with specific strategies to handle your child's tantrums, because quirky kids vary so widely. It is, however, worth the effort to figure out what your child's triggers are and to try to address them. The AAP recommends a method for parents called Antecedent-Behavior-Consequence (ABC) where parents observe a given behavior to determine what preceded it and what followed it. They look to understand over time what tends to set the behavior off and what function it may be serving for the child. The ABC charts to help parents plot this out are available online.

Behavioral therapy is directed at exactly this type of analysis. Maybe it's all about frustration at the things they can't do that other children can. Maybe there are certain variations in their routines that they just can't handle. Maybe it has to do with sensory sensitivities such as noise or crowds. Knowing some of the triggers doesn't necessarily mean you can head off every tantrum, but it helps you understand what's going on with your child and offers possible strategies to consider. One rule of thumb is that it's best not to intervene *during* a meltdown, which can cause it to escalate, but rather to wait until the child has calmed down to address what provoked the storm and what might help in the future.

> **Chrissie had these paint-peeling tantrums from very early on—at the least provocation. She still has several major meltdowns per year at school, and she will insist that I be called and that she must go home. She also misunderstands people's motives. If another kid says, "Can I help you with that?" she thinks the kid is making fun of her, and she cries.**

Major rages at home and the occasional terrible tantrum in public can make you feel like a failure as a parent, especially during those moments in public when people seem to be coming from miles around to express unsolicited opinions about how to handle the situation. Even in the privacy and safety of your own house, as you watch a tantrum develop and deepen, you desperately feel that there must be *something* you can do to get your child out of the cycle, to solve the problem, to make things better. Remember, parents don't create the rage in their quirky kids. Tantrums, in most quirky kids, are a combination of their developmental differences and consequent frustrations, sensory problems, inability to express themselves well enough, and peculiar emotional wiring. You can help your child progress developmentally, filter and accommodate the sensory stimuli, and handle the emotional impulses, but you must do it without placing blame, either on your child or on yourself.

That highly cranky, oppositional, nonverbal, rage-prone child is also a child who may provoke a lot of anger and even violence from even a loving and tolerant parent. These kids can drive their parents crazy, and parents may feel pushed toward physical discipline and displays of uncontrolled anger themselves. *It's important to recognize the danger signs and know when you're getting near the edge.* Know whom you can ask for help—someone you can trust to take care of your child and give you a respite or to listen nonjudgmentally to your lamentations and offer an honest opinion or just take you out for a little fun when you need it most. And that may mean—and we'll come back to this topic—that parents can benefit from therapy too.

A pediatrician may be able to schedule a longer appointment, perhaps with the parent only, to discuss strategies and referrals and community resources that are appropriate for your family. Some child specialists are trained in therapeutic techniques, such as parent-child interaction therapy or parent-child psychotherapy, that address difficult behaviors, and these therapies have helped many families in our practices develop strategies to cope with extreme and difficult behaviors.

The Vulnerable Child

In pediatrics and child psychiatry, we talk about the *vulnerable child syndrome,* in which parents worry excessively about one particular child, usually because that child has been severely ill or badly hurt in the past. Quirky children can be vulnerable in a variety of ways. The quirky child is often seen as the family problem, the child who is somehow in jeopardy, about whom everyone, especially the parents, is always worried. Because their development may be less regular and less predictable, they may remain dependent on their parents longer than other children, sometimes into adulthood. Because parents love their quirky kids and worry about them, they may identify with a child's every disappointment or difficulty and try to protect that child from all the hardships that they fear may lie in wait.

A parent's sense that one child in the family is especially vulnerable and in need of protection may translate to the other children as a lack of attention or a lack of caring. "You can ride the school bus, but your brother gets driven to school." "I'm sorry we had to come late to the school picnic, but your sister had to go to her language group." One persistent theme in this chapter is the importance of building in family time that is *not* centered around one child's quirkiness.

> If I followed all the recommendations that various people have given me, I would be out every afternoon and every night doing something that might help her, and we would have no family life— never have dinner together, never be lounging on the bed reading aloud. So there are times when I've decided that something had to give, and it's usually the special therapy appointments. I resent the time they take away not just from the other kids but also from my daughter herself and the normal things in her life. We all deserve a little down time as a family, to just hang out and enjoy each other.

Siblings and Only Children

Plenty of quirky kids are the only child in the family, which can be both a blessing and a curse for parents. It is easier to manage the day-to-day life of the family when you have only one child's behavioral issues to contend with. Without siblings competing for time and attention, it's easier to maximize the interventions and available help without guilt and remorse about other children. But that same sibling rough and tumble can teach a quirky child some important skills that may be more difficult for an only child to acquire. A family with more than one child requires more flexibility from everyone, including the quirky child, who may end up learning a variety of adaptations and coping skills from the sound and fury of sibling relationships. When the temperaments of siblings and parents need to be considered, the quirky child has more opportunity to interact with others and resolve conflicts. This can help a child prepare for the real world, where little is tailored to any one person's temperament. Parents of only children tend to look for social opportunities in the extended family or community so their kids can interact with other kids and practice the give and take of family relationships.

Everyday Life

Life at home is complicated, often chaotic, and a particular blend of the routine and the wildly unexpected. To keep a household chugging along requires logistical balancing and managerial organization. The volume of detail involved in keeping everyone clothed and fed, as well as making sure they're present at the appropriate activities with the appropriate equipment is enough to make all parents feel at times like just pulling the covers up over their heads, hoping they aren't found. Add a quirky child, and everything becomes that much more complicated. On the other hand, quirky kids make life interesting, and there will be fun times together inside and outside, unexpected moments of affection and positive reinforcement, and plenty of wonderful memories.

Mealtime

All sorts of behavioral and emotional issues come to the fore at the dinner table. For many families, it's the one time of the day when everyone sees one another, although in other families, people eat in shifts according to their schedules and preferences.

I do have the wish and the expectation that our family will sit down together for dinner—all 3 kids and at least one parent—and the reality of what happens when we do has been kind of hard for me to take. I think this was a very important value of mine, in my fantasy of how my family life would go.

But just getting dinner on the table with these kids who need my constant attention is a challenge. I tell Sam to get the milk and the butter and the grated cheese and put them on the table, and on the way to the refrigerator, he gets distracted and notices something on the bulletin board, and I either yell at him or I get it myself or I tell John to get it. So I have special little occupational therapy knives for John, but he's not strong enough to cut anything, and Sam is such a space shot, I'm afraid to let him do anything with knives.

Next: the getting-ready process. Everybody has to wash their hands, and usually they balk. And now, the moment you've all been waiting for: I bring the big bowl of pasta to the table! During dinner, I want them to leave their butts in a chair for 10 minutes, and it's really hard to get them to do that! Sometimes I turn the timer on and time them. John gets so distracted and he's not that much of an eater. There's almost no conversation. Basically, though, there are no reciprocal conversations, the kind we would like to be able to have with our kids. Sometimes we'll ask a direct question, one will start to answer, one will interrupt, and the other one will start screaming.

And then, of course, something will get spilled. We're trying to give John a cup with no lid at the table, so it always gets spilled. And then everyone will get up and leave, and that's that.

Reasonable expectations

All parents learn, usually the hard way, what can be expected of young children in this most primal social setting. A quirky child, who lags developmentally and socially, is going to tax your patience well past those early years. Adjust your expectations given what you know of your child's abilities and temperament. Those harmonious family dinners may come, but it's probably going to take a while. You cannot make your child typical. You can't make her someone who easily fits in. Your role is to support who she is, not to make her into someone she isn't. You also need to help her acquire the essential skills she'll need, and that's going to take a lot of patience on your part. This goes well beyond mealtime; awareness of what she can and cannot manage will help you avoid environments in which she cannot function and help you decide what truly are the essential skills. It's OK, for example, for a child not to ice-skate if it's impossible for her to lace up her skates and manage on the ice. One less thing to worry about!

Mealtime routines

Some children will drink from only one particular cup. Some can only sit comfortably in a certain chair. Some eat their foods in a ritualized order, get upset if any food is touching any other food on the plate, or will not eat in another person's presence because they cannot tolerate the sound of someone chewing or the scrape of a knife or fork on a plate (a condition called *misophonia*), and they want to be fed before or after dinner or in a different room. Pick your battles carefully. Go ahead and label the cups or the chairs if that makes for a peaceful evening. TV-dinner-style plates with compartments that prevent food touching other food have saved many a family dinner. Increasingly, kids are wearing noise-canceling headphones at the dinner table, as well as in other overstimulating environments.

Picky eaters

Many parents complain that their children are picky eaters, and the pediatric response generally is that as long as the child is growing normally and is not anemic or deficient in vitamins or micronutrients (which would only be tested in a child who is not growing normally), you should choose your battles carefully. Quirky kids, however, can have very restricted preferences, which can create a lot of angst for parents. We know kids who will eat only crunchy or soft food, or food that is white, and they live on rice, white bread, plain yogurt, and pancakes. Food and feeding issues can become a major battlefield, and given the risk of eating disorders, this is not a place where we want our children feeling that they need to exert more control. It's the rare toddler or even 4- to 7-year-old who eats what parents consider an ideal healthy diet. Most children do just fine even if they restrict the range of what they are willing to eat for some stretch of time, but it's important to keep suggesting other choices and not assume that children will never eat the foods they don't like when they're young; there's good evidence that it can take multiple tries to acquire a new taste. If children restrict their diets so severely that it actually does affect weight gain or growth, consider an evaluation by a pediatric nutritionist, gastroenterologist, or a feeding team that has experience with quirky kids, which virtually all do. Your pediatrician should be able to refer you. A restricted diet can eventually lead to overweight as well as underweight; for kids with a strong preference for breaded fried foods, for example, weight gain can become a problem in adolescence, when kids control most of their own intake, and they can become undernourished yet overweight.

> Megan stopped eating meat when she was 3 years old because she made the connection between the cute little animals in her books and the food on the table. She has never eaten meat since. She has a lot of aversions and particular likes and dislikes. For example, she will eat green but not red grapes.

To preserve your own sanity, we recommend setting limits: "This is what I am making for the whole family, and if you don't want to eat it, you can have a peanut butter sandwich" or some other basic food that the child will accept. It's usually a bad idea to get pushed into catering individual meals, although certainly there are parents who make macaroni and cheese every night for the kids and save the real dinner for themselves. If your child's diet is clearly deficient (no fruits or vegetables ever), add in a chewable children's multivitamin and, above all, keep offering. Many picky eaters, as they grow, expand their repertoires by suddenly accepting a taste of some unlikely food and discovering that it's OK. As much as you can, don't allow a picky eater's preferences to dictate the menu; if everyone else likes take-out Chinese food and one person just eats plain rice, so be it.

Slow eaters

Because their motor control is poor, simply getting the food to their mouths can be a challenge for some quirky kids. They can be distracted or dreamy and far away, or have obsessive rituals around food. These behaviors can drive everybody crazy at the dinner table, but it's the slow eater at breakfast who is often the most problematic. Some quirky children have to be reminded to take each new bite and then, sometimes, chew and swallow it. And there's many a quirky child (and, for that matter, many a nonquirky child) who finishes breakfast strapped into his booster seat in the back of the car on the way to drop off an older sibling, which is why God made bagels and protein bars.

When my son was a preschooler, every meal revolved around how many bites of food he ate. Once we were told that he had "oral-motor-planning difficulties" and declined the surgical solution of putting a tube though his skin into his stomach to feed him, we took on his meals with a vengeance. This involved sitting in front of him, offering him a bite, and then singing our "chew-and-swallow" song to the tune of a song we'd learned at his music therapy. Everyone else who might feed him—his grandparents or his babysitter, for example—had to know the song. We cheered when he swallowed something and then started the whole routine over again. Meals took forever, but we didn't know what else to do. We worked with occupational therapy and a feeding team, but none of that really made all that much difference. Now he's 10 and still doesn't have a great appetite, but he does eat enough to grow and has his likes and dislikes. It's not extreme, and we are less worried and know he will just be a skinny guy.

If you're living with a truly slow eater, don't get too obsessed about it. The last thing you want is to find battle lines drawn at every meal or to make your child more self-conscious. Try feeding him when he is really hungry. If a kid comes home from school ravenous and consumes a big bowl of macaroni and cheese, you can relax when that kid dawdles over his dinner. And by all means choose those hungry moments to offer healthy alternatives—it's a great time to introduce baby carrots with humus or cream cheese, or celery with peanut butter, or favorite fruits. And the quirky slow eater should also be able to eat without being pressed to hurry by siblings, so don't expect the rest of the family to stay at the table until that slowest eater has finished. Maybe one parent will stick around for company, but it's also OK to go ahead and start doing the dishes and excuse the other children who have sat at the table and (on a good day) behaved. And, as with the picky eater, if you can find a couple of reasonably nutritious foods that your slow eater likes enough to gobble down, don't feel bad about serving him those foods over and over. As we said earlier, keep offering new foods, don't give up, and if a diet is really restricted, make sure the child's growth is being monitored and give him a multivitamin.

Many quirky kids have such restricted diets that tend toward carbohydrates and fried foods (chicken nuggets and French fries, anyone?) that they are prone to constipation because of a lack of fiber in the diet. Be mindful of any opportunity to get fiber into a child's diet, and if it cannot be done with diet (for example, high-fiber frozen waffles or chopped-up apples), talk with your pediatric provider about a daily dose of a mild laxative to keep things moving along.

Table manners

This issue looms much larger for some families than for others. What we mean here is not just saying "please" and "thank you" and pass the butter, but helping a child learn to eat without making a complete mess. This can be a tall order, but it's worth the effort because a huge part of social life at home, at school, and in the community revolves around meals. Because quirky children are at high risk of being socially marginalized, teased, and ostracized, anything you can do to help them learn good manners early on is extremely important. Yes, the toughest jocks in middle school may belch at the table or spill (or throw!) their food with total impunity, but that doesn't mean that your quirky child is going to get away with the same behavior without being teased or shunned. How can you teach manners? By continually praising the child who remembers proper manners, promptly correcting the child who forgets, and repeating, over and over, the order of steps in cutting food properly. As we discuss in Chapter 9, this is an area in which a relationship with an occupational therapist (OT) can be of real help.

Make mealtimes potentially less difficult by serving easy-to-manage food sometimes, especially when company is there, but serving harder-to-handle items also is important, on the assumption that a child might as well wrestle with that first solo steak in the privacy of home. This means that family mealtimes will include that constant repetitious dialogue: *Watch your elbow—you're going to knock over your milk. Close your mouth when you chew. Say "excuse me" when you burp. Use your knife as a pusher, not your finger. Use your napkin. Cut smaller pieces. Take smaller bites. Chew before you swallow! Also, say "thank you." Say "please." Don't say "yuck" when you don't like something. Ask politely to be excused.* It's not pleasant all the time—and the special problem with a quirky child is that because of fine motor issues and social dislocation, this process can go on long beyond the point at which you might reasonably have expected a child to need such constant correction. As with food preferences and picky eating, try to do the best you can without letting it dominate family life. So it's important to let the subject go sometimes and concentrate on letting people relax and have fun at the table, and that may mean serving something for dinner that is obviously finger food, with juice boxes and not a fork or a napkin in sight. Oh, and don't forget to go out for a pleasant adults-only dinner every now and then. When you do, resist the urge to criticize each other's posture or behavior or cut each other's meat.

Dinner conversation

Some parents of quirky kids, especially as their children grow older, feel that poor language skills are their child's most significant problem. And it's true that as most children age, parents who emphasize the importance of the family dinner table are rewarded with the occasional episode of civilized discourse, which can certainly make it all seem worthwhile. Quirky kids, with their obsessive tendencies and poor social and fine motor skills, can make for fairly agonizing dinner table conversation.

> Occasionally, our daughter will come up with something sort of gross, but we just tell her it isn't appropriate. "Nice people don't talk about that stuff at the dinner table." Which is pretty much the way my parents brought me up. It's sort of hard to keep her on topic, but she is getting better.

Sometimes it helps to talk about what you're going to talk about at the table, to make family rules, and set guidelines: 5 minutes a night of conversation on each child's favorite subject and then on to something chosen by the presiding parent. Don't try to do this more than a couple of times a week; it's quite an effort for all involved. And, once again, you need to reward yourselves with some adult meals in a sane, pleasant atmosphere—at which you will inevitably end up discussing your children!

Playtime

We hear over and over from parents that they began to notice that their children were different because of the ways they played—or didn't play—when they were young. Some children showed no interest in toys or games but preferred some particular random-seeming household objects to which they became attached; the child's toys sat on the shelves, perfect and untouched, while the anxious parents kept bringing home new ones.

> We had a playroom at home that looked like a toy store. In my quest to find something that Abby would play with, I acquired a huge number of toys that were never touched. Then, by the age of 1, she developed overwhelming fears and anxiety. She threw things around rather than play. Her fine motor skills were bad, so she couldn't hold a crayon. She became overstimulated easily. We had an infant seat with colorful plastic toys on a bar at the front, and I had to remove all but one because it was too much.

Other quirky kids are willing to play with toys but only in ritualized and unusual ways, such as lining them up or arranging them in particular patterns. What most of these kids *don't* do is the standard symbolic play, in which they pretend the doll is a baby or the toy truck is a real one. The quirky child may be more likely to line up all the dolls, head to toe, or set up the cars and trucks in an unalterable grid, or spin the wheels on the trucks for long periods of time. Parents and therapists can try to help a child expand his repertoire of play skills by getting down on the floor and interacting with the child in a playful manner, with a lot of repetition, engaging her around her special toys or interests.

> My son liked toy cars, but he just lined them up around the edge of our guestroom bed in a "U" shape. We would get on the floor and try to show him where the driver was, where the children were, but he just didn't care.

All children nowadays are growing up in homes with screens—phones, tablets, laptops, TVs—and all parents have to give a little thought to screen time. It's a widespread concern these days in pediatrics, and quirky kids are especially prone to spending long hours staring at screens. According to the American Academy of Pediatrics (AAP) guidelines, kids younger than 18 months should avoid screen time, with the exception of video-chatting with family. If parents want to introduce digital media, the recommendation is that from 18 months to 24 months of age, it should be of high-quality content, and the parent should watch with the child. From age 2 years to 5 years, the recommendation is an hour or less per day of high-quality content and, again, as much co-viewing as possible. Many parents of quirky kids may find this unrealistic; screen time is how their children occupy themselves, and it may eventually become a way to play with other children. We would say that it's important to keep these recommendations in mind and, above all, remember that parents have a responsibility regarding time, content, and interaction. You may decide to allow a little extra screen time for a child who has difficulty with other kinds of play and with other children, for example, but you should still set limits and pay close attention to the content of what your child is watching or playing, and one way to do that is by viewing the content together. Even if you relax a rule or a standard, there still should be rules and standards. No child, quirky or not, needs to watch television while riding in a stroller, when there is so much to look at and learn about. But we are parents too, and we know that there are days when a little screen time babysitting is the best we can do.

Indeed, as kids grow, screens are usually a required part of the school day, and almost all parents find themselves negotiating the question of how large a role they should play in children's lives more generally. Problems arise when kids spend all of their down time on a screen, watching videos, playing online games, or chatting with friends. People have worried for years about the phenomenon of screen addiction, and in 2018 the World Health Organization recognized *gaming disorder*, a syndrome in which gaming (digital games or video games) takes over someone's life to the exclusion of other activities and interests. This is a phenomenon that can loom large for some quirky kids, especially boys. If you have children who are particularly drawn to screens, you need to stay engaged. Know what your kids are doing online, how much time they are spending there, and with whom. Set some rules and limits around screen time, both for individual children and for the family as a whole. The AAP recommends designating screen-free times (eg, the hour before bedtime) and places (the dinner table) and, perhaps above all, keeping electronic devices out of the bedroom. Parents in our practices lock up the phones and tablets an hour before bedtime to keep kids on a schedule and encourage good sleep hygiene. Rules like these, for parents and siblings to follow as well, take into account that many of us are also tempted by screens, and we need to think about our own habits.

Parents of quirky children need to strike a balance between allowing their children the freedom to enjoy the things that give them pleasure and excite their interest and attempting to lure them into trying, and perhaps liking, some of the more typical pleasures that don't immediately attract them. Let him line up the trucks if that's what gives him pleasure. But by all means, try to expand the game a little, relating the toy trucks to the real trucks you see outside or talking about the driver and showing the child how to make sound effects. We firmly believe that children are entitled to certain domains of life in which their preferences, talents, interests, and inclinations are what count, even if those are eccentric. Don't turn every moment of your child's life into a therapeutic opportunity and don't press too hard for a specific kind of play. Children can often sense when their parents are disappointed in them, and there are plenty of disappointments in life without making a child feel bad that she isn't interested in dolls or in the train set. However, toys truly are useful tools for all kinds of therapeutic interventions that work well with young children. You may find yourself on the floor, teaching your daughter to roll a ball back and forth as a way of getting her to practice social interactions and develop motor skills.

Playdates

Unusual play habits make the idea of inviting another child over for a playdate seem complex and even fraught with tension. We suggest that you think carefully about why you are interested in setting up such playdates and whether your child is in fact ready. Many quirky kids are not socially ready by preschool age to play one-on-one with another child without adult help and supervision. Many are not particularly interested in kids their own age. Some quirky kids prefer adults or older children, who are more predictable and can adjust their reactions to unusual behavior, whereas others gravitate toward babies.

> When a kid would come over to play with John, we couldn't just
> leave the two of them alone. We needed a plan, such as, "We're
> going to play checkers and then build a fort and then go out for
> ice cream." John was always interested in his one thing, whatever
> it was—telling time, the weather—and he just couldn't shift into
> anything else. He was scared so easily. One friend used to like to
> play pirates and he would create these scary scenarios and John
> would get scared.

If your young child has siblings at home and attends some kind of preschool, child care, or early intervention group with other children, it may not be vitally important to arrange many playdates. Some parents find themselves doing it because they are aware that all around them, there is a busy world of playdates, parties, and sleepovers. But if your child shows no interest, you may want to wait a little while, keep an eye out for the best possible match in terms of playmates, and generally take it slowly.

For more thoughts on playdates and children at different ages, refer to Chapter 8.

Teasing

For many parents of quirky kids, the idea of teasing or bullying is a major concern. Quirky kids are different, which is exactly why this is a risk for them. These legitimate worries will be addressed head-on in Chapter 8, The Social Life of a Quirky Kid: Finding Friends and Making Connections. Here, though, we want to talk about something a little different—namely, how to handle the kind of teasing that routinely goes on among siblings. This kind of teasing is not happening just because a child is quirky. Siblings tease one another in pretty much every typical family, and instead of trying to protect quirky children from it completely, this may be an opportunity for parents to help them learn how it works and to respond appropriately.

Teasing requires a certain social sophistication, an ability to put yourself in the other person's place and figure out what would really touch a sore spot. This is precisely what quirky kids are lacking, and they do not understand that some teasing can be meant as a form of joking. They will experience it as criticism and actually be hurt by it. We have heard from adults about the teasing they were subjected to as children at home, which felt cruel to them, and how their parents did not protect them from siblings or others who teased them.

You might want to institutionalize a modicum of gentle family-style teasing, helping your quirky child understand that people do this, and it is not meant to hurt. For quirky kids, this may mean spelling it out: This is okay, this is friendly teasing, this is meant as a joke. So Mom can be teased about always forgetting where she left her car keys, Dad gets laughed at for not understanding social media, and big sister is being teased because she bumps into the wall while texting, but you need to be very gentle when attempting to tease a quirky kid. Alternatively, you can make general rules. No teasing anyone about any aspect of physical appearance. No teasing anyone who feels bad. No teasing at the table. Parents should consider making a commitment to monitor the teasing, explain the rules repeatedly to the entire family, and even help the quirky child respond in kind. For more information on teasing within a social environment, refer to Chapter 8.

Homework

We have come to the realization that many schools assign a lot of homework, especially in the early grades, that is meant in large part as discipline for the parents. Keep in mind that this may be one area where you can—and should—find common cause with other parents; typically developing children often struggle with the homework burden as well, and many parents dread the assignments. Schools may claim that they are building good study habits and helping children get used to the idea of working in the evening, but, quite frankly, we don't always buy it, especially when it comes to quirky kids. The kind of homework we are talking about tends to be profoundly repetitive: copying letters, words, and sentences; coloring in drawings; and completing worksheets. However, homework, as a child ages, can offer a real opportunity for a parent to help with study habits and academic strategies. It may not always be joyful for either of you, but keeping an eye on your child at homework time can give you a sense of what is easy for that child academically and what is difficult.

Homework was hell for Megan. It took so damn long to get anything done. She just couldn't focus. She would do a little, then she would rock back and forth like a human rocking chair; sometimes she'd flap her hands and that was always accompanied by running around in circles, usually around a piece of furniture. It really did upset me and I had no idea what it meant at that point in her life.

Lisa decides it's difficult beforehand, and she will have her good days and bad days. If I ask her to do her homework, she'll start crying sometimes. Even though I'm really pressed for time in the mornings, I find she's better after a good night's sleep. After school, sometimes she's overloaded, and everything seems overwhelming to her.

Aidan was such a perfectionist he would become paralyzed around homework, and ultimately he didn't do it, ever. Despite how bright he is, school has been a real challenge because his anxiety affected everything, including his ability to do his work.

More on homework

For many quirky children, a full day of school is pretty exhausting. Trying to wrestle with their attentional issues, the social matrix of the school environment, and the specific learning-related challenges of reading and writing and numbers can leave a child wiped out by 3:00 pm.

Many quirky kids already attend extra therapy sessions of one kind or another after the school day is over. It seems to us that these kids deserve to come home and relax. A 7-year-old who has spent a day in school trying valiantly to cope with fine motor problems and then gone to an OT session should not come home to struggle with a worksheet, handwriting, or more frustration. And if the therapy itself is part of the frustration, think carefully about how much it's really helping. Occupational therapy for handwriting, for example, may be exhausting and not likely to make much of a difference. A child might be better off playing at an after-school program where there's also the chance to get some homework done.

Quirky kids—like all other kids and most adults—will first do the things they enjoy and find easy. There's a real danger that at the end of the evening, when the child is most tenuously balanced, what will be left will be the hardest, most hated piece of work. Although the point of homework is supposed to be, in part, to teach independence, almost all parents of almost all children find themselves drawn in, supervising, policing, correcting, and helping until they cross the line and find the architect father sitting up all night making his fourth grader's ancient Rome diorama out of toothpicks! Homework is rough on parents and on families, too. When the tired, frustrated child, up a little past bedtime, is crying because the assignment still doesn't look right, while the parent knows that what the child needs most is a good night's sleep, there is no academic triumph for anyone. Be sure to partner with your child's teacher about what is a reasonable expectation for your child. This can also be written into an education plan if your child has one.

As children grow up, homework success becomes more and more about organization. If your child switches classes for different subjects, can he or she keep track of what each teacher wants done tonight and handed in tomorrow? Can he or she track the due dates of longer-term assignments and upcoming tests? Can he or she bring the right books and papers home from school and write down the correct pages to read, the math problems that are due, and the list of topics that are on the test? These organizational tasks can be real challenges for quirky kids.

In the older elementary grades and in middle school, homework becomes much more serious. Some schools pride themselves on assigning large amounts of homework, as evidence of academic rigor. A child's executive function problems or learning differences may really show up here; it may take much longer than it should to struggle through the history reading assignment or write out answers to 10 short-answer identifications.

Sacrificing sleep to do homework is a chronic problem in many high schools. Quirky children may be at special risk because of the learning issues that make homework hard, the organizational difficulties that make it problematic to structure their time, their overall lower stamina, or an obsessive perfectionism that gets in the way of finishing assignments. As many learning specialists have said, the perfect is the enemy of the good. Being tuned in as a parent (no, that does not mean doing the homework for your child) may give you a window on what are the most important academic struggles that need to be evaluated and addressed.

Homework strategies

Fatigue exacerbates attentional problems, learning difficulties, obsessions, anxiety, and social distress. On the other hand, homework can be of real benefit to the middle school or high school child who finds the social world confusing or intimidating or is bothered by the sensory overload of changing classes and worrying about class participation. Homework can be an opportunity to concentrate on academic issues without all these tensions and distractions. And some quirky kids are academic superstars, and homework is what they love to do to demonstrate their academic prowess.

It's worth considering whether homework is such a struggle that it is interfering with a child's well-being. If it is, talk with your main point of contact at the school to see if an accommodation can be made in an individualized education plan or a 504 plan that reduces the homework load (we discuss these plans in more detail on pages 149–152). The following strategies may also help mitigate any frustrations or bouts of anxiety in your child when tackling homework:

- *Consider your child's daily rhythms.* Most children, especially those with attention-deficit/hyperactivity disorder, do much better if they do their homework relatively early in the day—maybe not immediately on coming home from school but certainly before supper. Everybody deserves a break, and these kids, in particular, may need a chance for some physical activity before they have to sit down again. Some quirky kids are notoriously early risers, and that can be a terrific time to get homework done. Kids who have poor handwriting usually find that it deteriorates over the day and looks best first thing in the morning.
- *Have a specific place to do the work.* How can you minimize distractions if that's an issue? How available do you, or some other supervising adult, need to be? You can try to set up a dedicated homework place, which can be in the child's room or, if that is where there are the most distractions, in some boring adult setting, such as a little desk in the living room or some space on the kitchen table.
- *Organize.* For many quirky kids, just keeping track of papers and assignments is a big task, and their backpacks can be a jumble of everything that comes home from school. Organizational issues are major developmental tasks for all kids, especially in the later elementary school years. Quirky kids will be in good company. Still, as with other tasks, getting organized may take longer and require more help for the quirky child. Whoever is picking your child up from school may need to review with the child or the teacher whether there is homework, and whoever is taking your child in the morning may need to check to be sure that the completed assignments are packed and ready to

go. When assignments are given at school, your child should know exactly where to put them to be sure to bring them home. After homework is done, have your child pack it up in whatever folder or backpack is going to school the next day. No matter how carefully you plan, every parent has made a late night call to another parent for a scanned and emailed copy of homework instructions. You just don't want to have to do it every day.

- *Have a plan of attack.* Sit down and strategize the day's homework with your child: How much has to be done? What looks easy? What looks hard?
- *Use tools to plan.* Help older children plan their time—not just for any individual evening's work but for the bigger, longer-term assignments. Some quirky children are unable to understand how to break these assignments down into manageable steps, and a chart, checklist, or calendar with separate due dates for each task can be very helpful.
- *Don't overschedule.* If you fill up every afternoon with therapies and activities, then homework will have to wait until later, and that may be hard. Consider moving some of these activities to the weekend or helping your child become accustomed to bringing some homework to the physical therapist's office if you know there's usually a wait. Some schools send home a packet of assignments for the week that is due on Friday or the following Monday. This allows for more flexibility in planning, and the final product is more likely to be relatively neat and well thought out.
- *Plan for supervision.* Think about homework supervision as you make your child care arrangements. If you have a babysitter overseeing some of these after-school hours, give her clear instructions for helping with homework and make sure she understands that, if possible, it needs to be done before dinnertime. If your child spends time in an after-school program, find some provision for homework, if possible. Many of these programs offer a supervised homework room, where kids can work in peace and get help if they need it.
- *Reward accomplishments.* We are big believers in small, tangible rewards for small, tangible accomplishments. Finish your worksheet and you'll get a cookie. Finish all your homework and we'll go to the playground for 15 minutes before dinner. For younger children, there's nothing wrong with offering an M&M, a grape, or a gold star for every successfully completed task.
- *Bend the rules.* By far, our favorite homework activity for young children is reading—reading together, letting a child read to the parent, and, of course, letting the parent read to the child. We'd like to express the hope that homework reading programs will recognize the pleasures and comforts of reading aloud and allow children to select the books that interest them. If you find yourself with a homework reading program that is taking all

the fun out of reading, you may need to make some discreet alterations at home—with or without notifying the school.

- *Find ways to compensate.* If you think your child is struggling unduly with a particular kind of homework, be ready to reopen the possibility of a learning evaluation. Remember that smart kids can compensate amazingly for all kinds of learning disabilities, and it may only be when all the other kids catch up and become fluent readers, for example, that your fifth grader's language-processing differences come to light, because they have more to do with understanding complex paragraphs than they do with decoding words and sentences. Talking with your child's teacher can help you develop strategies: Maybe your child can listen to audiobooks while reading along. All kids for whom handwriting is laborious should be provided laptops by their schools.

- *Check with other parents.* If it seems to you at some point that too much homework is being assigned, talk to other parents. You may not be the only one who feels this way. When children have multiple teachers for different subjects, it's important that the teachers connect with one another and synchronize so that everyone doesn't load it on the same night.

- *Check in with the teacher.* If the assignments are not always clearly specified, or if your child has trouble figuring out exactly what is expected, check in with the teacher on a regular basis or establish a connection with another parent who seems relatively clued in, so that you can, in a pinch, call for advice and instructions. Some teachers are available by email, and some even post homework assignments on a school intranet or web page.

- *Evaluate the type of homework assigned.* If it seems to you that the assignments your child brings home are not particularly helpful, bring this up with the school. As we said earlier, our basic prejudice is that homework in kindergarten through third grade should be minimal—a 15- to 30-minute assignment that reinforces what's going on in school and teaches the habit of, well, doing homework. We have seen children sent home with assignments that seemed, quite frankly, completely useless: filling in coloring-book pictures of Disney characters, copying words over and over in different colors—first red, then blue, then green, then yellow. These assignments may be reasonably easy and entertaining for some children, but if they play right to your child's most distressing challenges, then you need to go in, meet with the teacher, and try to negotiate an exemption. No one ever experienced major consequences in later life from not coloring in a drawing of Minnie Mouse.

- *Consider homework groups.* Some families we interviewed told us they use this approach to help motivate their kids and make homework more fun. Invite one or two kids from your child's class to come over and do a little homework together. It can be an effective way to get a look at other children's studying strategies, and if there's a chance to play for a while when homework is done, that's a strong incentive to do the work more efficiently.

- *Remember the power of praise.* Try to make homework time a period associated with a certain amount of praise, some physical comfort, and even the occasional treat. It won't make your child love worksheets, but it may start to feel like a familiar and relatively pleasant interlude in the day—or, at least, like a doable assignment.

If your child receives additional services in school after an evaluation, or if you find yourself hiring additional private tutors or coaches, make sure to discuss the homework issues with the people your child is working with and make sure that homework strategies are included. You can also ask the teacher whether the school has a specialist who might have something to offer a child who is struggling with homework. For some kids and families, homework remains an Achilles' heel, and the happiest day for them is high school graduation.

Personal Hygiene and Good Grooming

Personal hygiene is a big deal for a lot of quirky kids. The tensions and strains around using the toilet, keeping clean, wiping runny noses, and getting dressed can be fraught with tension for lots of parents. As a child ages and still doesn't seem to comprehend basic self-care, a parent can foresee future social disasters. For some of these children in later elementary school and middle school, the personal hygiene issues do become the focus of teasing, bullying, or social ostracism. The eighth-grade girl who picks her nose all the time is going to get noticed and probably will be shunned, and this should be a priority for treatment, because it may be a kind of tic disorder. A second-grade boy who's been running around outside for hours will smell of dirt and dust and energy, but an eighth-grade boy better understand about taking a shower and changing his clothes. Even for their parents and other relatives who love them dearly, it's just plain easier to cherish a relatively clean, unsnotty, pleasant-smelling child.

These issues stress out almost all parents: the daily maintenance and supervision of small children's bodies and the need to civilize them and teach them self-care. It's a long journey from the cuteness of that first newborn poopy diaper to the 2-year-old—or 3-year-old or 4-year-old—who can reliably pee and poop in the potty, and quirky kids are notoriously late potty trainers. Then you still have to know about it and hear about it, not to mention help wipe! And once again, parents of quirky kids experience it more intensely and for a longer duration. These children need more supervision, and they need it further along in life, which contributes to that vulnerable child syndrome in which parent and child feel more tightly tied together than is usual. There's nothing like handling someone's bathroom behavior and nose wiping to give you certain kinds of boundary issues. In general, when it comes to self-care, parents of quirky kids are going to need an extra supply of patience and good humor.

> John has never been able to stand water in his face, especially in his eyes. We remember watching his very first bath through the window in the newborn nursery. He was screaming and arching and so clearly miserable. At the time, we thought that he must be cold or that all babies must hate their first bath. The fact is it hasn't changed much in 10 years. He completely hates taking a shower if he needs to wash his hair. He seems to lose his sense of himself when his eyes are closed, and the sensation itself drives him nuts. We started having him shower with goggles on, and that does help. But, if the goggles are too tight they hurt, and water gets in if they are too loose. It's always a struggle of some kind.

With a quirky child, it is important to have patience, organizational abilities, resilience, a sense of humor, and, of course, love for your child. You may find you learn strategies from other parents or from your OT. The following subsections offer some specific suggestions that may help make situations run more smoothly.

Using the Bathroom

Quirky kids are often notoriously late to graduate out of diapers. Some are generally slow developmentally or at least verbally. Others seem to be out of touch with their bodies and physiological impulses. Your child will have to be ready in order to take these steps. If that's later than you would like, be aware that while it's fine to encourage progress, there are real risks in turning potty training into a struggle or a test of wills. It's not uncommon in pediatric practices to see children of many ages who develop constipation or continue soiling their pants as toilet training goes awry.

Even after quirky children have managed the great transition, they are likely to need more teaching, not less, about the mechanics of using the toilet, wiping, flushing, and washing hands. Some children find damp wipes easier to use than toilet paper. You may find yourself repeating simple instructions over and over or posting signs to remind a child to wash his or her hands after using the toilet. You may find sticker charts valuable: a star for every dry night (or for every poop in the toilet, depending on the issue) and a reward for an entire week of stars. Gizmos are available to attach to the toilet that can make the cleaning up and wiping process easier for older kids who have trouble managing the motor skills of bathroom hygiene.

Personal Grooming

Personal hygiene rules, like many other social customs, may never come easily to the quirky child. They won't make sense to many quirky kids or fit in with their view of the world. A child with fine motor delays or weaknesses may have trouble with the details of dressing or grooming and may need help or at least careful inspection long after other children the same age can button their shirts, comb and arrange their hair, or get the spinach out of their teeth. What you probably *can't* do is depend on peer pressure to convince your quirky child that these issues matter. You'll hear parents say from time to time, "Oh, when he starts to care about girls, then he won't want to have spinach on his teeth." This is much less true with quirky kids. They have trouble decoding the social rules and therefore can't quite make the connection, or they just don't seem to notice or be bothered that there is spaghetti sauce on their sweatshirt.

Morning washing-up routines, in particular, need to be kept to the bare minimum in most families, simply because of the realities of trying to get out of the house. Frankly, as pediatricians, we recommend to parents of young children that they teach detailed teeth-brushing skills in the evening.

> I use a lot of bulletin boards and dry-erase boards to keep up with Trevor's lack of organization. Mornings can be really hard, especially if he senses that I am losing patience, and I am not a patient person. I take a train to work, and there is very little wiggle room. If the morning isn't going well, it can be a disaster.

Keep an eye out for modifications that make life easier: a toothpaste that your child likes—or at least dislikes less—is more likely to get used. Occupational therapists sometimes recommend shower chairs for children who have difficulty keeping their balance. A handheld telephone showerhead may be easier than an overhead shower for a child who hates getting water in her face. Goggles may keep water out of the child's eyes and help make shower time tolerable. Search until you find the right soft towel for a child who is sensitive to sensory stimuli. You may want to keep hair short, especially if washing or brushing feels unpleasant to your child.

Clothes

Many quirky kids are slow to dress themselves in the sense that they can't do it till they're older than you might expect; they're also slow in the sense that it takes them many minutes to get ready. Choose clothing that is easy to manage—elastic-waist pants, shirts without buttons or snaps at the neck, and jackets and shoes with Velcro fasteners. Tying shoes is a complex motor skill and comes late indeed to many quirky kids. Fortunately, we live in an era of slip-ons, all-terrain moccasins, and Crocs. Also, dealing with clothes that are a little bigger is usually easier than dealing with clothes that are a little smaller. Many children have strong preferences about the textures they can tolerate next to the skin; when you find the perfect seamless socks or the ideal cozy and warm sweatshirt, buy large quantities. Try to budget time in the morning so that a child who dresses slowly gets woken up first and there isn't as much pressure. And no matter how much we want to foster independence, there are always going to be morning moments when you just grab your child and stuff her into her clothes and run out the door. One mom we know put her son to bed in his clothes for years, so he would be dressed and ready to go in the morning.

Continue to praise and congratulate and reward—recognizing that even if you feel these behaviors should be completely routine by this age, your child may be struggling. Finally, be aware that your child may not perceive the social implications of clothing—that is, may happily dress in outfits that other kids find odd or even ridiculous. You can help by making sure that his dresser drawers are stocked with standard-issue kid clothes in the appropriate sizes. Keep an eye out for what other kids are wearing, and don't hesitate to shop the big chain stores: the more generic, the better.

Chrissie's clothes are often crooked, and sometimes she doesn't realize exactly what she is wearing—you know, striped tops with flowered pants. I tell her she needs to change because the colors clash. And she usually does it, after I explain why she needs to do it. Her wardrobe is pretty limited because she hates wearing jeans and pants that snap or button. She prefers elastic waists. I've told her it's OK by me, but as her tastes change, she's going to have to adjust her preferences if she truly wants the latest clothes. I'm thinking I might want to take mother-and-daughter sewing classes with her at some point.

Ben is very particular about his feet, especially his socks. If his feet are sweaty, he will not touch them to put on his socks and needs me to do it for him, even though he's 8 now. He has slip-on shoes, and

I went out and bought the next three sizes, now that I've found a
shoe he will put on and wear.

If there is some part of your child's bedtime routine that he especially looks
forward to, make it conditional on getting through the appropriate evening
bathroom ritual. Have him say out loud what he has completed: "Yes, I went to
the bathroom, I flushed the toilet, I washed my hands and my face, I brushed
my teeth, I took off my clothes and put them in the hamper, I took my shower,
I put on my pajamas." Once he has mastered the bathroom ritual, then you can
move on to his favorite part of the bedroom routine.

Bedtime

Quirky kids can have profound difficulty with sleep. Some are historically
bad sleepers, especially as infants and toddlers. These are the ones who can
never seem to settle down; who could never be counted on to sleep through
the night, no matter what techniques their parents tried; who can't sleep
in any unfamiliar place; who toss and turn and fret. Maybe it's an early manifestation of the sense that many quirky kids seem uncomfortable in their
own skin. Maybe it's separation anxiety or some other anxiety. Maybe it's
just bad luck.

Parents of quirky kids often find bedtime even more difficult with a child
who may experience more than the usual dose of fear and anxiety, or more
intense attachment and great trouble separating from the parent for the night.
On the other hand, some parents have told us about their experiences with
quirky kids who just love to go to bed! The effort to make it through the day
can sometimes leave a quirky kid exhausted and eager to sleep. Some remain
restless or light sleepers, and may wake in the night, needing reassurance. Talk
this through with your pediatrician—sleep problems are a common topic in
pediatric primary care. You'll probably end up trying some behavior modification strategies, which work for many children, though rarely as a quick fix. If
things don't get better, ask for a referral to a pediatric sleep specialist; you and
your child shouldn't suffer with this for years.

Occasionally, when he's in bed, my grandson Max will permit a back
rub, but more often than not—more now that he's 9—he does not
want me in his room at bedtime.

The following are some special quirky-kid issues around bedtime and some coping strategies:

- **Screen time.** Beware of screens before bedtime. Quirky kids are drawn to screens and often use them to wind down. The reality, however, is that screens are activating for the brain and make it more difficult to fall asleep. We suggest following the AAP guidelines about this: no TV in the child's bedroom, no screens of any kind for at least an hour before bedtime, and phones and other devices should be stored (and recharged) somewhere else overnight. If you start this strategy early in a child's life, it will be easier to manage at a later age. Apply this rule to everyone in the family.
- **Anxiety.** Think about what can make the separation at bedtime easier for an anxious child: a night-light, an open door, the promise that a parent will come in and check on her, or a favorite book or song by which to fall asleep.
- **Rigid rituals.** Indulge bedtime rituals, but keep an eye on time. You don't want the whole evening to be taken up by the many elaborate steps of getting a child into bed. And don't allow the ritual to require only one particular adult. Mom, Dad, Grandma, or a sitter must be included and allowed to participate.
- **Consistency.** All the well-worn comforts of transitional objects and familiar bedtime stories or songs may be even more important to a quirky child—and may continue to matter even after other children have outgrown them. Never disdain any strategy that helps get your child happily into bed. Many children (and adults) with sensory sensitivities like to sleep in the cocoonlike environment of a sleeping bag or under a heavy comforter or weighted blanket, which are readily available. This anchors them physically, comforting them by enclosing or pressing down on their bodies. Be open to the idea that a child may want to sleep in a sleeping bag, zipped up tight, all year round.

John sleeps in a sleeping bag 12 months a year—he likes the feeling of closeness. And he likes the room to be absolutely dark. You'd think he'd want a light on because he gets frightened so easily, but, no, it has to be totally dark.

There were a lot of things I used to fight with Lisa over that now I understand—like the heavy blankets she liked to sleep with even in the summer. It was a nightly battle, that and all the toys she wanted to sleep with, and how they had to be in certain positions. I thought she just didn't want to go to sleep, but with her sensory stuff, she likes the weight of the blankets. She needs those animals so she can find her place. It was so much easier once I understood it.

- **Medication.** If your child is taking medication, any abrupt change in sleep habits should be discussed with the doctor in light of the medication, the dose, and the timing. We often move children's dosing regimens around, giving them the same medications but at different points in the day, trying to help them be awake and alert at school and then able to relax and fall asleep at night. Medications can also help a child who struggles to stay asleep. Most pediatricians will start with melatonin, which is effective for many kids and has minimal side effects. Talk with your child's pediatrician about melatonin, and if it is not sufficient, a child and adolescent psychiatrist should be called upon to help. You can read more about this in Chapter 10.

Life with a quirky child can be wearing. As a parent, you are entitled to factor in your own need for a little break in the evening, a little adult time to pause and regroup and think about what comes next, or maybe enjoy a glass of wine and a good novel!

> I was a maniac about bedtime. We followed the rules for how to
> make sure they know how to go to sleep by themselves—and they
> all learned. Sam was my most challenging. He would stay up later
> and set himself up in any number of places around the house.
> Sometimes we'd find him under the piano or the dining room table.
> He liked the feeling of the hardwood floors against his skin. He told
> me, "I just need to hear the sound of your voice." For the most part,
> he would manage by himself, so it was OK. I just needed that break.
> As he has gotten older, I see that he has lots of anxieties about
> other things, too. I just didn't know it at the time.

Babysitters

Every parent of a quirky kid ends up with a babysitter horror story or two, although, to be fair, so do many parents of all kinds of kids. And, most babysitters have a couple of good stories of their own. But here you are, thinking of leaving an unusually challenging child with another caregiver, and you would really like it to work out, so that you can do your errands, hold down your job, see your friends, or just enjoy time away from the house. Depending on your family resources, babysitter time may be an occasional luxury or a regular necessity, but sooner or later, most parents need someone to cover.

What are your expectations of your babysitter? It's one thing to be hoping for an occasional evening out or a free Saturday afternoon to run errands, and it's another thing for a babysitter to pick up your child from school 5 days a week and spend the afternoon supervising homework.

Let's consider the more serious, longer-term babysitter first. Are you expecting her—or him—to be your child's playmate, tutor, or therapist, or will you be happy if she keeps your child safe and relatively clean until you get home?

Toddlers and preschoolers who are involved in early intervention programs or behavioral programs need a babysitter who understands the program. A babysitter might take turns with you accompanying your child to the early intervention playgroup or might participate in a behavioral program with a home-based therapist. For the more intensive behavioral approaches, usually reserved for younger and more severely affected children, the therapist will insist that any regular babysitter be involved in the program so there is consistency.

A babysitter who is doing school pickup and afternoon hours is going to be faced with homework supervision and perhaps with getting the child to and from appointments. These responsibilities and expectations need to be clearly explained. You should not assume that just because someone is in college that that person can supervise a child preparing a second-grade book report or doing fifth-grade math. You need to clearly explain to your babysitter what you mean by helping with homework, both in terms of the help you expect (eg, show him how to look up the words in the dictionary, correct her when she reads aloud and makes a mistake) and the help you don't want (eg, do the math problems for her, color in the Minnie Mouse for him). Here, as elsewhere, you also need a clear set of instructions for what the sitter is supposed to do if she runs into a problem. No parent is happy to learn that the babysitter has invented a new punishment or restricted a privilege without asking.

The issue of punishment and expectations brings us to perhaps one of the most complicated questions that comes up with babysitters: how much do they need to know? If a sitter is going to supervise the end of the child's school day and be there for homework time, she probably needs to know everything she can about how your child functions and learns. However, if she's going to babysit for the occasional evening and that's it, you might just give her an orientation about the child's evening habits and bedtime behaviors, and leave it at that.

You do need to warn babysitters if there is any chance they may have to deal with any dramatic or potentially dangerous events, such as seizures or major tantrums. Fortunately, we live in the cell phone era and sitters can easily reach parents to ask questions. Babysitters who are asked to give medications need to know what they are giving and whether there is any possibility of a reaction.

Babysitters vary enormously in their experience of the world and with children. Just as you may have relatives who refuse to believe that there's anything different about your child (except, maybe, a lack of parental firmness!), you may encounter babysitters who doubt your interpretation. Experience and attitude are by no means tied to age. We have heard stories of older babysitters who did not believe that any of these syndromes exist or that anything was going on that couldn't be cured by a little discipline, as well as stories of older babysitters who brought a kind of wisdom and experience to handling quirky children that made everyone's life much easier. We also have heard stories of younger babysitters who were completely overwhelmed by the oddities and pressures of quirky children and about others who brought energy and sympathy—and sometimes recent training in child development or special education—to certain lucky families.

> We had one babysitter who thought it was all total nonsense and there was nothing wrong with any of my kids except that I'm too indulgent with them. Now we have a new sitter who understands it and has strategies to help deal with it. At one point, she had two of my kids playing a card game and one building something, and I was in awe, because they weren't screaming at each other.

> We hired a young woman to help with our kids after school. She came with solid references and a lot of experience. We went to great lengths to explain the issues of our kids and how we expected her to deal with them. When I came home the first afternoon, she met me at the door and said, "I cannot do this." When we spoke about it, I realized that she was too high-strung and inflexible to manage with our kids. I was grateful to her for figuring it out so quickly and moving on.

Look for a babysitter who seems to genuinely like and appreciate your child, however she may formulate her understanding of the quirks. Quirky kids, as we all know, can be endearing, eccentric, and exasperating, sometimes within the space of about 5 minutes. A sitter who can't indulge and appreciate your child's intense feelings—about baseball statistics, beetles, batteries, or bus schedules—is going to miss all the fun of getting to know a remarkable kid. A sitter who thinks that allowing your rigidly unbending child to follow set routines and rituals, or offering your child with motor planning problems extra help with dressing and personal hygiene, is just spoiling the child is going to communicate that attitude and is unlikely to bond successfully with her charge.

When you think you've found that sitter who likes and appreciates your child, treat her—or him—well. Just as your job is harder than the average parent's job, her job is harder than the average sitter's. Acknowledge it when she goes the extra mile, pay her well, and thank her often.

Of course, many children behave differently with the babysitter than they do with their parents. In many families, babysitter nights are understood to be nights when the familiar routines are varied a little, the rules are relaxed, and a good time is had by all.

Going Out in Public

Young children, by and large, typically do not know how to behave in public places. One of the great joys—or one of the potential burdens—of child-rearing is the chance to spend time in playgrounds, theme restaurants, creative puppet shows and theatrical presentations, water parks, cartoon matinees, and places where you pay good money to climb around in a great bin full of colored plastic balls. Most parents begin by taking their children to these child-centered places and then, when their child seems ready or when the parent absolutely cannot stand to listen to another repetitious, squeaky-voiced song, they try, somewhat tentatively, a real restaurant, a show that isn't just for kids, or a bigger concert.

With a quirky child, you have to take things a bit more slowly and carefully. Even the usual child-friendly activities can prove highly unfriendly or highly challenging for quirky children, and their reactions can attract attention and censure even in places where routine childish misbehavior is going on all around you. Every parent has a story or two of a child who misbehaved so outrageously that they can never go back to the restaurant or the store. Parents of quirky kids have more of these stories, and the stories are more extreme. The sense that other people are judging you and your child really hangs over many parents.

You're not the only one who's ever been publicly humiliated. To give you the courage to venture out again, we offer some strategies for coping in public.

There are a growing number of friendly spaces for kids with sensory-processing difficulties and autism spectrum disorder issues. Many YMCAs have sensory friendly spaces for kids to play with minimal noise, no flashing or bright lights, and a relatively serene environment. Autism-friendly spaces not only dial down the sensory stimulation, but also provide information and prompts to help kids navigate social issues and make the whole setting more predictable. You may find such spaces at restaurants, hotels, and resorts, as well as in airports and sometimes at theaters or at parades. Some hospitals are developing autism-friendly initiatives, training all staff members to make individuals with neurodevelopmental differences more comfortable in the clinical, and often overstimulating, environment of a hospital. If you find yourself in an emergency department with your quirky child, ask if the hospital has an autism-friendly program, and even if it doesn't, it's worth letting the staff know what your child finds difficult in medical settings.

Think carefully about the activity in which you are engaging or the event you are attending. Are you taking your child to *The Nutcracker* because she has expressed an interest, loves music, or watches ballet dancers on TV, or are you taking her because it's always been part of *your* fantasy to have a daughter with whom you could dream that Sugarplum Fairy dream? Generally speaking, your chances of success in public endeavors are much, much higher if the child has expressed an interest. In fact, many quirky kids do just fine at more adult-oriented activities, such as *The Nutcracker* or the symphony or a major league baseball game, if that's what they like. They will be riveted and you can relax.

Rehearsing a scenario with your child can be helpful. This is exactly what Social Stories are intended for (we discuss them in detail in Chapter 9). A Social Story allows you to anticipate what may be tricky moments—loud noises, tight crowd scenes, scary sights—and it helps your child understand step-by-step exactly what is going to happen and prepare for it. But just because you have described the restaurant scenario or the birthday party scenario, don't assume your child knows it and will remember it for next time. Remind her each and every time and accept that going over the scenario itself is probably reassuring, a familiar prelude to what is becoming an increasingly familiar activity.

Make sure to keep your sense of humor. Yes, we know we keep on saying that. But the truth is, there is nothing that ages as well for most parents as the memory of a public disaster. You may find yourself telling the story to other parents to console them for the disasters that they've been through or offering it up at dinner many years later to the howls of your entire family. Identify a few good friends who can listen to your stories and are guaranteed not to respond with accounts of their own perfect children at the all-county deportment awards ceremony, and then you need to keep laughing, even if it's sometimes through tears. Find other parents of quirky kids. They are the ones who will truly understand your stories and sympathize with you in a way that parents who haven't walked the walk will never be able to do, even though they are very close friends.

Restaurants, Movies, Public Life

Start slowly with restaurants, and take it easy—basic common sense advice for all parents of young children. Go at hours when things aren't too busy and go to places that aren't aiming for a hushed and romantic atmosphere. This doesn't mean you have to sacrifice good food. There will be great informal ethnic restaurants everywhere you look, good restaurants dubbed family friendly in many cities and towns, and any vacation destination is likely to have casual joints with great food.

As for the quirky child who eats only the same 3 things? Well, if you want to take him out to a restaurant, you'd better pack up thing 1, thing 2, and thing 3 and bring them along. Confide in a server, request an extra plate, and then order plenty of food for those of you who *are* eating.

Being in a restaurant with your quirky child may make you acutely aware of how different your child is developmentally from other children the same age. Even if your child isn't self-conscious about table manners or about needing you to cut the meat, *you* may find yourself smiling nervously at other adults—or even other children—and wishing that your child could grow up a little.

> **Last night we were at an Italian restaurant with friends. He was sitting next to this little girl, and they brought hot rolls. My son hands one to the girl next to him and says, "Can you butter it?" I mean, he's 11 and he can't butter his roll.**

Restaurant trips are an excellent opportunity for the kind of scenarios we previously mentioned. Go over with your child the specific mechanics of a trip to a restaurant: "We'll arrive after driving for 20 minutes. We'll park in the parking lot and go in. There will probably be music but it's not too loud. We'll choose our food. I called and know they have macaroni and cheese and chicken fingers. You'll tell me what you want to eat, and someone will come to take our order." This continues right through to paying the bill and saying "thank you." By scripting out the trip in this way you should have as few surprises as possible.

Similarly, a trip to the movies may be easier for a quirky kid who knows exactly what to expect—from the concession stand in the lobby, to the coming attractions, to the credits, to the movie itself. For most quirky kids, you would be better off starting with movies that are more or less known quantities rather than expecting them to be surprised or delighted by movies they are unfamiliar with. You don't want to have to deal with the consequences of a scene that is too scary or disturbing, and you don't want to have to answer loud, persistent questions in a public place. Movies can be very loud and overwhelming for kids with sensory-processing difficulties, and the right pair of earplugs can make the difference between pleasure and pain. All quirky kids should have some good earplugs for those moments when life is louder than is tolerable, which can be as routine as a subway ride or a movie.

Again, with any new outing, any new activity, take it slowly. Don't let yourself be carried away by the experiences of the typical kids who are the same age as your child. There's an awful lot of variation among children, and one child's favorite movie is another child's screaming trauma. Some kids think Ursula from *The Little Mermaid* is simply hilarious—so horrible she couldn't possibly be real. This is less likely for an anxious child or a child who can't make the imaginative leap into that Disney world. For that kid, Ursula is absolutely terrifying and a source of nightmares. Just about every Disney movie has an Ursula-like character. Learn as much as you can about the movie before you go and tell it to your child, breaking the whole thing down into a scenario or script that lays out exactly what's going to happen. And then go and try to have fun, but stay ready to bag the whole thing and get the hell out of there if it starts looking like a disaster is in the making. And despite all your preparations, that can happen.

> **We took Aidan to the Christmas tree lighting ceremony. Lights came on and music started playing at the same time. It was just too much for Aidan. He was way overstimulated, and we needed to get out of there pronto. It made us very sad we couldn't do this special thing.**

If you have other children, being ready to make a getaway often means having two adults present so that, in an emergency, one can take the unwilling child out in the lobby or out of the restaurant for a walk without ruining the activity for the rest of the kids.

And here, as elsewhere in public life, you may occasionally have to deal with officious strangers. Try not to be unduly rude to these people, but remember that you owe them no explanations and no information, only a polite apology if your child has in any way intruded on them. To the kind stranger who crosses the street to tell your child, *"If you would only stop covering your ears, you would really enjoy the parade,"* you need only reply, "Thank you so much for your suggestion."

Activities and Sports

Life, of course, is not all restaurant trips, movies, and parades. There can also be team sports, music lessons, religious school, skating lessons, gymnastics, dance, and practically anything else you can think of. And for a given quirky child, any one of these may be a good activity—or even *the* activity, the be-all and end-all. Be careful, though, about overscheduling the quirky kid or filling the schedule with activities important to you but not to your child. The child who faces additional struggles in school and with homework, and who also might have a couple of extra therapy or special-help sessions every week, is unlikely to thrive on the addition of violin lessons (*because every child should play an instrument*), ballet (*because it will help her with grace and coordination*), soccer (*because team sports are so important for teaching kids to get along in life*), and religious school (*because it's so important to know one's heritage*). That regimen leads to overscheduled children and the perils of pushing too hard. For a child who is already struggling to meet academic and social expectations, it's out of the question. Choose activities that really matter. Ideally, they are the activities that really matter to your child, not to you. In the words of one elementary schoolteacher:

> I look at Annie—she has ADHD and ASD—and I think that her parents, who are very success oriented, were expecting a perfect child: you know, one who comes home and does a wonderful job on her homework, practices the violin, works on her community service project. And you know, it just isn't like that.

Giving up your fantasies can be painful for parents, but it shouldn't be painful for the child. It's important not to restrict quirky children's activities completely and to allow them to pursue their interests. It's also important to keep in mind that if a child is truly determined to play baseball—or the piano—that determination may accomplish more than years of OT.

Children's team sports are a big deal. There are towns where every girl plays soccer on Saturday or where spring is heralded by the appearance of Little League T-shirts. Your child may want to be part of the action. It's best to give team sports a try while your child is young. The youngest divisions in these leagues are rarely intense or highly competitive, which will give you a chance to assess your child's skills and pleasure in the whole process.

On the other hand, many quirky kids prefer individual sports that don't involve cooperation with other team members, such as swimming, tennis, or even rock climbing. And someone who takes tennis lessons, or becomes a good swimmer, may have the opportunity to be part of a team later on. Some children are not going to find it easy to participate in regular community teams and leagues. There are recreational leagues for children with developmental disabilities that can provide accommodations. There are summer programs and activities staffed with counselors with special training. Some children will thrive and succeed in these settings. Physical activity is important, and as pediatricians we are always advising more of it, but finding the activity that will keep your child engaged, preferably outdoors, can be a challenge. Keep trying!

Logistics of a Hectic Schedule

We can't stress enough the importance of logistics, the details of getting from place to place. With all their extra appointments, quirky children can end up with complex schedules. Certainly, anyone who has more than one child is faced with a great deal of detail in masterminding daily life. Similarly, a single parent is going to be more stressed by logistics and perhaps face even more difficult financial and work-related decisions. And, of course, some quirks can make the logistics that much more complicated. Many parents need help from another adult, if not a spouse then a grandparent or babysitter, to help manage the schedule and the special issues that arise.

For example, some quirky children simply cannot handle the school bus. It's too noisy or crazy, or they get bullied. Whatever the reason, you may be faced with the need to drive your child back and forth, which can greatly complicate your own life and excite the envy or scorn of less quirky siblings who did, or do, just fine on the bus.

Wherever possible, opt for integration, folding therapies into the school day. For many families, this is ideal, and it's generally much more possible than it used to be. However, it's still true that parents often find themselves coordinating additional help for children outside of school, between medical issues, therapies, and, of course, the regular activities that come up in the lives of quirky kids and their siblings. With all the therapies and appointments, life gets more complicated. Someone is always schlepping a kid here or there, trying to remember what to bring along, running a little late. This may have financial implications for the family. Is someone going to cut back on hours at work? Does someone else need the car so Mom has to take the train to work? There also are time and stress implications for all concerned. Inevitably, siblings find themselves getting dragged around to therapy appointments as well as one another's music lessons or sports events. The result can be a great deal of groaning and complaining and also a certain amount of teasing, as your quirky child's siblings look around at the other children in the physical therapy waiting room, or the kids attending the social skills group. It would be easy to say that it's best not to bring siblings along to these appointments, but it's just a fact of life for many families. Parents have an obligation to teach the sibling how to behave. Although some offices have toys or puzzles, these will rarely satisfy week after week. Bring activities—books, toys, homework—for the children who will be doing the waiting and thank them (and maybe reward them) for their patience.

If you sometimes feel as if you're slogging, it's probably because you are. Get help if you can afford it with housecleaning, laundry, or shopping, and forgive yourself if your standards slip a little. Keep your eye on what really matters— your child, your family, your partner. Cut your losses when you need to. And remember that you are doing a challenging and important job. Logistics matter because they get the children to the activities they enjoy or to the special help they need. All this detail, schlepping, and exhaustion will make sense as you watch them grow and learn and progress.

If anyone had told me 5 years ago, when we first got his diagnosis, that George would have perfect pitch and would be playing in the high school band and dancing with girls at dances, I would never have believed it. He's come a very long way!

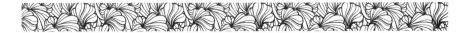

5

Family Life: Siblings, Parents, and Extended Family

In this chapter, we look more closely at the relationships that family members—both immediate and extended—have with their quirky brothers and sisters, nieces and nephews, grandchildren, cousins, and all the rest. Of course, we recognize that there are all sorts of family configurations. Our goal is to point out some problems that may arise, and suggest some strategies and approaches, but we also want to celebrate the wonderful and positive effect that a supportive and accepting family can have on an eccentric child's life, and the joy that a child who knows everything there is to know about volcanoes or climate change can bring to the family. We also look a little more directly at how parents can take care of themselves and everyone else.

Siblings

The siblings of your quirky child are probably much on your mind as a parent. Are they getting their fair share of attention? Is the household so focused on one child's needs that the less needy are sometimes left to fend for themselves? Do they feel ashamed of a weird brother or sister or cringe inside when someone at school laughs or teases—or are their own social situations compromised as they rush to defend or explain or intercede? Sibling support groups are increasingly available, and it might be worth asking your specialist if there is one that would work for your family.

Nina is the oldest child with two very impaired younger siblings and has adopted a caregiver role with both of them, especially her autistic brother. When other kids come over and see him doing his self-stimulating behavior, she just says, "That's my brother who is autistic. He doesn't talk, but he goes to a special school where they are going to teach him to talk." When she sees him after school, she greets him with joy and affection. We worry about her, though, because she assumes this role both at home and at school. There is a child in her class with autism, and she reaches out to him and takes care of him, too. We worry she is growing up too soon, accepting too much responsibility for her age. So we brought her to the school counselor and asked her to work on this. We want Nina to have a childhood.

My granddaughter Sophie is very strong and protective of her brother Max. But one night, as I was sitting on her bed as she was falling asleep, a soft voice came up from the pillow and said, "Sometimes I think it would be so nice to have a brother who didn't have autism." I nearly cried.

Some children grow up with a special kind of assurance, a confidence that can come from knowing you are the nonquirky, high-achieving child, whereas others grow up feeling ignored and neglected. All we can do here is suggest that you think through the decisions you make about your quirky child from the perspective of how they affect siblings and try to be sure that the quirkiness and accommodations do not become the all-defining features of your family life.

The nonquirky sibling needs the following:

- *To be sure of a certain amount of privacy and protection from the more extreme moods and behaviors of your quirky kid.* It's not fair to expect a sibling to sleep through nighttime crying or to manage a tantrum. No matter how supportive and helpful, other children need to know that when things get extreme, it's not their problem or their responsibility—and that they have a place to go and get away, in their rooms or some other reasonably safe and private spot, while you deal with what's going on.
- *To be able to keep important possessions and school stuff safe.* Young children with autism spectrum disorder (ASD) can be highly destructive. Children with good intentions and poor fine motor skills can inadvertently spill or rip things or knock things over. You want to avoid the scenario in which the nonquirky child is always angry at the quirky sibling, always screaming, always upset. One way to do that is to make sure that her stuff is safe and she knows that if anything does get damaged, you will do your best to replace it. Everyone can benefit from a general family rule: All children can keep important possessions in their rooms—or in their special drawers—where they are absolutely off-limits to other family members. Anything left out in

the common space may be handled by all comers. After all, it might easily be the quirky child who is profoundly distressed by having a sibling touch or move or wreck her stuff. Maybe the trucks got moved out of formation because a younger brother wanted to drive one across the floor. Maybe a precious spatula (oh, yes, there are children who bond to spatulas) actually was used to flip the pancakes. In this case, you have to try to protect the quirky child's rights: "OK, this will be your special spatula, and your sister can't use it." "If you set up your trucks in your room, we can close the door so your brother won't touch them."

- *To be encouraged to help—and acknowledged for helping.* You may find that a sibling has the ability to comfort, soothe, or engage a quirky child who is generally harder to reach. At the risk of sounding trite, siblings can be great for quirky kids and vice versa. Sibling relationships provide models for friendships and present ways for kids to try to live harmoniously with others, life skills that they all need. Quirky kids usually need extra practice, and brothers and sisters can help a lot.

- *To find ways to deal with the embarrassment of having a brother or sister who sometimes behaves strangely.* A sibling support group can be very helpful for a child with a sibling who draws a lot of attention, not always in positive ways. You can also help your child by acknowledging the embarrassment or the distress without making a big issue out of it. Help your child find an easy way to explain what's going on. As long as the diagnosis has already been disclosed to the child, a sibling might say, "My sister has autism and gets upset when she hears loud noises because her ears are so sensitive." "My brother really needs to do everything a certain way. Sometimes it's a pain, but we can just go do our own stuff and my mom will take care of it." Make sure the sibling has protected space to have a friend over. Don't expect your quirky child to be included or insist on a game that everyone can play. Consider distracting the quirky sibling or even taking him on an excursion for a different activity or a treat, so that, at least occasionally, the other child and friend(s) can have full run of the house.

There is one rule that applies in any household to any set of siblings: There may be squabbles at home, but when you are out in the world, you take care of one another, protect one another, and stick up for one another. In the household with a quirky child, it goes a bit further: It is never OK to make fun of the quirky child to others or to initiate or join in any teasing or tormenting. This rule is inflexible.

The way that you and your family deal with your quirky kid, and the way that you feel and convey that feeling will have a great effect on siblings. Many children with more severely quirky siblings are acutely aware that as certain parental fantasies and ambitions are given up in the face of the other child's development, those same parental fantasies and ambitions may attach with even greater strength to the more typical, higher-achieving brother or sister. This may be a considerable burden to carry, and, occasionally, there are even children who, in one way or another, crack under the pressure.

> I worry about Sophie forming attachments in the future, in terms of letting Max go and in terms of what her expectations of herself will be. I worry about Sophie feeling free enough to make independent decisions for her own life. I worry about Sophie developing resentments of all sorts, directed at Max, at her mother, and at her father. Her childhood has been limited; I hope somehow she will be able to fly free when she grows up.

Many children look at a quirky sibling and worry that they, too, will develop the more troubling behaviors or symptoms, whether severe anxiety, seizures, or tantrums. This concern can play into the preoccupations of parents, who may be unable to stop anxiously watching their other children for danger signs. We found this to be especially true for parents whose first child was the quirky one. Any mild variation in the second child's development or behavior will almost automatically be viewed as the onset of more serious and familiar issues. Parents do have good reason to be concerned and attentive, though. Children who fall into any of the quirky-kid categories *are* more likely to have siblings in these categories as well. As we've said, ASD, anxiety, attention-deficit/hyperactivity disorder, and mood disorders all have genetic components, although the genetics are not simple and straightforward.

Try your best to view each child separately, as the person he is, as her own unfolding individual. Comparisons are fruitless. Sibling relations are often awkward and touchy, even when everyone does everything in strict birth-order chronology, is equally high-achieving and sunny tempered, and is aware of receiving an equal and fair share of parental notice and appreciation. Actually, this has never once happened in recorded history, but we suspect that even if it *did* happen, there would still be some touchy intersibling issues. When one child is on a genuinely different developmental trajectory, sibling relationships become more complicated and touchier. The less you measure your children against one another, the harder you come down on anyone who does, and the more ways you find to distinguish and celebrate each one, the better off you'll be when the crunches come.

One common issue you may face when one sibling is quirky and one is not is the situation in which a younger child surpasses an older child. There's no easy way to deal with it when a younger sibling achieves a developmental milestone first, masters a skill that the older one still struggles with, passes the older one academically, or even reaches a social landmark (eg, a sleepover party, a first date) that the older child has not yet reached—and may never reach. This situation is awkward for everyone, unless your older, quirkier child is genuinely immune (eg, uninterested in the sport, the skill, or the social scene). It would be a noble younger child who could refrain from remarking on having gotten ahead of the older sibling. You have to remember that birth order often seems like a mandated footrace to young children, and it's only natural to crow when you pass the person who started out ahead.

Parents have to be matter-of-fact and frank about this, and they can't let their concern for the quirky child's feelings stifle whatever celebration or congratulations are warranted for the sibling. You certainly don't have to compel the quirky child to participate, but you can't downplay the achievement itself. So, no, don't drag the 10-year-old boy who is physically awkward and uncoordinated to his 8-year-old sister's gymnastics championships. Don't compel him to come and cheer because it's such an important day for her. But make sure you are there, and hang that picture of her with her team, and everyone wearing rosettes, up on the wall. Then look for something to celebrate with her brother.

Although her father tries to give Sophie "special time" and enrolled her in gymnastics classes, Sophie is free to do "her own thing" only if Max is involved in a program that takes care of him.

By far the most basic and widespread issue for the siblings of quirky children, however, is the constant daily rub of being in a situation in which one child is unusually needy, and the parents have to arrange life so that those needs can be met. Anything that parents can do to address this imbalance is helpful. Special time scheduled with each child, whether formally or informally, is important. Kids need to be with their parents sometimes and have their parents concentrating fully and solely on *them*, not on the family conundrum. Rotating choices (eg, what to pick up for dinner Friday evening, what to do on Saturday afternoon) so that everyone gets to choose, rather than catering only to the person with the most restrictions (even if that sometimes means that the restricted kid can't participate), can help siblings feel that their own lives aren't being shortchanged by preferences and dislikes they don't share.

By the time John was about 5 or 6, I started planning these mom/
son weekends away with each child alone. I felt each deserved
some of my undivided attention, and I wanted the chance to truly
revel in being with one of them at a time, without constantly
feeling guilty that I couldn't meet everyone's demands all the time.

Now that Megan is away at college, it's really nice for us to have
time with our son, because so much of our energy has always been
taken up trying to help Megan out. There always seemed to be
some kind of crisis, and he honestly did not get the attention he
should have.

Above all, remember that the complexities of family life, and of rubbing up against siblings, can be the best thing in the world for a quirky child. A child who needs help with social dynamics will find plenty in the direct speech of her siblings. The home environment should be a safe place to relax and have a little fun, free from some of the anxieties and strictures of the school day. The love, understanding, and tenderness of siblings at different points over the life span can mean a tremendous amount to your quirky child, and the returned affections of a quirky brother or sister can enrich siblings' lives.

Our son is a pretty understanding sort of kid, which isn't to say that
his sister doesn't drive him crazy from time to time. But I've always
had one rule: You don't even have to like each other, but you must
be polite to each other. That means, no name-calling, no excessive
teasing, and especially no hitting or shoving.

The Extended Family

For some parents of quirky kids, it is in their extended family that they find help and support and acceptance. For others, the most difficult, most tense, and most unpleasant day of any season is the family gathering.

Our relatives think, "She's just a wacky kid and will outgrow it." But I
thought she needed more help, because I knew that day-to-day life
with her was not just "wacky" but painful.

Extended families will react according to their own histories, expectations, wisdom, and experiences.

> My brother has a son with ASD, and he and his wife basically locked themselves up. For years, they didn't come to any family celebrations because Paula [his wife] couldn't tolerate the way people looked at their son. She thought she saw reproving looks—that everyone thought it was all her fault. They wouldn't go to the beach with the family in the summer anymore. That created a big rift in the extended family. Nobody could understand, and she just wouldn't come. Since she wouldn't tell them, the family interpreted it as Paula thought she was too good for them, or she had something better to do. They didn't know it was painful for her too.

Think carefully about how you want to discuss your child's issues within your family circle. Of course, keep in mind that in most families, news travels. Because many extended families have more than one quirky kid in the mix, it can be helpful to share a diagnosis and the plans you have put in place to help your child. You may learn something about another child you love in the family.

Some problems—such as many learning issues—really don't need to be discussed in great detail. Your child may be asked to explain why he's reading easier books than his younger cousin, but chances are, that's a familiar question for him, and he should have his answer ready. (A simple "Because she's a very good reader" is often effective.) Major social oddities are obviously going to be easier for people to take if they're prepared, as are any really noticeable speech or motor delays. If your extended family doesn't see you or your child regularly, the more you can prepare them for what he's going to be like, the easier you'll make it. Autism spectrum disorder is known to be an increasingly common diagnosis in childhood, and naming it is the right thing to do: "He has autism. You'll see that he's obsessed with dinosaurs and simply doesn't know how to make conversation about any other subject. Yes, his table manners are still pretty lousy. I'd really appreciate it if you could sit him next to me so I can help him cut his turkey."

Family Gatherings and Celebrations

Every child has at some point or another disgraced herself and her parents at a family wedding, Christmas party, Thanksgiving dinner, bar mitzvah, or christening. Thank heavens, you do get some slack in the family circle. Parents tend to remember these disgraceful events that starred their own children more clearly than anyone else does. Family events are, after all, highly charged and often emotionally complex, and they are rarely attended by people behaving only as their most adult selves. However, you probably want to take part in the family traditions, in some form or other. You may also find that both you and your child receive special help and acceptance there. Most parents want their kids to be familiar with their cultural rituals, and most extended families think children are an important part of landmark events such as weddings and even funerals.

However, there also are some activities you should reconsider: your quirky, difficult, obsessional screamer of a 3-year-old as the ring bearer at your sister's long-planned, formal evening wedding for 500 of her closest friends. Or a raucous and hypercompetitive family game of charades for your extremely anxious 9-year-old with sensory issues around loud noises.

The following are some general tips for strategizing your way through family gatherings:

Anticipate the event as much as possible. Think about things that might set your child off: loud music, camera flashes, crowds. Talk it through with the child, bring essential supplies (earplugs, a familiar and comforting book), and praise good behavior lavishly.

Talk in detail about the rules of behavior in an unfamiliar setting: the getting up and sitting down in a church or synagogue, the need to be quiet while a ceremony is going on. If you know a big event is coming up and your child is unaccustomed to religious services, it might help to go once or twice before-hand, so the overall atmosphere is somewhat familiar.

> We took John to this big bar mitzvah in Chicago. The music was so loud, he just started crying, so it was good we were staying in the same place, and we could take him up to the room. It turned out that there were lots of little boys who were not exactly interested in the big party and would rather play Pokémon cards than eat a big dinner. Now when these events come up, we plan an escape route so we can all enjoy ourselves.

As a general rule at family-only celebrations, the custom is that you put up with everyone's quirks and peculiarities, but at big formal events to which many people are invited, different rules may apply. If it's a highly elegant dinner, and a child who can't manage a knife and fork is going to give offense, then you might want to think about whether it would be kinder to your child and to you to arrange things differently. Your decision may depend, at least in part, on whether your child actually wants to go and will feel bad about missing the event. Don't start a family feud over an invitation that means nothing to the child.

Plan who is going to be with your quirky child the whole time you are at the event. These are, by and large, not the kids you blithely send off to the children's table and never think about again. One of the parents, or a genuinely dependable older sibling, has to pay attention to how things are going at all times, interceding at danger signs, making sure that food and drink are manageable, and generally troubleshooting.

> **Right around now, I'm anticipating the holidays and the get-togethers. I feel we shouldn't expect to eat anything because we will need to help Aidan through the events. We don't expect him to play with the other kids, but we always have to worry that he could become overstimulated and start one of his tantrums.**

Think about who might be able to help your child enjoy the event. Is there a special relationship with Grandpa or a cheerful aunt who seems to enjoy listening to your daughter talk endlessly about cats? Ask ahead of time if that person can pay some extra attention. Sometimes there is a quirky adult in the crowd who is just as interested in iguanas as your child or who will play chess or otherwise engage a child to your utter delight and relief.

Prepare your child for any questions likely to be asked. Children with social difficulties may find it intimidating to have lots of people coming up to them and asking questions. The fact is, adults tend to ask the same questions over and over of children: "How old are you?" "What grade are you in?" "What's your favorite subject?" Or they make even more personal remarks that aren't really questions: "Isn't that a pretty dress you're wearing?" If you can rehearse your child in giving a few simple answers and even make a little game of it ("Let's see how many people tell you you've gotten taller!"), you can ease a lot of the tension. Absolutely stereotyped repetitive conversations, after all, can play right into a quirky child's social style, and you should take advantage of this. Many children love being let in on the joke of adult predictability. For some, it can be a real social lifesaver to know they have pat answers ready for the most common questions.

> **Sam should be going into fourth grade, but he's going into third. He's very aware of this, so when people ask him what grade he's in, he says, "Well, my school doesn't have grades," and he kind of goes on from there about his school. I didn't teach him this, but it works, it distracts people. "If we had grades, I would be going into fourth, but we don't have grades."**

Make an escape plan. Who's going to be responsible for taking the child out if things don't work, and what's the first-line destination? Playing with his tablet in a quieter setting? Some people swear by some quick physical stimulation. Try 20 jumping jacks in the lobby or running around the block. Try anything! Work it out and agree on it, so you don't end up in a big marital argument in the middle of somebody else's event.

Think a little about what you're going to say if people make any comments. Sometimes just naming what your child has will silence the critics and educate them at the same time—assuming that you have a name for what is going on. But if you don't, or if you don't want to go into detail about any aspect of your child, especially at a large event where many of the people are not close to you, then don't. Even if your child acts up and has to be taken out, you still don't owe people anything more than a prompt and heartfelt apology—a specific apology for the behavior, not a general apology for your child.

Aunts, Uncles, and Cousins

In many families, each new generation of cousins serves as a kind of field of comparison. Adult brothers and sisters who are close may find themselves feeling pleasantly supported or miserably competitive—and sometimes both in syncopation. How are you supposed to cope with your sister's absolutely perfect gold-medal children? How about your brother's youngest, who looks suspiciously like your own quirky child at that age? Or what if there's already another quirky child—or quirky adult—in the family?

> My sister started giving me all kinds of diagnoses of my daughter Lisa. When Lisa was diagnosed with sensory processing disorder, she kind of descended on me: "You gotta call this person and get this done and call that person and get that done." And when Lisa had a febrile seizure, she said, "Oh, that isn't a febrile seizure, that was something else, and you're going to have to deal with all these seizures." She really terrified me.

People need to be sensitive about the differences among children. Everyone is aware of the comparisons, and the parents of an obviously way-ahead-of-her-age, brilliant, and socially poised 10-year-old have a certain obligation to roll their eyes and complain about her bad moods at home or her terrible taste in pop music. Of course, your sister or brother may not adhere to the sensitivity rule, in which case you have little recourse other than to smile, praise the child in question, and absolutely refuse to be drawn into any comparative conversations. "He's doing really well, and we're proud of him" is a perfectly adequate remark to make about your own child. It is by any reckoning better manners than making everyone listen to a long list of prizes and achievements.

> People looking in from the outside—grandparents, aunts and uncles, classmates' parents—they think they have some advice for you. They think they have an answer you haven't found, because they were successful with their kids and you may or may not be. It's like people without kids giving advice about kids, only worse, because I know that their experience was nothing like mine in raising her. None of that advice applies, and it's infuriating to have to listen to it sometimes. I always feel that the subtext is that she would be more normal if only we did this or that.

In a large family with many cousins of similar age, the quirky child may appear as an outlier. Maybe some kids are out on the lawn playing touch football, and your child is lining up his cars or reading that book about Hawaiian tree snails that he already knows by heart. It's your job to stick up for him, stand by his preferences, and help him find an identity within the family. Maybe you can teach him a little about touch football so he'll feel comfortable playing or keeping score. If not, maybe you can include him in the adult conversation or link him up with one particular relative who is in no way interested in the football game. Maybe he can help Grandma put the marshmallows on the sweet potatoes. Finding a task or an activity that your child likes can help him feel included and help you as the parent feel less concerned about his well-being during family functions.

> My sister-in-law has three kids, all high-achieving in every sport. Each plays multiple instruments and practices them every day. She's got it all planned out for them to go to a good college. Sometimes she asks why my kids aren't playing an instrument. She just doesn't get it! She doesn't understand that it's all we can do to get through homework.

Think about your quirky child in relation to some other quirky relatives. It's reassuring and even delightful to look at a beloved, if eccentric, aunt or uncle who has created a good life. If Aunt Molly also loved astronomy as a child and could name all the constellations too, and now she's an aerospace engineer, that's exciting for a child to see. Regardless of whether your son has much in common with Aunt Molly, thinking of her may make it easier for family members to see and accept his peculiarities. Maybe there's a family member—an artist or a musician, a software developer or a gardener—who has followed a creative but nontraditional path. There are lots of ways to live a life, and quirky kids need to know that adult life comes in many forms.

Once again, cousins and aunts and uncles can mean a lot to a quirky child. They are a built-in social network, a group of people guaranteed to turn up over and over who will, with luck, accept, embrace, and acknowledge this fellow member of the tribe. Quirky children, who sometimes seem to be outsiders in any group in which they find themselves, need that feeling of belonging and family connection.

Grandparents

Most of us grow up with the certainty that despite what our parents may believe, our grandparents think we are perfect. It can be particularly valuable for a quirky child to experience that kind of unconditional adoration, that sense that just by coming into the world, the grandchild has accomplished a miracle. Many grandparents need education and support from family and peers to understand the developmental trajectory of their quirky grandchildren, but once they are armed with that education, they are the best allies a parent and child can have.

Unfortunately, it's not uncommon for grandparents to find a quirky child's eccentricities or developmental slowness difficult to tolerate and, maybe in part because of a child-rearing mindset that developed before many of these diagnoses were commonly known, some may be inclined to blame everything on parental laxity or other aspects of the way you are raising your child.

> My parents are very clear that the problem is child care. They never put their children in child care and can't understand how anyone could do it. This is their way of understanding her developmental delays—that she doesn't get enough of our attention, and that it's because we put her in one of "those places." In other words, we brought this on ourselves.

Grandparents can mean a tremendous amount in the life of a quirky kid. They can be the child's biggest and most sincere cheerleaders, your absolutely lifesaving babysitters, or the people who provide a little family context and perspective. After all, they knew *you* when you were young, and they may see some connections. Obviously, this is all highly dependent on whether they see you every other day, every month, or once a year, as well as on their situation in life and state of health. But for many families, even the grandparents you see only every so often are eager to help in any way they can. However, depending on your relationship with them and their beliefs, they may be the very last people you want to let in on the details of how you are managing with your child.

> My mother-in-law doesn't know John is on meds. I feel it's none of her business, and I guess I'm not entirely immune to other people's opinions. I just don't want to hear what she might say about it. When John was little, her take on him was, "He's fine; why are you taking him to all these appointments?" But now she'll say, "Oh, that was so awful when he wouldn't eat and he wouldn't talk!"

> My husband's parents are very supportive of everything with Jack and Rebecca; in fact, they're in a grandparent support group. For a while, they were bringing home articles about crazy diets and nutritional supplements, but I don't go for that stuff, so I asked them to stop. Now they share different kinds of information. My mom, on the other hand, has the "he'll outgrow it any day" attitude toward Jack and thinks there is nothing wrong with Rebecca at all.

Many parents with quirky kids speak about a grandparent who refuses to believe that anything is wrong or of concern or even different. If the children are academically smart, and especially if they have prominent splinter skills, such as strong math abilities or perfect pitch, many grandparents will define them as geniuses and accept them—and boast about them—in those terms.

> Aidan's paternal grandparents are very interested in learning— Grandma is a teacher, Grandpa is a librarian—and they are so pleased with how bright he is and how early he knew the alphabet. He can do no wrong.

Allow grandparents the pleasure of believing—and boasting—that their grandchild is gifted, while presenting the very real problems and your concerns. The grandparent who believes that he or she is nursing a budding Einstein is a grandparent who will be able to provide the unconditional love that can mean so much to a child, especially one regarded by others as the family problem.

With children who are more delayed and less readily seen as eccentric geniuses, grandparents, just like parents, have to confront the loss of their own fantasies. Many grandparents are heavily invested in the dream of their grandchildren following certain paths or mastering certain skills. You need to remember the evolutionary process by which you modified some of your own expectations so that you can be tolerant and helpful as your child's grandparents modify theirs. Try hard not to get too angry at a grandparent who perhaps does not see your child every day and who seems to be persistently puzzled by some lack of developmental progress. It's a difficult personal journey, and a little sympathy and support will go a long way.

Familial reverberations are another interesting issue that often arises with grandparents. Many a parent has been astonished to learn that he himself (or maybe his brother) was highly quirky in his youth, in ways that perhaps did not have a name back then but that resemble, shadow, or interestingly contrast with the ways in which his child is now developing. Other grandparents, having staked their claim in some way on their own children's normalcy, and having refused to acknowledge problems and eccentricities the first time around are not about to open that retrospective can of worms now.

> My husband's older sister was very developmentally delayed, both speech and motor, as a child in the 1950s. I remember their mother telling me things about her, but she never related it to my kids being the way they were. She never wanted to go that far. Her daughter had had both speech and motor delays and some significant learning difficulties that must have been simply impossible to deal with then. You would think there would have been all these bells and whistles when they saw our son and all his delays, but no. It was like there was something in their family code that kept them from talking about it.

> My husband is one of three kids. His brother was very "hyper" as a child but became very depressed as an adult and committed suicide in his 30s. My mother-in-law recognizes her deceased son in her grandson, Ben, and is very supportive of me and my husband for all we do to help him. She says she wishes she had been stronger to have gotten her son the help he needed when he was young.

All kinds of complexities can be involved in negotiating the emotional balance among the three generations, but grandparents and grandchildren are generally held together by strong bonds. Grandparents, like parents, are in this for the long haul, and for many families struggling with complicated quirky children, grandparents provide some welcome help, hope, and respite. Grandparents are often the babysitters who aren't really babysitters because it's a treat to visit them or to be visited by them, or simply because they're the ones doing this for love, not money.

Some general points about grandparents as babysitters:

- Teach routines, but it is a time-honored truth that at Grandma and Grandpa's house, or when they are babysitting, all bets are off, and all kinds of treats happen. As long as your child is happy, relax and enjoy it!
- A grandparent who is going to do any significant amount of babysitting needs to know how to handle peculiar or alarming behaviors, though don't be surprised if you come home to the serene report, "He's always good as gold with me!"
- If your child is engaged in an intensive behavioral program, anyone who spends a significant amount of time with her will need to be educated in the system you are using. This includes grandparents, who often find it especially difficult to respond as the program has prescribed.
- Make reasonable allowances for age and health. Some difficult quirky kids really require a lot of running, a lot of lifting and carrying, and a high level of energy. If you have a grandparent who is eager to help out but may be limited in terms of health or energy level, keep those babysitting visits short and sweet—or ask for some late-night hours, after your child is asleep, and go to a late show or dinner. A couple of families we talked with have used a younger teenager and a grandparent together as a babysitting team. This can take the pressure off grandparents for tasks requiring a lot of physical stamina and provide some good on-the-job training for the teenager at the same time.
- Grandparents can help you make sure all siblings get some special adult attention. Don't let the problem child monopolize all the babysitting time that grandparents offer. Make sure siblings get some time alone at Grandma's house or a special outing once in a while.

We hear again and again in our pediatric practice about grandparents who refuse to acknowledge that anything is wrong or different. Every parent needs to decide whether to pursue the issue. A grandparent who blames your child-rearing practices for any problems your child encounters can eventually wear you down. You may find yourself wanting to do some educating—or some screaming. But grandparents who let you know that as far as they are concerned, these issues don't require diagnoses and their grandchild is his own special self who just needs to be loved and appreciated are expressing the thinking of their own parenting days and are to be cherished and appreciated.

Parents—Taking Care of Yourself

It may come as no surprise that life with your quirky child can affect your life, spirits, and relationships (ie, spouse, partner, good friends) and you will need to decide how you go about protecting and cherishing them, so that you can do as good a job as possible at everything that matters most—including taking care of your quirky kid.

Single Parents

Single parents have it a lot harder, no question about it. All the additional pressures, sorrows, and tensions of life with a quirky child devolve on that one parent. There may not be another adult easily available with whom you can discuss the child at length and strategize, and from whom you can receive help and comfort. Try to develop a community of friends or relatives who know your child (or children) and can offer support and respite when you need it. You'll need a regular break from rearing a quirky child on your own. Don't wait until you've completely lost your cool before setting up some time just for you. Do it regularly. Most communities have support groups for single parents and some even have groups for single parents of quirky kids. This is a long haul. The more support you garner for yourself, the better off you and your children will be.

In the following points, we talk about the ways that being parents of a quirky child can stress a relationship between spouses or partners; if you're doing this on your own, you may sometimes feel that you experience all the stress and receive none of the support. Single parents may also be under more economic pressure and be less able to modify their work schedules; everything is riding on that one person. We know people can be very resourceful about finding support and community, whether through their faith or through parent advocacy groups. If you're feeling overwhelmed by the demands, consider finding a therapist who is a good fit and "gets it," and who can help you as you process the emotions of this journey over time.

You and Your Partner

A quirky child can stress a relationship mightily. We have seen couples become polarized and even split up over the disagreements and logistical pressures of child-rearing, especially when it comes to disciplining a behaviorally challenging child. Other couples are simply so stressed by the rigors of life at home that one parent starts spending less and less time there, the other resents it more and more, and the couple's relationship ends up in trouble.

> What created marital tension was this: My husband believed Jacob
> was normal and didn't agree with me about an evaluation. I was
> very concerned. Now my husband and I have separated, and the
> stress around Jacob and his issues was one of the main factors.

What can you do to prevent these problems or deal with these disagreements and the additional stresses of daily life?

- Go together to a parent support group and meet a community of other parents. Try attending educational sessions or conferences together, so you are on the same page with your knowledge and strategies.
- Don't designate one partner to cope with this while the other one concentrates on other things; that may drive a deeper wedge between you. You are in this together—for yourselves, for each other, and for the child. A partnership will make a world of difference.
- Acknowledge the stresses and their dangers. Help each other through the process of acknowledgment and/or diagnosis. Talk about your hopes, disappointments, and fears.
- Work diligently at finding common ground. Seek out expert assistance. Fights and even divorces can happen over the anger that is generated when one parent is more concerned than the other. One may think something is really wrong, while the other thinks it's nothing and the child will outgrow it. You cannot raise a child together unless you find a way to make sense of what your family is going through and understand your child in a way that makes sense to both of you.
- In a marriage, as in all partnerships, nothing is ever completely equal; one of you is likely to do the lion's share of the work involved in parenting a quirky child. Be careful; if the division of labor regarding your child is too rigid, the more involved parent can end up feeling isolated and overwhelmed, while the less involved parent feels excluded and marginalized.
- Pay careful and respectful attention to each other's opinions, both about what's going on with your child and about the best way to address special needs and issues as they arise.
- At the beginning of any new therapy, parents should meet the doctor, therapist, or teacher and agree that they feel comfortable with the person and the plan.
- Pay serious attention to the logistics, the who-is-going-to-pick-her-up-after-physical-therapy-when-it's-also-Peter's-Boy-Scout-night questions. It's rarely possible for one parent to handle the logistics unaided, whether that means getting help from the other parent, a babysitter, or a friend.

- Talk frankly about your financial situation and the implications of your child's issues. If one parent stops working or cuts back on hours, discuss the effect on the family finances. Many extra expenses come along with quirkiness—therapies, special after-school programs, medications, private schools, tutors, babysitters, and so forth. How can you budget for these additions?
- If you are considering relocating, do you agree on a town that you think has good public school programs that might be right for your child?
- Take care of each other. You love each other and you both love your child, and your child's best bet in life is for you to keep loving each other and taking care of the family together. This is a hard road to go alone. Aim for some conversation every day that is not purely logistical in nature and that does not focus on your quirky child's issues.
- Don't let your sex life become completely swallowed up by the busyness, fatigue, frustration, and possible depression that can accompany life with a quirky child.
- Pay attention to the adjustments and efforts your spouse is making, such as the endless patience with which your husband practices questions-and-answers with your daughter or the clever way your wife has reorganized the bathroom so your son can reach everything he needs.
- If your own relationship is under severe stress—if you're fighting all the time, not talking at all, or never having sex—see a therapist. Get help as soon as you realize there is a problem.
- Be on the lookout for signs of emotional overload in your partner and yourself. Depression in parents of quirky kids can go unrecognized because it seems reasonable to be sad. Depression also can wreak havoc on your family, so if you are worried about your partner or yourself, seek professional help.

Other People's Children

Many parents find that in the course of watching their children at school, sporting events, or other activities, or in spending time with friends, they become at least periodically possessed by envy of parents with so-called normal kids. You may watch your best friend's son hit a home run or play his violin and think, "Surely this is the child I was meant to have." Or you can listen to another parent complaining at length about her obviously typical daughter's obviously typical whininess and think, "Honey, you have no idea!"

> Family vacations with Caitlin and our extended families are very difficult: There are multiple families with about 15 people, lots of kids. I usually become very sad and realize all over again how much easier it is to raise "regular" kids.

Almost all parents go through various disappointments and challenges to their most precious heartfelt fantasies when they watch their kids grow up. However, when you find daily life overshadowed by ugly moments of resenting other parents whose kids seem to be just fine, as well as resenting their typical, normal, perfect, high-achieving kids, remember the following:

- Find your people! Join a support group of other parents who will understand your feelings and not judge you.
- Remember that every family has issues. Every child has issues. They may not be as apparent, but no family or child is perfect.
- There are going to be moments when you feel yourself ready to burst with the emotion that arises from seeing what seems to come easily to every other child or from hearing the complaints of parents who have no idea what life is like on the quirky side of the playground.
- Come up with a couple of basic strategies or statements that explain what you're feeling, but don't upset anyone else. You are entitled to a rueful smile and a wistful comment: "I look at those kids and I really, really wish my daughter could enjoy the beach, but that's who she is and there's no changing it."
- Do not, under any circumstances, rain on another parent's parade. When someone else is glowing with one of those proud parental moments, dizzy with the joy of a child who has just hit a ball, spoken to the company in Chinese, buttoned himself into his first tux and gone off to the prom, or been accepted into college, congratulate her.
- Perhaps the hardest moments for many parents are not the achievements of someone else's child. What can actually be much more difficult are the public moments (eg, at the pool, circus, playground) when it can seem that every other child knows how to be a child and have fun—except yours.
- Practice reality. Make a joke of it when you can. Relish your child's quirks and eccentricities. As long as you can find pleasure and joy in the child you have and the life you lead, by all means give yourself permission to feel sad sometimes for the child you don't have and the life you didn't get.
- We'll say it again—if you cannot escape the regrets or the envy or the anger, find someone to talk to. Maybe there's a parent support group where you can finally say some of the things you've been keeping to yourself.
- Be open to the idea of therapy, and even of medication. You are doing a very hard job, and you need to take good care of yourself, body and soul.
- Take a day off to go to the beach with your partner. Join a chorus, take a swim class at the YMCA. By all means, take care of yourself so you can care for your child; just like on an airplane, put your oxygen mask on first.

You and Your Job

What about your career, your job, your professional future? Some parents' work lives continue on much the same trajectory, quirky kid or no. Some parents make modifications. Some give up their jobs. Some change jobs and end up devoting their lives to some particular aspect of the quirky-child universe.

> I am an artist, but my work schedule had to change because of having a child with so many needs. I have spent so much of my life in doctors' offices and waiting rooms, and so much of our money has gone to getting help that our insurance doesn't cover. But the fact is that we believe that we have helped her, that she is doing as well as she could be doing, and she could be doing much worse.

> For me, I find my job is very grounding, and I like the job. I know that if I didn't get to get out of this house and go to my office, where I feel like a grown-up and have a certain amount of authority and control, I wouldn't be able to come home and take care of my kids.

Plenty of parents, usually but not always mothers, end up scaling back their jobs or quitting altogether because of the demands and stresses of caring for a quirky child. This can happen because one parent has a job that he or she is not particularly attached to, or because the logistics of family life become too complicated to accommodate more than one parent with a demanding job. Clearly, this has financial implications for the family. In addition, it may mean that that parent becomes increasingly tied to the child.

It is, of course, true that tending to a quirky child can take a tremendous amount of time—as can tending to any child. Many parents, most often but not always mothers, quit their jobs and devote themselves full time to tending to typical children, too. Some quirky children may have such complicated needs, or some situations may be so difficult to manage that a full-time parental pilot is the best—or only—solution.

> I quit my job for a while to spend more time with Jacob and to get him the help he needed. I am now trying to restart my career. It was the right thing to do at the time, and I do not regret it.

Other parents, with high-powered or demanding jobs, sometimes use those jobs to escape their less-than-relaxing homes, their demanding and puzzling children. When one parent does this, the quirky child—and indeed, the whole family—loses a necessary balance. When both parents do it, the quirky child is given over to therapists, babysitters, doctors, and teachers, all of whom may be dedicated and loving, but none of whom can take your place as parents.

Let us confess our own frank prejudice as pediatricians and mothers. If you can manage it, it's generally better for both parents to keep their jobs, however modified, and to avoid that strict division of labor that so often occurs when one person earns the money and the other cares for the kids. Parents who work and like their jobs should not be pushed or shamed or harassed into quitting them to become full-time advocates, therapists, chauffeurs, and tutors for their quirky children.

By keeping your job, you bring in more money, and you maintain more balance in the relationship. All the financial clout isn't on one side and all the parental clout on the other. You also protect yourself from becoming completely identified as the parent of a quirky kid. You will have someplace in your life where you can go and be someone else.

> **I love to go to work. Sometimes I get so entrenched in the appointments and evaluations, I forget that I have another life. It's such a relief to go to work and talk with other adults about anything. I find there is more of me to give when I get home, because my universe is greater than the "mom of a child with differences."**

There are lots of ways to balance your children and your professional ambitions and opportunities, your finances, and your marital and family logistics. Speaking as mothers who have found it worthwhile and psychically necessary to pursue reasonably demanding careers while rearing our own children, we appreciate firsthand the rewards of taking your work seriously, even while you take your children seriously.

Making It Your Mission

And then there are the parents who take on their children's issues and needs with such energy and thoroughness that they end up turning some aspect of having, or being, a quirky child into their lifework. Sometimes an unexpected twist in the road of your life really does show you the way to a larger destiny. Some parents have taken on ASD or school issues or sensory processing disorder and found ways to use their own knowledge and experience to help other parents and children and even to change the world a little bit. We salute them and honor them, and we cite many of their books, websites, and organizations in this book, hoping to introduce you to people who will understand all the different aspects of the parental journey on which you are embarked, because they have been this way themselves.

We do offer a brief caveat: Making your own single quirky child into your life's mission can be dangerous. If your whole life is taken up with and taken over by the needs of your child, by fighting her battles and ferrying her to her appointments, if you're in school almost as much as she is, and you spend your spare time surfing the internet for more information on her disorder, this may become unhealthy—for you, for your primary relationship, for your other children, and even, perhaps, for your quirky child.

This may sound harsh or unsympathetic. But we have observed that when a parent becomes almost obsessed with a quirky child, the family ends up off balance, and the child has to bear the burden of that parent's full-time concentration. It's not easy being another person's cause or the object of another person's every thought or another person's reason for living.

One Final Note to Parents

Family life is challenging at times for everyone. Making a marriage work is hard. Figuring out how to blend careers, adult ambitions, and children's lives is hard. Being a single parent is hard. And taking care of a quirky child is hard in itself and can make all these other jobs that much harder. Some parents realize that they themselves are probably on the autism spectrum but were never diagnosed. As a result, some people find themselves with both a quirky kid and a spouse on the spectrum—or maybe even two quirky kids and a spouse.

> This past year, I realized that I was doing too much alone. My husband's work schedule required that he travel a lot, and I was home trying to keep everything going—school and homework, piano practicing for my other kids, various appointments and medication evaluations, the works. I gradually became overwhelmed and had real trouble getting pleasure out of anything. I found some help, but, more important, I realized that I need to set limits for myself. I can only do so much for my son, and sometimes that means I just can't do everything.

We say this again: If you find yourself in trouble, get help. Relationship counseling, pastoral help, psychiatric help—whatever you need to make it through. Do not think of the responsibility of caring for a quirky child as something that you are going to tough out. Don't feel guilty that you have needs of your own. Talk with your friends, your spouse, your doctor. Call a hot line or join a parent support group. Check to see what you or your spouse's insurance covers for counseling services and research low-cost counseling programs run by charitable and civic organizations. Take a credit-union loan at work, but get help. Everyone feels overwhelmed and depressed at times, but if you're chronically overwhelmed, chronically sad, and unable to take pleasure in the things that usually make you happy—or if you even *fleetingly* contemplate hurting or killing yourself—please, get help. You will be glad you did, and you will be able, once again, to be what you need to be, to help the people depending on you, and to enjoy another day.

The people with whom you are most closely connected, and who, after you, feel the strongest sense of family attachment and communion with your child, can greatly help you along the way. If you can garner support and a helping hand at critical moments from aunts and uncles and grandparents, you will have made the world a more connected, more welcoming place for you and your child.

Many parents worry about what will become of their children after they die or if they are unable to care for them, and this worry can start very early in a child's life if the child is really struggling. We recommend facing this issue head-on: meet with an estate planner who is familiar with making plans for a relative with a disability. Many are lawyers or financial planners who are parents themselves and are familiar with the laws and options available. You'll need to think about what resources you have, both in terms of people you can depend on and financial resources. You'll also have to consider some questions that probably can't be answered yet: Will your child be able to live independently and work, and, if not, what will be the most important types of support? You're not going to know yet what your child will need and want as an adult, and the range of possibilities is large and complex, but facing your worries and beginning to make plans should make it easier in the long run.

Parent support groups can also be a big help. This is a conversation that will continue as your child grows and as you get a much clearer idea of where things are going; the information you've acquired and the connections you've made will be more valuable than ever.

Involve older quirky children or young adults in this process, ask them about their own plans and preferences, and let them know what options for adult living are available to them.

Having a quirky kid is an adventure, for you and for your whole family. No one can tell you exactly how it will evolve over time, but more is known now than 20 years ago, and more support is available to help you—and your family— along the way.

6

Educating the Quirky Child: Every Year Is Different

As pediatricians, we look at life at school and school performance as essential measures of whether our patients are able to manage in their worlds. A child who is physically healthy but seriously unhappy in school, academically troubled, struggling to get by, or actually failing is a child we worry about. We often ask parents to bring a child's report card along to the annual checkup because it contains a lot of information, not just in the grades but in the comments, about how a child is managing at school. It's a lot easier than trying to reach a teacher on the phone.

Making decisions about educating your child may present you with some of the most difficult hurdles you'll face as a parent. Making those decisions means tailoring children's every-day, all-day settings to help them function, adjust, and learn. We start from the assumption that a quirky child's experience in school has enormous potential to help him learn to use all his skills, but we also realize that both the academic and social aspects of school can be terribly hard on these kids. Decisions about the type of setting that is most appropriate can change over time, like everything else with regard to your child. Be prepared for the possibility that a good year might be followed by a miserable one. Here are some general thoughts on the process:

- *Take it slow and be open to change.* Don't let yourself be convinced that you have to make a permanent decision right at the beginning or that a "wrong" decision in kindergarten will have lifelong implications. All children grow and change, and quirky kids change in very unpredictable ways.
- *Be realistic and know her needs.* Educational planning works best when you are looking realistically at where your child is and what she needs right now. You can think about the longer-term future, of course, but don't set your

heart on any one school or program. Plan for the next year or two, stay alert as to how things are going, and be ready to reconsider.

- *Know your child and how to advocate for your child and know your school.* The more you know about how your child's mind works and about how the school year is going, the more likely you are to become aware of a problem early—and be able to address it. You will be a more effective advocate for your child if you understand the various roles of the people at the school, if you've taken a good look at the school's resources, and if you've figured out who makes key decisions.
- *A rough few months in school—or even a rough year—is not the end of the world.* Almost all kids, quirky or not, have a rough year or two somewhere along the way—a poor fit with a teacher, a difficult social situation, or just a period when the child's individual learning style and interests didn't fit well with what the school requires. Changing schools immediately or even assuming that all problems are the school's fault is not necessarily the correct response. A rough year can be a growth experience for a quirky child, or at least a valuable lesson in how to take certain setbacks in stride and keep on going.

There is no tried-and-true educational program that works for all quirky children, and most families don't have much choice about where their children will go to school; even so, you will come across parents and teachers with very strong feelings about what is right and what is wrong. Your job as a parent means taking into account individual learning styles; developmental, social, and interpersonal differences; and, in some cases, mental health issues. And even if you've found a good fit, you'll need to stay in close touch to make sure things keep working as your child grows and changes.

Some parents looking at schools will need to focus on academic programming, the style and structure of the classroom, the backgrounds and orientation of the teachers, the academic philosophy of the school, or the availability of special education resources. Others might feel that their children will do fine with any good standard academic program but have special concerns about social or athletic expectations or about the size or general atmosphere of the school. The group of children we're discussing here, after all, includes children with learning differences, children who shine in various academic areas, and children with a wide variety of behavioral and social issues—and all these may describe a single child! The parents' task, then, may be to take into account all these factors while being realistic about what is available, affordable, and practical in the family's real-life situation. We also want to acknowledge that working with schools is often more challenging for families of color, immigrant families, and non–English-speaking families. These children—especially Black and Latinx children—may be more likely to be viewed in school as misbehaving, when they are actually struggling. These parents may experience language and cultural barriers or feel intimidated or sidelined by school processes. We want to emphasize that schools are required to provide advocates and translators if these are requested, and there are community resources available to help families who need support navigating the school system.

Where to Start the Search

- Know the territory. Learn what you can about what's available to you in your school district. Go to whatever your community offers in the way of a school fair, collect information from the school district, and visit the schools that interest you most. Learn whether there is a collaborative with other school districts that serves different types of learners.
- Contact your school district's special education office and request an evaluation in writing, if one is necessary for your child.
- If you are considering private schools, you may have to collect information school by school, or there may be an independent-school fair or you may find yourself contacting a consultant.
- If your child is already in child care, preschool, or early intervention, talk with the teacher about your concerns and about elementary school recommendations. If your child is receiving therapy in early intervention or elsewhere, ask the therapist for ideas about schools that might work well for your child.
- Talk with other parents. You'll get useful information and may well discover options you hadn't heard about anywhere else. If you can find some parents who have quirky kids a few years older than your own, they will be a valuable resource.

Some of you will be looking at only one possible school—perhaps because it's the only one around—and trying to tailor an educational program for your child within that school. Others will consider a few schools, and some parents, especially in urban areas, may feel there are too many choices. Whatever your range of school choices, we want to help you think about a program that works for your child. Finding the right school is a hard job, but it's a job that has been done successfully by parents working under all kinds of constraints.

> **Brian went to a private progressive elementary school. He went to a school for special learning for seventh and eighth grade—a very small class size, a lot of social support, lots of tutoring, and the capacity to individualize curriculum beyond what a resource room would be able to do. Then he moved back into a regular private high school, and did fine.**

Gathering Information

Examine your own assumptions about how you want your child educated. You may be a staunch believer in public education—with fervent political and social convictions—only to find that there is no public school nearby that fits your child. Parents who believe devoutly in the advantages of private schools may come to the conclusion that this particular child would be better served in a public school, where certain services are legally mandated and where the teachers might have lots of experience with different learning styles and quirky kids. Or you may have cherished the hope that your fantasy child would thrive in parochial school but come to the conclusion that, for your real child, it would be a disaster. Obviously, your family's financial resources are a major factor here, and for many families, private school tuition is not a realistic possibility, but we do want to repeat that if the public schools are simply not meeting a child's needs, it is worth thinking about whether the public school system can be asked to pay for that child to go to a private school, which will provide the necessary supports.

Some families have used educational advocates who act as consultants and are knowledgeable about school options in the area. If you choose to go this route, interview a couple of potential advocates first to be sure you can work together and ascertain that they have worked with other children with similar needs.

> **We found a school for Abby after long consultations with an advocate and the school itself. The school identifies itself as one**

for mild-to-moderate learning disabilities. We spent 3 years there struggling because it turned out that the learning disability the school is most comfortable with is dyslexia, and Abby is not dyslexic. Her nonverbal learning issues affect every aspect of her being, and trying to learn in an environment that is devoted to something else has been too hard. For middle school, we are moving on to a school that, for right now, seems to understand her issues and embrace her anyway.

What Are the Options?

Whatever type of school you are considering, approach the school with a consumer's attitude: Are you offering what my child needs? Here are some questions to address as you look the school over:

- Does it provide specialists to help kids with learning differences or with physical therapy (PT), speech and language, or occupational therapy (OT) needs? Although all public schools will, in some form or other, many religious, charter, or nonspecialized private schools may not. Is there a resource room? A reading center? A counseling service? An on-site school nurse?
- Will your child require a behavioral analyst to help with behaviors that interfere with learning or social life at school? Find out if the school has dealt with these situations before, and if there is someone there who can work with you.
- If these resources and specialists are available, just how available are they? Full-time? Once a week?
- What do parents think about the skills and flexibility of the specialists? About their accessibility and availability to discuss children's progress?
- How successfully does the school cope with children who don't fit into neat categories—those who need special help in some areas but may have strong skills in others? You can describe your child's strengths and weaknesses and ask if they have children with similar profiles.
- Can the school foster a special interest or talent? Is the curriculum for math or music (or whatever your child's skill) adequate and engaging enough to keep your child on track?

Your Child's Social and Sensory Needs

In addition to your child's learning style and academic needs, you have to pay attention to what's going to happen outside the classroom. Because many quirky kids are of at least average intelligence, academic demands are often the least of their worries, especially in preschool and elementary school. Sometimes it can be the challenges of the playground, the gym, or the cafeteria that makes a given school a good possibility or an impossibility.

> John's experience in first grade was colored by the size of the school and the noise level. He found the cafeteria especially difficult because there were hundreds of kids. The noise level was very high, and he had trouble supporting himself on a cafeteria bench.

The following issues are of general concern to many quirky children:

- What is the size of the school and, therefore, of the crowds at recess or lunch? How many children are enrolled in the school? How many children are in a classroom? How does your child cope in a gymnasium or cafeteria with hundreds of kids and deafening noise levels?
- How about the playground at recess time? How closely are the children supervised? How much organized activity versus how much running around? Will that fit with your child's activity level, social skills, and attention span? Do the teachers seem to be aware of the social dynamics, and will someone reach out to a child if he is unhappy?
- What's the general noise level? Is there a public-address system with frequent, loud, and sudden interruptions?
- How big are the classrooms? How crowded? Are there enough classroom staff members to manage the needs of the kids or help negotiate conflict? Does the classroom seem organized, as if there is a system and the kids know what it is?
- How are the classrooms set up? Desks in rows? Small groups of tables pulled together? Is there a range of configurations? Are some kids in socks or slippers in a cozy reading corner with pillows?
- Is there a policy regarding teasing and bullying? If so, what exactly is it and how seriously is it adhered to? This can be a critical conversation for parents of quirky kids, because they are more frequently victims of bullying behavior.

Armed with your notebook, it's time to venture out and visit as many schools as you can.

> David's school, which is a small private school for children with special needs, does not have kids with behavior problems, which is good for David, who gets very distressed and anxious when kids are causing trouble. They have very clear and direct expectations about

what they do and how they do it, and David likes that. There's very little wiggle room. He attends a sensory motor group where he is learning about himself, his likes and dislikes. For example, he will now comment, "I don't like this kind of shirt. I don't like loud noises." And he will come up with strategies to help himself when he feels uncomfortable.

The Individualized Education Plan

If you know, or think, that your child needs some additional help—academic, social, attentional, or related to learning style—you have the legal right to request a full evaluation performed by the school and its team of experts, which will generate an individualized education plan (IEP). The following are some key points regarding that evaluation and plan:

- You can do this before your child starts school or at any point throughout the educational career.
- If your child hasn't yet started school and is older than 3 years, call the special education coordinator of your local school district and ask to begin the process.
- If your child is already in school, speak to the classroom teacher, the special education coordinator, and the principal about your concerns. Make a formal request in writing with a date on it; the school is legally obligated to complete the evaluation within a specified time frame.

An educational evaluation done through the public school system involves a number of specialists evaluating a child's achievement, potential, and areas of academic difficulty. The evaluation identifies problems, sets goals, and makes recommendations for services (ie, occupational, physical, or speech and language therapy, or time in the resource room for extra academic support in a given area). In some cases, for children with severe behavioral problems or serious academic weaknesses in several areas, the evaluation may lead to a recommendation that the child be in a special needs classroom, probably with a higher teacher-to-student ratio and various other modifications. If the process sounds intimidating, ask the school district to direct you to a parent advocate who can attend the IEP meeting with you. This may be especially helpful for non–English-speaking families, but anyone who feels uncertain about the process is entitled to this help. The IEP is a legal document. Parents are asked to review the plan and sign it to show agreement. Review the IEP carefully before you sign it, and ask for clarification if needed. The language itself can be difficult to understand and sometimes seems downright silly:

Student will be able to write a cohesive story 80% of the time. Student will be able to catch a ball 50% of the time.

For most families, the only IEP they ever see is their child's, and so at the outset, at least, they are reading it without a lot of experience and expertise. Before signing it, we recommend reviewing it several times, asking questions of the team, and perhaps going over it with your pediatric primary care provider or another specialist involved in your child's care. If you do not agree with the assessment or the recommendations, hold off on signing it and discuss this with the evaluators at your child's team meeting. These meetings are educational for most parents, and even if you disagree with some aspects of the school assessment, it's important to try and keep these meetings cooperative in tone and not let things become adversarial. It is in your child's best interest to have his parents and the school working together in a reasonably cordial way. Although you have rights under the special education laws of your state (and may need to lean on those rights), you also want to keep a positive working relationship with this team.

Creating a Program

Once an IEP has been developed and accepted, the team will offer a program aimed at helping your child meet the goals that are spelled out. We've already mentioned some of the possible options:

- A standard classroom with no additional supports (this isn't exactly an individual program; however, this is what typically happens to some of the more functional quirky kids because their academic work is on grade level and the school doesn't see any need for extra help)
- Inclusion in an integrated classroom mixing typically developing kids and kids with a variety of special needs or learning disabilities
- A separate classroom designed for kids with more challenging learning and/ or behavioral concerns

Within any of these types of classrooms, a child who needs special education services might receive that help in one of several ways:

- Services and therapy delivered in the classroom to small groups of children. This has the advantage, when it works well, of integrating the extra help with the other activity in the room.
- A "pullout," in which the child leaves the classroom to receive the services. This can provide a resource room teacher, for example, the opportunity to work intensively with one student or a small group in a setting designed to encourage concentration, which is important for many quirky kids.

- An increasingly popular option, albeit expensive from the school's point of view, is an aide in the classroom devoted to the child or children with additional learning needs. An aide can make or break a child's ability to function in a public school setting. This is a wonderful option for many quirky kids.

Though the IEP is a legal document, many parents find that putting its recommendations into effect can be challenging. In areas where school districts are enduring budget cuts, special education services are often the first things to go after art and music.

The team agreed that Sam needed intense speech and language intervention as well as help from the resource room teacher, but the aides had no additional time in their schedules to take on another child. So where did that leave us? He had done OK without it, so I know he was not a high priority for them, but I also know that he was slipping in his schoolwork and it wasn't going to get any better until he got the help he needed and deserved.

This mother's frustration echoed time and again throughout our interviews. Our experience in pediatric practice has been that it is often difficult to obtain the services a quirky child may need in overburdened school systems, especially if an evaluation determines that school achievement is adequate, which usually means on grade level.

The Individuals with Disabilities Education Act, usually referred to as IDEA, is a congressional act mandating that all states provide services for children with disabilities. All states must adhere to this law, although there can be tremendous variation in its interpretation. The standard is a Free Appropriate Public Education, which means that the school is required to provide just that—a free and appropriate education—but it does not necessarily mean the child is entitled to the best possible education that will foster the best possible outcome. Each state is also required, according to the same law, to offer a resource to parents to help them navigate the special education system. If you need an advocate to work with you, ask for one; this service is free of charge and should give you additional support.

There is nothing easy about accessing or implementing special education services, and it is a rare school year in which a quirky child will be on autopilot. Keeping track of your child's progress requires considerable energy and effort. Parents of middle schoolers and high schoolers have commented that once a child has multiple teachers—different teachers for different subjects—it is the parent's job to be sure all of them have read the evaluations and are aware of the necessary accommodations.

An IEP generally is in effect for 3 years, and then the child undergoes a complete reevaluation by all the specialists on the team; they determine how much progress the child has made toward reaching the goals that were set and whether there is still a need for the services described in the original plan. Less formal ongoing assessments and evaluations ought to take place as well, and you may request a reevaluation at any time. Some kids truly outgrow the need for certain kinds of help.

The summer John became interested in baseball, he played every day with the zeal he had previously reserved for schedules and clocks and calendars. He had had some significant motor issues and we'd been told that his visual perception was off, so we didn't have great hopes that his interest would go very far. In fact, I was kind of heartbroken for him. What could be harder for him than swinging a bat and trying to hit a ball, or catching a ball that could be coming from any direction at any speed? I was also exhausted from all the baseball playing he demanded of me! When we headed back to school and PT in the fall, his PT asked how he did it. He had improved dramatically in virtually all the areas she had been working on, and she couldn't believe it. She told him he had designed his own PT program and was doing a lot better with it than he would do with her. He beamed. That was a few years ago, but I'll never forget it, and not just because it was two appointments a week I could cross off my calendar.

Public Schools

The vast majority of quirky kids are served quite well by the public school system. Some communities have special education services at all of their schools, some have them only at a select few, and some have none at all. In the last case, children who need those services are usually educated in a neighboring community at the home school system's expense or in a collaborative school shared by several communities. Virtually *all* quirky kids spend at least part of their school years in a public school setting, and it's probably a good place to start.

Chrissie started kindergarten in a public school program that worked well for her. She had a great teacher, and she made friends.

> In fact, I wanted her to repeat the year, but she couldn't because
> she was at the age to move on. I think this is a downside of a public
> school system; they insisted on moving Chrissie through the grades.
> She is smart, but she's also very immature. Now she's in the fifth
> grade, and she has an aide in the classroom whom she shares with a
> couple of other kids.

Because public schools must cope with a wide variety of kids, they often have good resources and generally a more inclusive attitude. Almost all public schools have some staff members trained in special education. There are reading specialists, speech and language therapists, counselors, and psychologists. Many schools have access to a psychologist specifically versed in the issues of the quirky-kid population. Virtually all public schools have a nurse on staff at least part of the day—a distinct advantage for children with medical concerns such as seizures or complicated medication regimens. Keeping this in mind, you should look for someone within the school system—teacher, counselor, nurse, special education coordinator—who seems to understand your child and with whom you can connect. Many families do better if they find that one crucial ally who can keep an eye on things within the school.

Many families also find that the public school experience is valuable for their quirky children for other reasons. They get to know the other kids in the neighborhood, and they go to school with what may be a more economically and ethnically diverse group of children than they would find in private school. In general, the public school experience may be closer to the real world; a quirky kid who can thrive, or survive reasonably intact, is well prepared to take on the challenges of adulthood.

Sometimes families move to particular communities specifically because their public school systems are better equipped to handle quirky kids with their many potential educational and social concerns. Although this is a major undertaking and a big life decision with implications for the whole family, the fact is that many families *without* quirky kids do exactly the same thing for the same reasons: They look for communities with schools that will be good places for their children. As long as you keep in mind that what's the best course of action now may not always be the best, and as long as your other children are faring well, this is sometimes the best possible decision a family can make.

> We looked around a lot, investigated various communities, talked
> with parents we knew through EI and speech therapy groups, and
> decided we needed to move. We moved to a community known for

its great schools (for typical kids, of course) that had wonderful special education services. We are lucky to have been able to do it. Our daughter is thriving, we are more relaxed and more available to each other and to our kids, and our other two children seem to have weathered the move reasonably well.

Alternative Public Schools

Charter schools, pilot schools, alternative education programs—communities are increasingly offering publicly funded but more progressive or nontraditional schools and programs. Because they tend to be founded and directed by idealists and visionaries who aspire to education outside the box, they may look appealing as possible places for the child who is clearly outside all the usual boxes. Be careful about assuming that a quirky child and a quirky school will automatically be a good match. The occasional good match is possible: the music-oriented charter school and the intensely musical quirky child, the small alternative progressive program and the child who can't face the bustle of the regular big elementary school. But the fact is that most quirky kids require and are comforted by a lot of structure and very clear expectations, which isn't always the case in alternative settings.

By all means, check out the nontraditional public school offerings in your area, but keep in mind that most quirky kids need a certain amount of stability and do well with more experienced teachers and specialists.

Private or Independent Schools

Sending a child to private school may be a major financial commitment for some families, an expected and planned-for expense for others, or an impossibility for many.

When looking at private schools, you face certain important considerations. Private schools are under no legal obligation to provide any special education services, and the vast majority do not. They are not required to do pullouts or provide an aide in the classroom, and they receive no funding from the state to do so. Therefore, for the more needy or impaired children with autism spectrum disorder, a typical independent school is not likely to be a great match.

Many private schools do not want to admit kids with special needs. And, for the most part, if the school doesn't want someone with your child's issues, then you and your child probably don't want that school. You can apply without specifying the issues, but if the school offers you a place, it may be unable to meet the needs of your child. Before applying to private school, you must carefully consider how you feel about disclosing your child's particular issues to the school.

Certainly, there are parents who apply to private school without mentioning, for example, that their child receives speech therapy or is prone to extreme tantrums. You dress the child in his casual best, take him to the interview, and hope that he enunciates clearly and refrains from attacking any of the other children.

We're not saying you have to tell the school everything. Small problems that seem to have resolved or behavioral eccentricities that don't prevent your child from functioning in a preschool class may not be relevant. However, it makes no sense to pursue admission knowing that your child will need a lot of speech and language help but then keep it from the school; you really can't get upset when it turns out the school doesn't have the relevant specialists at hand. If your child's behavior is so explosive that he's already on his third medication and his second anger-management group, it's not fair to the school to give the staff no hint of what they're taking on. Getting your child into private school can feel like a high-pressure and somewhat unpleasant game. Certain parents are determined to win at all costs, but the real object of the game is to find a good place for your child to learn and grow.

> **We applied to a number of private schools for our son for first grade. By then, we were pretty sure he could no longer survive in our public schools. We decided to be completely honest about his "stuff," hoping that one of the schools we liked would work out for him. One school did work out, and he has done wonderfully there. Of the ones that didn't, I most remember the admissions director who said, "This is not a good place for your son. He will not do well here." She was so clear, so honest, so direct—in very sharp contrast to the others who kept beating around the bush—and we were so grateful to her. It was painful to hear but so much easier to deal with, and it has become much less painful as time has passed. I remember her with a lot of respect and admiration.**

Some families we know have developed programs for their kids that include a private school education with extra supports outside of school and school hours. Some have even put in place an aide for the classroom (at the parents' expense). One mom commented that this worked well for her son and minimized the attention to his differences.

> Once we got an aide in the classroom for George, he seemed to settle down, he was less anxious, and he was able to learn better. He needs her pretty close by most of the time, but she floats about the room and helps other kids occasionally as well. This has been a great help to him, and to his teacher, and has enabled him to stay put in a school where he feels comfortable and where his brother goes. The only downside is the expense.

Some parents prefer to separate school and supplementary therapies. Sensitive about how other kids see them, many children prefer to keep their therapies outside of the school experience. Of course, such a program is highly dependent on parental resources, knowledge, initiative, time, and money. Someone has to assess the child's needs, find the specialists, put together the program, pay the bills, and bring the child to the appointments.

Parochial Schools

Parochial schools offer specific benefits that may make them absolutely terrific for some quirky kids—and out of the question for others. Most are fairly traditional in their approaches to teaching and learning, demanding that students wear uniforms in many cases (which quirky kids and their parents often like, as long as there are not too many belts, buckles, or snaps!), expecting even young children to sit still in class and pay attention, and requiring good behavior and a high degree of respect for the teacher, who may be a figure of some religious significance. Disturbing behavior in class is not tolerated, and punishments tend to be fairly traditional. These schools pride themselves on being academically rigorous and may assign a good amount of homework from the early grades on. Most require some course of religious studies in addition to the regular curriculum, which may involve something as extensive as learning another language from a young age (eg, Hebrew at a yeshiva, Arabic at an Islamic academy). This may add hours onto both the school day and the homework evening. It is worthwhile to think about the homework load for any school, and we discuss this in more detail later in the chapter.

The quirky children who do best in these schools are those who thrive on routine, who need a structured environment with clear rules and an emphasis on discipline and order. Some quirky kids find the whole business of clothes and the social pressure of knowing what's cool to wear difficult, and for them, uniforms are a real blessing (no pun intended). Some anxious children are troubled by any alteration in the daily routine. Parochial schools have for years offered parents a high degree of tradition, discipline, and order, combined with firm academic standards and, of course, a certain amount of ritual. These schools may be a real haven for the quirky child who responds well to clearly stated expectations and whose anxieties are allayed by the hierarchy of parochial school and even by the religious and social certainties on which the school and its curriculum are based.

Like private schools, most parochial schools have few resources for students who need extra help. A parochial school is definitely not the place for the quirky kid who cannot sit still or who needs individualized teaching. Classes tend to be large, and the expectation is that children sit still and behave or face the consequences. Choosing a parochial school should be based on the belief that it can meet your child's needs. If it does, the added comfort for you and your child of being in a familiar social group with familiar rituals will be a bonus. Some quirky kids take a special interest in their religious beliefs and history, and they want their families to move toward stricter religious observance. Can you imagine the positive attention they receive from the rabbi or the nun or the imam?

Schools for Children With Special Needs

An increasing number of schools—usually private but sometimes publicly funded—are specifically intended for children who are not succeeding in more standard settings. It is definitely worth knowing about these schools and keeping them in mind as possibilities for your child at one point or another.

Our experience suggests that parents often look to a specialized school for the slightly older child, and sometimes these specialized schools can be lifesavers. Sometimes the diagnoses and the learning issues have become clearer as the child grows up, or sometimes the later elementary and middle school years can be terribly hard on quirky children. Most such schools have academic curricula geared toward the learning profiles of quirky kids, with extra therapeutic services such as sensory integration, OT, social skills or pragmatic language therapy, treatment by social workers or other mental health professionals, and, in some cases, behavioral programs geared toward addressing undesirable behaviors (eg, aggression, self-harm such as picking or pulling at one's hair). A specialized school should do more than address your child's immediate learning needs; it should help you tease out important questions about the future and your child's potential for further education, work, and an independent adulthood. Vocational training and off-site job placements for those who are not college bound are important for older children struggling with special learning problems, social issues, and emotional complexities of the adolescent years from the quirky side of the aisle.

We talked with staff members at a number of such schools, including the admissions director of one school geared toward quirky kids who were not succeeding in their previous school placements and who in some cases had exhausted a number of less-tailored programs.

> When a family first contacts us about admission, we do a very detailed review of the child's educational and developmental history to be sure that our school would be an appropriate place and that they truly cannot find a less restrictive or less expensive alternative. Our goal is to work with a child and his family over a relatively short period of time so that he can return to a more typical educational environment. Most kids who come to us come at the middle school level, and many are able to leave for high school. The ones who do not are the ones who are unlikely to live an independent life, and we work with them to find job placements in the community, teach them daily living skills they will need to live in a group home, and prepare them for young adulthood. The admissions process is not usually a happy one for the families, because they have had to convince their local school department that it cannot meet the needs of their child. The cost here is so expensive that few school departments will easily accept that assessment without a fight. Families use mediators, advocates, lawyers to help them, and it can leave a lot of bad feelings all around.

Some specialized schools offer boarding as an option at the middle or high school level. This is a personal decision for most families and probably an easier one if others in the family have attended boarding school. In some cases, parents and siblings may need respite from the ongoing demands and emotional drain of caring for a child with complicated needs. A boarding school with appropriate staffing and supervision may meet the needs of the family while offering the quirky child a chance for independence and a new environment.

Therapeutic Schools

A child's depression or anxiety, obsessiveness or psychotic tendencies, antisocial tendencies or outbursts can make education—not to mention a social life—nearly impossible. A therapeutic school offers an environment of acceptance and a highly trained staff that works closely with the kids to address their psychiatric needs. Treatment usually includes individual and group psychotherapy, and schools are highly structured with clear expectations. The majority of therapeutic schools are boarding schools, and there are not many. They are tremendously expensive, and, unless you can convince your local school district to foot the bill on the grounds that the district itself cannot meet the needs of your child, most families simply cannot afford these schools.

Homeschooling

Homeschooling is clearly not for everyone. However, some kids at certain points in their lives thrive when social demands are kept to a minimum and they are free to concentrate on their academic progress—usually in anticipation of attending school at a later date. Some parents choose to homeschool their children *because* of the quirks. They may feel that none of the school options available to them meets their children's needs.

Homeschooling is a huge undertaking for any family. Regulations exist regarding homeschooling, and you need to be sure you meet your state requirements. Homeschooling or any approximation thereof requires a parent with the time, talent, and inclination to carry it out. You will find networks of parents in every state and often organized approaches to providing extracurricular activities and enrichment for homeschooled children. Even then, it may only be the right answer for a specific segment of your child's educational life. As pediatricians and as mothers who doubt seriously that we would have the talent or dedication to our own children, we do want to honor the dedicated parents who have made it work and emphasize that this is an option worth considering for certain parents—but it's an option that requires far more extensive guidance, tailored to your state, your child's age, and your child's needs, than we can provide here.

Making the Choice

So what are you doing as you look around for a first educational placement for your quirky child?

- If you are working with an early intervention program, speak to the public school liaison who can help identify programs in your district that may be a great fit.
- Write a letter to the local school department requesting an evaluation, preferably prior to your child's third birthday, when he is no longer eligible for early intervention services.
- If it's an option for you, check out some private schools and plan realistic strategies for what you're going to say about your child as you apply.
- Think about whether you're interested in parochial schools or homeschooling.

- Most important, talk with the people you feel have the best sense of your child's learning style: the preschool teachers, for example, and the speech and language therapist. By all means, talk it over with your pediatrician. We hear a great deal, good and bad, about families' experiences in the various schools available in the communities in which we work.

Sometimes a child's quirkiness doesn't become an issue until school problems arise. This scenario is more likely with children whose quirks are on the milder side, who make it through the early years at home but stumble when the academic and social demands of the elementary years hit. We've cared for a number of kids who weren't evaluated and/or diagnosed until fifth or sixth grade. As their pediatricians, we saw them year after year without suspecting that anything was up. When we talk this over with parents, they almost always say that they had worried, at least on and off, that something was amiss, but usually it was some worry so vague, so uncertain, so hard to explain that they never brought it up with us at annual checkups. After all, who brings up social awkwardness when a doctor asks if you have any worries about your child?

So it's not uncommon that children may reach the later elementary years without an evaluation of some kind, even though their parents have worried about them intermittently. For some, things may be going pretty well in general, but some recurring behavior seems, as one mother put it, "off the beam." Because some quirky kids are so bright or have a splinter skill that actually puts them ahead of the pack, their eccentricities may be viewed as charming or delightful, and there may be triumphs and pleasures that balance out their parents' worries about school function.

> John could tell time when he was 3 years old. We knew this was remarkable and were happy that he had an outstanding skill. One of his teachers, however, made such a fuss about how great it was that we felt she was missing all these other major red flags. It's one thing to be able to tell time, but it's quite another to have that ability take up so much of your time and attention. It got in the way of his doing other things he should have been doing at that age, and he used that skill to comfort himself and keep himself organized and in control. He continues, many years later, to be interested in timetables and schedules, but it doesn't take up so much of his energy.

In the elementary school years, most teachers are adept at noticing which kids in the class aren't keeping up academically and which ones may need a different teaching style. A good and experienced teacher will also easily pick up which of her students are socially isolated and anxious and which have peculiar habits or behaviors that make the others uncomfortable. Trust your child's teacher if she suggests taking a closer look at your child's differences, especially if her concerns make sense to you. A good and perceptive teacher, of course, can make a tremendous difference in a child's life—or even in a family's life.

> Brian was in the school where I was teaching, and third grade was a disaster from the first day. He hid in the corner, or in the bathroom. Within a week and a half, his teacher and some of the other teachers sat me down and said, "He needs to be evaluated. Something is not going right for him. You need to do something about this." And right then, I went on a mission.

On the other hand, when a teacher misinterprets a quirky child's behavior, the result can be a rough school year for all concerned.

> We started Caitlin at a small private school in kindergarten, thinking she would get more individual attention. She certainly did, but not the kind of attention we were looking for. She was just too different, too eccentric, too rigid to survive in that setting. The teacher called almost every week with complaints about Caitlin's "insubordination." When I asked for an example, she told me that when they were learning the letter "K," Caitlin turned her paper over and wrote the entire alphabet multiple times, omitting the letter K. I think this was her way of saying, "I can already do this. I'm bored. I'll show you!" She did not fit the profile of the compliant kindergarten girl, and her teacher wasn't equipped to recognize her behavior as anything but defiance. The director of the school called us and said she was not welcome back unless she had an aide in the classroom, for whom we would need to pay. We left the school at the end of the year.

The school-based evaluation is a good place to start for most families. Sometimes it's the expertise that is needed, both to determine your child's needs and then to meet them. It's the same process we discussed previously, in which a team evaluation yields an IEP, which the school is then obligated to fulfill. In good school systems around the country, with plenty of resources, schools are able to meet the IEP expectations and provide the supports kids need, and there's no need to switch the kid from school to school. Unfortunately, it doesn't always work that way.

Children in alternative schools such as charter schools, pilot schools, or private elementary schools face a different set of circumstances, which are usually more difficult logistically and emotionally. A school without the necessary resources is more likely to view a quirky child as a behavioral problem. If that is what you're hearing from school staff—especially if it's a relatively sudden change—it's worth considering what kind of evaluation might help tease out the problem, especially if you've had some concerns about your child's learning style or development. If it turns out that your child needs support and special education services, you have to think about whether it makes sense to stay in that school, even though it may have qualities you love. Sometimes it's just not worth the energy to put up a fight for services in a school that doesn't already have them in place.

Although this law is under some protest in certain states, your child is eligible to receive special education services through your local system even if he is not enrolled in the system. You may have found a terrific private school for your child that doesn't provide the OT he needs for fine motor skills or sensory processing disorder. At this point, you are entitled to request an evaluation from your local public school, and the school is required to do the evaluation and provide services if they are indicated. You may get some dirty looks, but you are within your legal rights. Most school professionals understand that families choose a variety of ways to educate their kids and that parents usually know best.

> Our son needed OT for many reasons, but his fine motor skills were probably his greatest area of difficulty. For several years, we have gone to our neighborhood elementary school in the early morning or the late afternoon for his OT sessions. This has worked well for him. He likes the fact that he does it outside of his own school, and they have a very nice relationship. His OT understands that his overall needs are better served in this way.

As you explore different options for your child and work to reconcile the impressions of the classroom teacher with the testing done by specialists, don't lose sight of the big picture. The point of all of this is to respond to concerns about your child and how she is doing in school. Your goal is to provide her with a world that supports her growth and learning and welcomes her every day into a place where she fits in.

Let's think about how children make their way through school, and the various ways in which a quirky child presents different challenges. The preschool years carry expectations for play and social skills as well as developing language, while the elementary years are when kids learn to read and read to learn, along with many other things. The middle school years can be particularly difficult for quirky kids, as the social demands of older kids become ever more complicated and often unspoken. And high school is often a time of reckoning with what adult life is likely to be like. Each stage has its own set of issues for both the children and the families who support them.

When we called this chapter, "Educating the Quirky Child: Every Year Is Different," to be honest, we had not imagined the 2019–2020 school year, the coronavirus pandemic, and the resultant school closures. In these chapters, we discuss school as an in-classroom experience with all students, teachers, and support staff able to interact in person. We want to acknowledge that the shutdown and remote learning has placed significant burdens on families of children with special needs and that many carefully arranged education plans were disrupted. Parents were valiant, and many kids managed to hold on to their progress, but many others have experienced the loss of their services or just burned out on the virtual learning and therapies. There have been some important lessons learned about how to manage learning and therapies remotely. We hope that by the time you are reading this, kids and teachers are back in school and there is a safe and effective vaccine (we do love vaccines).

7

Moving Through the School Years: Thriving and Learning in the Educational System

Your child is growing and learning and changing in school—that's why you've gone to so much effort to find a good fit. But as your child changes, you may need to revisit some of your decisions. Many of the families we have worked with realize over time that what worked well for a few years doesn't work well anymore. The wonderful school district that served your child so well in elementary school may become an unfriendly place in seventh grade. Or a specialized high school may start up near you and provide a great match for your musically or math-and-science inclined child. Take it as it comes, and ride the waves, and continue on your mission to find the best options available for every stage of development. In this chapter we take you from the preschool years through high school.

The Preschool Years

Many of the issues we may worry about in quirky kids are hard to test for in the very young. Learning issues and attentional problems may emerge as a child tries to cope with the demands of school. But parents who see clearly that something is different or challenging in a preschool-aged child may find themselves trying to determine the best educational setting for their child without having a clear statement of the problem or an "official" diagnosis. For those who have not been in early intervention (EI) programs, a regular preschool or playgroup in the neighborhood is likely to be the first school experience. As parents see their child in this context, new concerns may arise, and differences in development may become more apparent. Young children in a home-based child care setting may fly under the radar of concern, especially if the staff, however loving and dedicated, lack training in child behavior or development.

> We didn't know at the time what our son's problem was, but we knew that he was developing slowly and didn't eat enough to gain weight. He attended a small family child care program with a total of six kids when he was 1 year old. The child care provider, who had been revered by several of our friends for the care she gave to their children, clearly had no clue what to do with our son. She probably had never encountered a child like him. She insisted he was just fine, she didn't notice anything at all different, yet he never spoke a word and did not interact with the other kids. We believe she was just uncomfortable talking with us about his development and thought it would all come out in the wash. It made us slightly crazy.

While some teachers and child care providers are unable—or unwilling—to talk with parents when a child's behavior seems somehow problematic, others can be too ready to jump to a diagnosis on the basis of a few pieces of evidence. Both approaches can leave parents bewildered and sometimes resentful. Considering and comparing the impressions that these teachers form of your child is often the beginning of a long process of obtaining the kind of support that *will* be helpful.

> Charlie attended a pleasant private preschool in the neighborhood that did not offer any services, but the director was very open to welcoming his occupational therapist, who came in for occasional visits to observe and offer some advice to the staff. Charlie received his therapy at the local elementary school, which did not have a program for him because he wasn't "impaired enough." This system has worked OK for us, but it isn't ideal, and I hope we haven't lost precious time. Only time will tell.

Early Intervention

For children younger than 3 years, EI programs, federally funded programs available in all states, provide evaluation and therapy, usually in the home but sometimes in a center, in which developmental delays are addressed through games, songs, toys, and other activities. As we learn more about atypical development, children are being referred for evaluation by parents, early educators, and primary care providers and enrolled in EI programs at earlier ages. What used to be largely groups of children with neurological impairments resulting from preterm birth are now more eclectic groups of toddlers and preschoolers with a wide range of developmental differences and medical histories. Growing evidence, both scientific and anecdotal, shows that early intervention can make a difference in long-term outcomes, including in children with autism spectrum disorder.

Developmental Skills

For parents with children whose development is not precisely on schedule, there are all kinds of questions regarding the skills needed to participate in a typical preschool day. Because of speech and language delays, some 3- and 4-year-olds speak much less than other children their age, or sometimes not at all. Nonverbal children usually need a preschool setting with small groups and a high teacher-to-child ratio. They often do well in a program that incorporates a Picture Exchange Communication System, which involves the use of small cards with simple diagrams of items such as a pencil, a glass of milk, or a bathroom. Nonverbal children can use diagrams to communicate their wishes. We have seen remarkable amounts of communication with these cards, and that can often be a starting point for eliciting speech.

Think about the skills needed for your child to get through a preschool day:

- How is his receptive language–his ability to understand? It may well be better than his expressive language—the ability to speak.
- Can she carry on a conversation? (This is not the same as being able to talk.) Does she understand conversational turn-taking?
- How about gross and fine motor skills? Is climbing stairs an issue? How about putting on a winter coat? Can he sit in a regular chair? Can she hold a pencil, crayon, or marker, and can she write?
- Where does your child stand regarding potty training? Still in diapers, able to manage the potty with help, or fully independent using the toilet?
- Is he able to interact and play with other preschoolers?
- Can she follow directions?
- Does he have any splinter skills, such as a notably early ability to read (hyperlexia) or remarkable abilities in math or music?

Language-Based Programs

If your child has difficulty understanding spoken language or following directions, or she needs to hear things more than once or in several different ways, consider a *language-based* preschool program. Many such children benefit from this approach in preschool and beyond. Although not all teachers or schools use this term, look for cues when you visit a class: posted schedules so kids know what to expect as the day goes on; directions for a project explained in several ways; use of pictures or written words as well as spoken words to get a point across. Ask if a speech and language therapist is part of the team. This style of teaching and explaining comes naturally to many early childhood teachers but certainly not all. This kind of flexibility is helpful for many young children, especially the quirky ones.

The Right Classroom, the Right Teacher

Although it is virtually impossible to find the perfect teacher, the ideal speech and language pathologist, and the optimal occupational and physical therapists all in one place, it's worth looking at all your options and aiming for the best balance. The classroom teacher is the most critical. Put your energy into finding a teacher for the early years who will understand your whole child, not just her deficits. Early childhood teachers with special education training are often best equipped to do this, but many seasoned preschool teachers have a lot of experience with quirky children. What you want is a preschool teacher who appreciates your child in all her complexity. A teacher with a sense of humor, who delights in the child's quirkiness and makes accommodations for her differences without drawing too much attention to them, is a valuable guide on your child's journey through school.

For us, the decision about where Gabriel should go to preschool was pretty straightforward. We knew he needed every kind of service he could get, and there were only a couple of possibilities. The early intervention liaison was a great help, and we trusted her recommendation. Gabriel spent 3 really good years in an "integrated preschool" in a public school in the neighborhood. Half of the 14 kids in the class had some kind of special need. He got all his therapy in one place and had amazing teachers who were "on" to him. We learned a lot from them and still remember them with love and admiration for the work they do. It made a huge difference for Gabriel that he got off to such a great start in school.

Checking Out a Class

With the proper support in the preschool years, both preschoolers and their parents can develop strategies for school success, focus therapies on important skills at a time when there are no overwhelming academic or social pressures, and anticipate the coming years with their eyes open. This is the period to put as many supports in place as possible, helping your child make the transition to school as smoothly as you can. If, later on, it turns out that some of that help is no longer needed, more power to you, more power to the teachers, and more power to your child. It will mean that all the time you put into finding the right program made a difference, and all the supplementary therapies you pursued did what they were supposed to do: They helped shape her development and her school functioning so that life and school and learning could get easier, not harder, as she grew older.

> When Trevor started kindergarten, he spent half his time in a special education kindergarten and half in the regular education room. Gradually, over the course of the year, he spent more and more time with the typical kindergartners and eventually "graduated" into the regular class completely. He is currently in the third grade in a regular education class, with virtually no special education services. He is extremely bright in math and in an honors algebra class with kids from another school. He would be in an honors geometry class if his fine motor skills were not so poor.

The Elementary Years

Many experts believe the elementary years are the quirky kid's most important years. Elementary school is your golden opportunity to lay the groundwork for those future years. After all, as children grow up, parents have less control than they may want—over the school, over the peer group, and even over their child. It's usually easier to teach social skills to a 7-year-old, and help her practice, than it is to a seventh grader. Seize your moment when you can. All too soon, we all find ourselves standing around with the peculiar helplessness of parents of adolescents, wondering whether anything we say will ever again have any effect.

As quirky children age into the complexities of middle school and high school, the more coping skills and strategies they have acquired, the better off they will be. Approach the elementary school years not as a free-play zone before the serious work starts but rather as an opportunity to help your quirky kid learn how to learn, play to his strengths, and get along with other kids as well as with teachers and principals.

> When Lisa went into kindergarten, I was terribly worried about her, about how she would do socially with the other children, about what was going on at school. And she wouldn't tell me. She would

just burst into tears. The school helped me a lot with staff members' observations that she reacted in strange ways to different situations, that she couldn't seem to sit in a chair. She said the kids were yelling in her ears. She's easily distracted, and it's hard to sit her down and keep her on task. But on her last report card, the teacher said that she was making good progress, even though she still needed help with being organized.

What Kids Learn in Elementary School

We expect kids to learn to read, carry on a conversation, tell a story that makes sense, use language—both written and spoken—to expand their world, and work and play with their peers. We expect them to learn the basics of mathematics. We expect them to learn to write and draw using a variety of implements. We want them to be able to follow directions, take turns, and understand the rules of community behavior: raising hands, taking turns, not interrupting. We expect older elementary school children in fifth or sixth grade to be able to comprehend a variety of literary genres (not just science fiction or baseball stories) and write about them. We want them to be able to sit and eat lunch with a group of peers without grossing them out! Perhaps most of all, we want our children to make friends, have a social life, enjoy themselves on the playground, know how to play, and feel like part of the group. These are tall orders, and any one of these developmental or cognitive tasks can present a challenge for your child. Knowing which ones are most likely to be stumbling blocks can help determine the elementary school program most likely to work for your child.

George did OK in the early grades because he was a good reader. So much of the first couple of years is just getting kids to read and he coasted through. But once he hit fourth grade and needed to read literature, it was a disaster.

Typically, it is during the elementary school years that a child's difficulties declare themselves as real or not and as mild, more intense, or downright severe. Many families have needed to move their child from one setting to another as the situation became clearer.

John was assigned to a first-grade class in an integrated program, and we were thrilled. He would get all his therapies during the school day, and the teacher was certified in special education. It turned out to be a disaster. Despite her training, his teacher was very rigid and a screamer. This terrified him, and the sheer volume was overwhelming because of his sensory defensiveness. One day I went to pick him up and he was in "time-out" because he kept rocking his chair back and forth. When I spoke to the after-school-teacher, she said she just knew he was doing it to bug her. In fact, the chair had one short leg, and he couldn't keep it steady. His anxiety grew as the year progressed, and we finally brought him to a psychiatrist, who diagnosed him and said, "He's in the wrong school." That was just the catalyst we needed to get going. He ended up in a small, cozy private school with loving teachers who made allowances for his quirks yet fostered his education. The irony is that, on paper, that first program would clearly have been the right one, yet in reality, it wasn't. We learned a big lesson that year.

Learning Styles

Kids understand early on that they are in school to learn and that all around them other kids are learning. Children generally know where they stand with regard to their classmates and whether they are struggling with tasks that come more easily to everyone else or, conversely, when things are easy for them that are difficult for other kids.

If a child cannot learn, school becomes a repetitive exercise in failure. This, in turn, can get in the way of making friends, lead to all kinds of tactics to avoid school, or create serious anxiety or depression. Of course, learning disabilities and learning differences are in no way the same as intelligence. Many kids with major learning disabilities are extraordinarily bright. Ironically, their intelligence may make things harder for them, or at least more obscure, because these bright kids can compensate much longer in school, using their brains and the skills that come more easily to them to cover for the problems they can't solve.

We had always had some concerns about Debbie, but she did well in school so we didn't go looking for trouble. By high school, her grades slipped, and she was completely exhausted all the time. We thought she was depressed, and she was, but that wasn't the primary problem. The psychiatrist we took her to referred her for a neuropsychology evaluation, and it turns out she has a major learning disability. We were stunned at first but then realized that so many of her behaviors over the years made sense in this light. She

**is very bright and compensated with great effort for a long time,
until the volume and complexity of the work meant the strategies
she had developed weren't working anymore.**

Many quirky kids have learning issues that fall under the general category of
nonverbal learning disability (NVLD). For a description, refer to Chapter 2. But
any learning issues can turn up in quirky kids, from language-based learning
disabilities to executive function problems, to dyslexia—and these can also
coexist with NVLD. Because a child with NVLD has impairments in many
aspects of daily functioning, be sure the school you are considering understands what this means. Nonverbal learning disability is the most common
learning profile among quirky kids, although it is certainly possible to be
quirky without having NVLD or to have NVLD without another diagnosis.

The School Systems

Some experts argue that many children would do best in schools designed
entirely with quirky kids in mind, and there are a few around the country that
you might want to read about. You can find them, and find out about them,
through parent support groups or on the internet. However, these schools are
not an option for the vast majority of families with elementary-age kids; they
will attend regular schools of one kind or another, sometimes in special classes
or with special help.

Mainstreaming Versus Separate Classrooms

The most recent wave of special education laws has moved kids with atypical development into the mainstream. This concept that typical kids and
not-so-typical kids are best served together whenever possible is well known
to most parents. Plenty of controversy surrounds this idea, but at this moment
in educational history, this is where most quirky kids start. And indeed, with
resources and extra help, more mildly affected quirky kids can function in a
regular classroom.

Children can be mainstreamed in private or parochial schools, too, of course if
they can manage with the regular school program or if the staff is willing and
able to make some adjustments.

For some quirky kids, the ability to stay in a mainstream elementary school
classroom depends on having a dedicated classroom aide. If this is a possibility,
you should certainly consider it before moving your child to a different type
of classroom or an outside placement. Teachers are grateful for the extra help,
and kids can make great progress.

> Chrissie has an aide in her class whom she shares with two other kids, and this works well. The aide helps the kids interpret instructions they don't understand and helps to keep them on task. Chrissie has learned a lot more since the aide started and generally feels more successful at school.

Children with more significant delays, or whose behaviors interfere with learning, may need a substantially separate classroom. These children may require support pertaining to their language and communication, as well as their behavior in order to learn. If you believe your child might do better in a separate classroom, talk with the special education team about it. Speak with professionals who know your child best, such as the developmental pediatrician, occupational therapist, or psychologist to see if they agree with you. Sometimes a recommendation may come out of the IEP process, or it might be the parents or developmental pediatricians who feel that a child is not making adequate educational progress and will push for a separate classroom placement. These classes tend to be smaller, with a higher staff-to-student ratio, and with more attention directed toward individual learning styles.

> We found a "class within a class" for children with special needs right in our neighborhood. It was Jacob's OT who suggested it for him, and he has made a lot of progress. I don't know if I would have found it without her, and it is definitely the right place. I am doing a lot less traveling around to get him what he needs.

Gifted and Talented Children

The quirky kids with mathematical or musical ability and those with high intelligence may be well served in schools for gifted and talented kids, where there is a real premium on intellectual ability and less emphasis on social skills or sports. To a quirky child who's good at math, it can be a real joy to find herself in a place where math is the only thing that really counts (pun intended). There is less need to worry about your child's quirks in this environment because these places are full of quirky people. Your child is more likely to find friends with the same or similar interests—be it military history or Dungeons & Dragons—in a school for the gifted and talented.

The Middle School Years

For many of us, the journey from sixth to ninth grade doesn't take us through the happiest or easiest years of our lives. The goal for many kids in middle school, typical or quirky, is to make it to high school and get through puberty relatively unscathed. Anything more is gravy. Most kids have at least some difficulties with the educational, emotional, and physical transitions occurring at this time, as their bodies leap forward into the changes of puberty or lag behind their classmates', and as they contend with the personal, family, and peer-group implications of becoming teenagers.

Autism Spectrum Disorder and Middle School

This is by far the hardest developmental stage for most kids with autism spectrum disorder. Even as young children, they often feel uncomfortable in their own skin. As 5-, 6-, and 7-year-olds, these kids were more awkward, more uncomfortable, more wary, and more likely to be upset, injured, or frightened by the imperatives of their bodies, perhaps disturbed by sensory input that didn't bother other children. Throw in the physical changes of puberty and adolescence, the dazzling and confusing world of flirting and dating, and many quirky kids are overwhelmed. The social demands at this time tax exactly the areas these kids find difficult, if not impossible, asking that they navigate a complex and changeable—and often judgmental—social network, while adjusting to their own developing bodies and hormonally mediated mood changes. Most quirky kids lag behind their age group in terms of development and social maturity, making this time even more confusing. At the same time, increasing academic demands require an ability to integrate information that simply confounds many quirky kids. Gone are the days of straightforward math problems with a single answer.

If quirky kids ever need a specialized or separate school environment, even for a year or two, this is the most likely time. The middle school programs specifically designed with quirky kids in mind are generally set up with an explicit plan to reintroduce them to more standard school settings by high school, when their quirkiness is more likely to be accepted or even seen as a strength. Some sensible school districts devote most of their special education funds to the middle schoolers, because the payoff is the greatest when these kids can stay in their own communities and rejoin their classmates for high school. You should anticipate the middle school years, know your options, and visit a few places with your child's specific needs in mind.

Academic Issues and Middle School

For kids who had an individualized education plan (IEP) in place during elementary school, this transition is smoother, because the educational machinery should be updating the plan automatically, assessing your child's progress, and considering new options. For those kids without an IEP but who seem to have some learning issues emerging, the move to a new school is the time to reconsider whether additional services might help. Many quirky children have uneven abilities—strong in some areas and very weak in others—in an era when everyone is supposed to be well rounded. A smart quirky child, meanwhile, is more likely to fit the stereotype of the little professor.

> One child was sent to my school because he was kind of peculiar. He was continuously picking and rubbing his nose, and was chapped around the lips. He didn't want to do anything but read the dictionary or read about chemistry. He had the periodic table memorized in second grade. His teacher wanted to know whether what he was reading and writing about was correct. Did it make sense? We ended up spending an hour a week together for about 6 weeks, and did a little chemistry together. He was sent to me partly to support his individual interest and validate it and partly to gauge whether it was gobbledygook, and, of course, it wasn't. We did a nitrogen unit and we cleaned the fish tank, and I got him to join my fish-study group. When he did a chart and talked about the nitrifying bacteria and the nitrogen fixing bacteria, it was clear he was in heaven.

Smart kids can get away with a lot more in terms of their eccentricities. However, this is usually not an age at which kids in a classroom will make allowances for bizarre behavior.

On the other hand, kids who struggle academically need to be in a place where their disabilities can be addressed and where kids with similar profiles are succeeding. As with the elementary school–aged child, a good educational evaluation is an important tool for determining the right place.

Social Skills and Middle School

Almost no one remembers the social environment of middle school with tremendous affection, but there is no question that to get by, you need certain basic social skills. You need to be able to understand what's OK and what's not, what's weird and what's seen as normal. You need to understand and work within the various social hierarchies of early adolescence and find your place in the school's social networks. Finding that place means being able to participate in the activities that go with it, whether sports, friendly conversation, shopping, or playing video games. How a child succeeds in the middle school social world can have an enormous effect on his sense of himself and on his mental health. A kid who doesn't understand the give-and-take of conversation is more likely to be teased, ostracized, or banished from the social group.

These issues can be addressed with social skills training, which is available in many middle school environments.

> Michael has always been different but because of his high intel-
> ligence, he made it through elementary school without too much
> trouble. He hasn't ever really cared about having friends. He's
> physically awkward and shuns sports, and he engages in some
> pretty weird behaviors.

Depression and anxiety often begin or become more acute at this age, which is why a preexisting relationship with a mental health professional may really pay off now. However, a child who is in distress may need more than someone with whom to talk. You may need to rethink the whole school question and find a better fit. By this age, school and the peer group become something close to a child's entire world, and the right school at the right time can be a lifesaver.

> Our daughter became very depressed because she was so isolated
> socially. It didn't help that her older sister was so popular, could
> play every sport, and had loads of friends. The combination of her
> depression and her learning difficulties prompted us to look for a
> school that could address these issues. We found a private school
> for special education where she is thriving. She's learning and she
> has friends, and though she sometimes feels embarrassed about
> going to a "sped" school, most of the time she is pretty happy. She
> even went to an overnight camp for 2 weeks and survived!

The Buddy System

Many adults expect their children to help classmates who are in distress, but parents of quirky kids will tell you it usually doesn't happen on its own. A relatively mature child in the classroom with good social skills can be asked to buddy up with the quirky child for lunch or social activities. This can help to bullyproof the quirky child, especially if the buddy is a popular member of the group. Although kids (especially girls) of this age can be brutal to one another, they can also be remarkably receptive to having a little responsibility. Consider whether you want to discuss this possibility with your child's teacher at this stage. Be sure that he thinks it's a good idea and that there is a likely candidate in the class who could handle it. Of course, what most kids want is a real friend.

Ken has never liked sports, and once all the boys in the neighborhood stopped coming over for LEGOs and wanted to play sports,
he just couldn't get himself to do it. This year, he got interested in
Magic Cards, and there is another boy in his class who loves them,
too. This has helped a lot. He looks forward to seeing his friend, and
they can sit in a corner and play with their cards and enjoy themselves. They insulate each other from the eyes of the other kids.

For some quirky kids, being good at something or intensely interested in
something that happens to be of interest to the other kids can be life changing.

Once John got into sports, he developed a kind of persona at school
as the sports/math guy, and everyone knew him as that kid. Because
sports are so much a part of the life of boys, it created a social
world for him that he hadn't had before. Everyone talks to him
about the latest scores, and he engages in imaginary sports (like
making a three-point basket or catching a pop fly and turning it
into a double play). Kids invite him to play pickup games at recess.
Before the sports thing kicked in, he would motor around the edge
of the playground, observe the others, and wring or flap his hands.
We can hardly believe this has happened. I think he might have
needed a special school if it hadn't.

The School Systems

Although this is the exception rather than the rule, some school districts have
developed programs specifically targeting the quirky kid group, with the aim
of keeping the kids in the public schools. Other systems seem to think that
these kids are bright enough to function independently in a typical school
environment, perhaps with a little support. Certainly, this can be true, but
you know your child best. Your gut feeling about whether he can thrive (or
survive) in a given environment is worth a lot. Know your options, even if you
don't need to take advantage of them.

We visited a school geared toward kids on the spectrum just to get
a sense of whether our daughter would need such a place. It was
great to know that such a school existed. It was clear that a lot of
care had gone into the design of the building, the classrooms, and
the other common areas. The corridors were wide to minimize the
bumping and jostling that these kids find unnerving; the walls were

extra thick to contain outside noise and prevent distraction. Even the desks were designed with the physically awkward child in mind. The rooms for sensory integration therapy and speech groups were cheerful and inviting rather than a closet—literally—where she receives her OT now. The staff is all certified in special education and understands the learning issues of these kids. For the moment, we think she can survive where she is, but there is comfort in knowing other options exist.

Again, at the middle school level, many kids who can't quite manage on their own may do better with an aide in the classroom to translate or reiterate directions or keep a child on task. Of course, as a middle schooler, a child may be more self-conscious about having an aide than she was back in elementary school, but good teachers and a supportive school should help make it work. Keep in mind that your public school owes your child an *appropriate* education under the special education laws, and a classroom aide might turn an inappropriate environment into that legislatively mandated appropriate setting. Few schools will come forward to offer such an expensive addition to a child's education plan, but it has worked extremely well for some of these kids. It keeps them close to home, and it's a lot less expensive than a placement in a school outside the district.

Both typical and quirky kids who pass through this stage of development relatively intact have gained many of the skills they will use throughout young adulthood. You could argue that after adolescence, being somewhat odd gets easier and easier as you proceed through life. College is notoriously a time when kids who felt out of place in high school finally find their peers, and out in the adult world, quirky colleagues, neighbors, and relatives are everywhere. So if middle school is a hard row to hoe for your child, try to keep in mind that it will eventually get easier. But first, you have to get through high school.

The High School Years

High school was much better than middle school for Megan. She was fortunate to get a spot in a small program within the big public high school. There was a special education teacher in the program, and I gave her articles on classroom strategies for kids with ASD, and that helped. After the pilot program ended, Megan was in regular education classes at the high school and got involved in things like the science team. She worked as an apprentice at the aquarium

and went to biology camp one summer. I know there will be a place for her in the science world.

Older adolescence is a time when *all* young people are forging their individual identities and gaining a better idea of their place in the world. If you look at almost any high school class, you can see the extent to which many kids are actively trying to be different. In fact, declaring independence—from their parents, particular sections of their peer group, even their friends—is a developmental characteristic of this age group. Think back on your own adolescence. Were there groups of kids to which you knew you didn't belong and from which you felt you had to mark yourself off—that is, did you establish your own adolescent identity partly through the groups you belonged to and partly through the groups you emphatically did not join?

High school also generally offers a little more scope to pursue your interests and play to your strengths than middle school. High school offers most children their first serious chance to choose their own identities: the yearbook club, basketball team, chess club, jazz ensemble, and so forth. Even typical kids of this age are often interested in a special topic or area to the exclusion of all else.

In many places nowadays, geekiness is somewhat cool—thanks probably to well-known people such as Bill Gates and to the general awareness that in a highly technological world, geekiness can be strength. A bumper sticker we recently saw for sale in a store proclaimed, "Be nice to nerds: You'll be working for one someday." There are kids who are known by their peers and teachers as budding poets or writers and those who are brilliant in chemistry or applied math. Memorizing the periodic table can be seen as pretty cool at this age, at least by a certain select group. Spending 8 hours a day doing gymnastics or figure skating is not all that unusual in high school, and other kids may find these activities fascinating.

The fact is, if a quirky kid has made it to high school, he will probably find it more accepting and less stressful than middle school and may not feel quite so different anymore. His learning issues ought to be well understood by now, and strategies for coping academically, such as listening to audiobooks or writing on a laptop for assignments, are well developed. In fact, typing your assignments, which not long ago was a special adaptation for kids with terrible handwriting, is now pretty much the norm; virtually all high schools expect kids to have access to laptops, eliminating the drudgery of writing for kids with poor motor skills and making life much easier for teachers as well.

Academic Issues and High School

By the time quirky kids reach ninth or tenth grade, most of their families are knowledgeable about their learning profiles and what additional services are necessary to make things work in school. Parents also usually have some sense of whether their children are socially isolated, although that becomes more difficult to determine as children grow into adolescence and in many cases become much more private.

As in the middle-school years, schools devoted to kids with an interest or a particular strength in, for example, math and science or art and music can be wonderful places for quirky kids. Music and math are areas of strength for a subset of quirky kids and quirky adults as well. On the other hand, vocational schools can be terrific places for other quirky kids, lifting some of the academic pressure and giving them a chance to acquire skills that build their confidence and set them up for employment. For some parents who had more academic aspirations, sending their child to a vocational school can feel like a defeat. But remember, this isn't you; it's your child, and you want to give him his best shot at an independent livelihood.

By now, it should be pretty easy to decide whether your quirky kid can negotiate the corridors, move from class to class throughout the day, or find the gym or cafeteria. The degree of structure is a major consideration at this time. Does your child thrive on structure, as many quirky kids do? Does she need to know exactly what's next and where? Can he tolerate moving to a new classroom every 45 minutes? Is too much choice overwhelming? Look around at the other kids and their behavior with one another. Will your child's social behaviors be acceptable here? If many of the kids are wearing only black or have 10 piercings on their nose and eyebrows and total body tattoos, will your daughter's need to wear the same jeans and T-shirt every day seem so outlandish? How about the noise level? Will it be overwhelming? Are there options about where to eat lunch or do a study period? Are team sports required, or are other options available for the after-school hours? Make sure your child has a chance to look around as well, and see the students, physical facility, library, gym, and school auditorium. Meeting with the special education coordinator and school psychologist will be helpful for most families, and talking with other parents you've met over the years will help determine whether there's a good chance a particular high school will work for your child.

Separate high schools are also available for kids with special needs, although it's rare for a high school–age student who has not required a separate environment in the past to need one now. It's more likely for the situation to be the other way around; kids for whom a separate environment has been successful at the middle school level may find the transition to a more standard high school relatively easy. The anonymity of larger high schools is a bonus for a child coming from a more restrictive setting. Almost all kids this age are somewhat self-conscious about various elements in their backgrounds or their performance, and in a large school, there usually will be a mix of students from a wide variety of backgrounds and school experiences. Having attended a special school for a few years is probably not that interesting, and may not even be noticed.

Adolescent Issues and the Quirky Teenager

The developmental tasks of adolescence are challenging for everyone. As physicians, we are aware of what can go wrong during the teenage years and are on the lookout for struggles: mental health disorders for which the child is genetically predisposed, substance-abuse problems, eating disorders, high-risk sexual behaviors, questions about sexual identity or preference, reactions to longstanding family stresses. All of these problems exist in all high schools. In some ways, quirky kids are no better or worse off than any other teenagers. Those with very high intelligence or intense special interests may have an anchor that many of their peers lack. In the average public high school, most kids are able to find at least a couple of kids like themselves, and quirky kids may find themselves making social connections more naturally for the first time. As kids approach adulthood, their refusal to participate in certain activities has a lot less meaning. No one expects all teenagers—or adults, for that matter—to be the same.

Your High School Student's Mental Health

Your adolescent may communicate with you mostly in grunts, frequently look sullen, confine comments at meals to occasional sarcastic remarks, and shrug when you ask which teacher you should check with to see how she's doing. And this has nothing to do with quirkiness.

Indeed, with older children, it's not always easy for parents to tell how they're doing. There may not be one particularly involved or knowledgeable teacher to fill you in on your child's progress. Academic performance, of course, is one good indicator: A student who is failing in all subject areas is not in a good environment for learning, or something major is getting in the way. But academic success is not the only goal here; you also want to keep an eye on your child's mental health, and you want to do it while fostering independence, which can be a difficult balancing act for all parents. Because mental health issues such as depression, suicidal thoughts, anxiety, or obsessive-compulsive disorder often show up around this age, and because of the complex comorbidities of many quirky-kid syndromes, you should keep a close but not too intrusive eye out for any distress signals. Watch for increased isolation or for disturbed sleeping habits. Be alert for the adolescent who unilaterally decides to stop taking her medicine. She may be stopping because she's having a problem, or she may have a problem because she's stopped taking her medicine. Depression can manifest as a loss of appetite, unexplained crying jags, or *anhedonia*, the loss of the ability to take pleasure in the activities a child normally enjoys. If you think your child may be in trouble along these lines, don't depend on the high school faculty or staff to detect, diagnose, or treat the problem. You need the help of a psychiatrist or psychologist (preferably one who has known your child for a while) to work with you and your child.

Thinking Outside the All-or-Nothing Box

Adolescents can be excruciatingly self-conscious and self-critical, and dissatisfaction with themselves, their performance, or their place in the high school world can bring on powerful and destructive emotions.

Academic achievement can be an important factor here, and you know your own child well enough to think about what would be a good setup for school success and what might be major stumbling blocks. You may also have a sense, for example, of whether gym class is likely to be pleasure or torture. To make the best of your child's high school experience, a good recommendation from one of the mothers we interviewed is to "think outside the all-or-nothing box." Many systems are willing to make accommodations to keep children in their local schools, but you may need to suggest them. A child who simply cannot learn a foreign language, becomes anxious or obsessive in health education, or is too uncoordinated for gym class can still thrive with relatively minor changes in expectations. Think creatively. How about an extra year of high school, with fewer classes per year, or an independent study or a studio class for a child with special interests or abilities? Don't focus too much on graduation requirements or college admissions, especially during the first years of high school. Save those concerns for later, when you have a better sense of what the future may hold.

8

The Social Life of a Quirky Kid: Finding Friends and Making Connections

School may be more important for your child's future and family life more fraught with friction on a day-to-day basis, but it's probably the social life of the quirky child that most gnaws at parents. Over the short term, when parents worry about a quirky child's social abilities, they are worrying about whether their child will be able to participate in and enjoy all the various games, jokes, and friendships that are a big part of life for school-aged children. Parents may worry about the global picture: Will my child ever fit into the world? Ever have friends? Ever get along normally with colleagues? Ever find love? The social peculiarities can serve to isolate a child early on, perhaps even before the child has been evaluated, and can leave the adults around him bewildered.

> I'm Jewish, and Andrew's father is Christian. Andrew has decided he prefers Christmas. When a mother came into his preschool class to talk about the Hanukkah celebration, he yelled out, "I hate Hanukkah!" The mother thought he was an anti-Semite. Fortunately, I was there, and I explained that he was half Jewish himself. Recently, he said, "I hate Hanukkah; I hate Jesus. I only like the big bang."

Many quirky children struggle socially to one extent or another, and their parents struggle with them. You have a child you adore, whose challenges and triumphs you recognize and celebrate. You see all those lovable, if eccentric, endearing qualities. It can hurt a lot if your child's classmates seem to see only a weirdo, a freak, an outcast. And it can hurt even more if now and then you see your child through their eyes: a mix of off-putting personal habits and obsessive conversations.

Social Life During Preschool

During the toddler and preschool years, you have a certain amount of control over the child's social life. Parents arrange playdates for young children, make the phone calls, schlep the children back and forth, and supervise them as needed. Many children in child care and preschool-aged children are willing to go on any playdate with any classmate; if there are toys and video games and snacks, or some combination, it seems like a treat.

On the other hand, many younger quirky kids may not be ready for a lot of socializing. Early intervention offers some social contact, and that may be enough for them. Socializing can be fairly stressful for many of these children, and they may need to decompress and relax without the additional pressure of a playdate. Maybe your child would be better off if you took him to the playground and let him play alone with his favorite truck while he has a chance to observe the other children. Parallel play—playing next to one another without interaction—is normal in toddlers and often lasts longer in quirky kids. Many like being around other children but without getting too close or without the pressure of having to talk, share toys, or take turns. Don't let your own wish to see your child as "normal" or your hopes that playing with other children will somehow be good for her push you into setting up a social life that she's not yet ready to handle.

Quirky children may require more supervision than other kids to make sure that the playdate is peaceful, that the guest's wishes are respected, and that both children come away feeling they've had a good time. In fact, for some quirky children, playdates are essentially supervised parental project times.

What are some of the special issues to consider as you think about whether your preschool child is ready for playdates and, if so, how can you make them work? Play may be harder for a quirky child for any or all of the following reasons:

- Many have difficulty with symbolic play. Their imaginations work differently, and they just don't understand how to dress up or pretend to be pirates.
- Language delays or language problems can make it harder to play, understand, and be understood.
- Sensory integration issues may make it hard to handle loud noises or the touch and texture of something that's part of the game.

- Fine motor problems can make children less skillful at all kinds of games or frustrated by their own inability to do something that other children can do easily, whether it's dressing a Barbie doll or putting LEGOs together.
- Tantrums may be so severe that they scare the other children.

Negotiating sharing and turn-taking can be more complicated because of the following:

- Because of different developmental trajectories, a quirky 4-year-old may have as much trouble sharing toys as a more typical 2-year-old. This isn't selfish or bad behavior; quirky kids may be much slower to develop the ability to see the world from someone else's point of view, and at the same time much more rigid in their habits.
- The more typical 4-year-old with whom your child is playing is not going to have a whole lot of patience if she doesn't get her turn. Preschoolers, when they do master the sharing concept, turn into real sticklers about rules and fairness.
- A particular toy or game or object may have extra meaning for the quirky child: a truck that has to stay in the lineup or a stuffed animal that always sits in a particular position on the pillow. Put away any objects that you think your child may not want another child handling or playing with.
- Children with rituals may have trouble changing their rules and routines when another child is around. Talk it through in advance: "We're going to have a snack together, and *you* can eat all your raisins before we open the box of Goldfish crackers, but Susie might want to mix them up."
- Keep these early playdates as brief as possible. This is more reasonable if they don't involve long drives. In fact, this is one situation in which a multifamily house or a congenial city neighborhood offers real advantages.

A lot of John's early social experience was with the boy downstairs. They would have short, sweet interactions, and when things started to escalate, it would end. That's the great thing about a multiple-family house: You don't have to go to any trouble to set this up or cart them for miles. I think it's much harder in a suburban or rural area where everything has to be arranged in advance.

Tailor the playdate to your child in the following ways:

- Ask your child: "Who do you like spending time with at school?"
- Ask the teacher about your child's interactions at preschool or child care, and find out with whom your child most often plays, talks, and eats.

- Think about an activity your child enjoys that you think would work well with another child: a trip to the playground (outside time is often much easier than inside time), a game that you know your own kid understands and can play competently.
- Make a plan and walk your child through it. Quirky kids often do better if they know what to expect: "Susie will arrive with her mother, and you'll play hide-and-seek. And then we'll have a snack, and then we'll let Susie choose which video to watch. Then her mother will come, and we'll say good-bye." This lets you make bargains in advance, if necessary: "Susie chooses the video when she's here, then you choose one after she goes home." It's not a guarantee of good behavior, but preparation and rehearsal really help these kids.

When your child is invited over to another child's house, be realistic.

- Keep it short, especially at the beginning.
- Consider whether you want to stick around for at least the first part of the visit. This probably depends on how well you know the other child's parents and how concerned you are about how your child will do. When inviting another child over for a playdate, many parents have in mind a couple of hours of relative freedom for themselves, with their child happily occupied with a friend. They aren't necessarily expecting to have to entertain another adult during that time. On the other hand, if you know your child may not make this easy, and may in fact need extra supervision, you might want to explain this and offer to at least be on call and available.
- Be easily reachable and don't be too far away.
- It is perfectly acceptable to call halfway through the visit and ask how things are going. Be prepared to pick up your child early if necessary.
- Tell the other child's parents anything they absolutely have to know (eg, there may be a tantrum or a seizure or an episode of tics; your child is phobic about water or dogs or vacuum cleaners).

Whether the playdate is at your house or at someone else's, if something goes awry, do your best to figure out what happened. You may be able to avoid that particular trigger the next time around or talk it through with your child. Don't assume that anything that goes wrong was necessarily on account of your child's quirks. It takes two to tango. Part of the give-and-take of playdates for children is figuring out what to do when your guest acts rudely and won't play any of your games, mixes up all the Play-Doh colors, and says she wants to go home after 5 minutes. This is a parent's cue to be gracious and under-standing toward the other parent and make it clear that you understand that all children have their good days and bad days.

We don't mean to make this sound as if playdates are all hard work and always poised on the edge of disaster. In fact, plenty of quirky kids start having playdates during the preschool years, enjoy their friends, enjoy themselves, and go back to school with special bonds to the children with whom they've played. So as you sense your own child's interest and readiness, it definitely can be worthwhile to enter the game.

You should also have some scenarios in mind that take into account the less successful turns that a playdate can take—not to mention the disasters. You know your quirky child, you know what to plan for (eg, an episode of stereo-typed repetitive behavior that will bewilder the other child, a tantrum), and you should have some options in mind, from a reliable favorite board game to a second adult available if the kids need to be separated. And just in case you do encounter a disastrous playdate (eg, your child bites her guest, the guest bites your child, a favorite and irreplaceable toy is destroyed, both children end up in screaming fits), comfort yourself with the knowledge that most children have a few calamitous playdates along the way. Then think about what you might arrange differently next time.

Elementary School Social Life

Caitlin developed a phobia about flowers on fabric, clothes, curtains, etc. If we went to a restaurant that had flowers on the china or even the furniture, we would have to leave because she couldn't tolerate it. And because her social skills were so poor, if anyone at school wore clothes with flowers printed on them, she would tell them they were ugly and she hated them.

Social life in elementary school is highly dependent on the school's schedule and the general school attitude. Some elementary school children have large amounts of essentially unsupervised, unstructured time—on the bus, on the playground, even at times in the classroom—whereas others are much more tightly regulated. Unstructured time is notoriously tough for the quirky child. A seasoned elementary school teacher will have a pretty good sense of what is going on socially among the children in the room, although this may be more true in first grade than in fifth or sixth.

David likes rules and doesn't understand the gray areas. At school, he couldn't understand why the other kids didn't behave properly and would tell them to behave themselves or he would tell the

teachers what they were doing. This became annoying to the kids
and teachers, but his motivation was more that he just didn't get it
rather than wanting anyone to get into trouble.

It is to your advantage to befriend your child's teacher, especially in the early
grades, and to feel you can check in occasionally about social issues as well as
about academic progress. Don't overwhelm the teacher with your expertise
without showing respect for hers. Some parents come in on day 1 with an
enormous pile of information about their child's issues, the most approved
techniques for dealing with any eccentricities, and social needs and emotional
requirements without giving the teacher any chance to observe the child in the
context of the classroom and draw some conclusions. You want the teacher as
a partner, an expert observer, and an interpreter of the academic and social
scenes during the school day. Keep in mind that he or she will have a different
perspective on your child's functioning and perhaps be more attuned to how
your child reacts to the social exigencies of a boy—or a girl—of a certain age in
a classroom group.

Boys and Girls

Boys and girls move through elementary school on substantially different
social trajectories. These are generalizations, of course, but for the most part,
girls are much earlier to develop complex social webs, cliques, interlocking
nets of friendship and best friendships, and intricate systems of in-groups and
out-groups. Boys, at least in the earlier grades, tend to be less socially aware,
more physical in many of their activities, and more willing to consider other
boys their age in the general category of friend. This can make the early years
of school somewhat easier for a quirky boy than for a quirky girl. Chances
are that in the second grade, a boy who pays no attention to his clothes and
sometimes says some pretty weird things will be included in a general pack
of second-grade boys, whereas a girl the same age might already be clearly
marked as an outlier. It may also mean that the gap between a quirky girl's
social perceptions and social skills and those of her peers will be much bigger
than the comparable gap for a boy.

Rebecca misses social cues. She wants to have friends, but she
gets into struggles. She doesn't understand the rules other kids
want to play by; she's extremely literal; and she pulls phrases
right out of cartoons and uses them pretty appropriately, but they
are not her words. One day, she screamed, "You don't love me
anymore!" I thought, what is this? Then I realized she had heard

it on SpongeBob SquarePants. She is impulsive and recently got
into trouble for stealing in her class. She was sent to the principal's
office, where she said, "I'm so bad. Please give me another chance. I
won't do it ever again." Once again, totally scripted from something.
The principal interpreted this as very "high-functioning," when in
fact it was scripted.

All of this can make life pretty tough on quirky girls. As a parent, you may
be able to help at this age by keeping a careful eye on what the other children
wear to school and use to carry their books or lunch or protect themselves
from the rain, and helping your child get it right. You can support any friendship that seems to be developing and try to cement it a little by becoming
friends yourself with the child's parent.

Peculiar Habits

As children grow, both boys and girls become more aware of any behavior that
marks a child as different. By third or fourth grade, the child with some repetitive personal behavior, an obsessive school routine, or some personal hygiene
black spot is going to be noticed and possibly teased or even shunned. And a
teacher who draws attention to this habit as well, even in trying to be helpful,
may increase the degree to which the other children pay attention.

My daughter has trichotillomania. She picks at her scalp, pulls her
hair out. We were trying to help her with this, and I mentioned it to
her teacher, thinking, of course, she must have noticed this, so I was
going to tell her some strategies that the behavioral psychologist
had suggested. She said, "I hadn't noticed." But then, apparently, she
constantly told my daughter to stop twirling her hair, and all the
kids in the room knew about it. I had to tell her, "Could you lighten
up on the head thing?"

All you can do is try to spot those possible troublesome habits well in advance
and target your behavioral modification at home, your work in therapy, or
even your medication trials. Even so, there will be visible quirks, and other
kids will point them out.

Is it ever worth visiting the school, explaining the situation to the other children, and asking for their tolerance and good manners? Absolutely. Children
have been known to rise to the occasion, and we have patients whose parents
have repeatedly visited the school, explaining a young child's severe skin

condition or the sometimes frightening aspects of a tic disorder or the absolute rituals of a child with obsessive-compulsive disorder.

> **When Brian was in fifth grade, they did a skit about differences, with a friend saying he didn't like the way Brian had to take a snack first and Brian explaining to the class that it was just his OCD; he couldn't eat something if someone else had touched it.**

Teasing and Bullying

A certain amount of teasing is a fact of life, but teasing in school can get out of hand, and it can be a parent's difficult and thankless task to assess the degree and intensity of teasing and respond appropriately. Elementary school is probably the time when your child is most likely to talk openly with you about being teased and least likely to forbid you to interfere.

> **Other kids teased me when I was growing up. I cared, but I didn't care. Nothing could stop me. I always thought I was the greatest painter in the world, even when I wasn't. I stopped caring whether other kids liked me. I would put it out of my head.**

When teasing passes a certain point, when it becomes ganging up or happens so regularly that the child is unhappy in school, or if the teasing reflects racial differences, the child's physical traits, or social and behavioral difficulties, it's time for the parent to talk to the teacher and time for the teacher—and the school—to do something. That kind of teasing amounts to bullying, and bullying needs to be taken seriously.

What the School Can Do

Schools *can* do something about this problem. Don't ever let anyone tell you they can't. At the elementary school level, at least, the tone set by the teachers and the administration, and their response to teasing that gets out of hand, can make an enormous difference. It is not impossible to create an atmosphere of censure in which the child who starts teasing will be shunned by other children who don't want to get into trouble (or don't want to have to meet and discuss it once again with their teacher). As with everything else, addressing this problem gets harder in middle school, but that doesn't mean it's a futile effort.

Where your child goes to school does make a difference. With Sam, at his first school, he was getting teased because Cinderella was his favorite movie. I brought it to the attention of the school staff, and they basically said, "We have enough on our plates. We can't take this on." You know, "Kids will be kids." But at his current school, they take it on. They process it, they meet, they discuss how it makes the child feel, and they say, "It's not OK"—and that makes a big difference.

Danger Signs

What danger signs should you look for if you think your child might be getting teased or bullied?

- Tears, fears, anxiety about going to school
- Asking to stay home or pretending to be sick—any school-avoidance behaviors
- Worries that seem to be directly connected to the less-supervised parts of the day: the bus ride, the playground, the lunchroom
- General signs that your child is upset: increased anxiety, sleep disturbances, unexplained crying

If you think something is going on, ask your child about school more broadly, ask whether anyone said anything to him that he didn't like, and then ask specifically about the less-supervised moments of the day: With whom did you sit on the bus? Play at recess? Eat lunch? Anything unusual happen?

Bring up the subject of teasing and discuss it before it gets to be any kind of problem. You can discuss what teasing is—saying mean things to make other kids feel bad—maybe with reference to what goes on between siblings, and you can tell your child:

- Never tease anybody, because teasing is mean.
- If anybody ever teases you, that person is doing something wrong.
- We should get help from a teacher. Teachers and principals don't like teasing.
- Please tell me if there's too much teasing in school.

What should you do if you think your child is being teased or bullied?

- Talk to the teacher, the bus attendant, or the lunchroom monitor.
- Do a little reality testing. Does it seem as if this is happening on a regular basis, or was it a one-time thing?
- Think about whether the problem could be addressed logistically. Could your child sit at the front of the bus, near the monitor? Would adding an extra lunchroom aide help, even if it is only for a week or two?

Involve the Teacher

If you think that something bad is happening, ask the teacher to take action. If the teacher isn't sure how to handle it or hasn't handled anything of the kind before, suggest a consultation with the school counselor or a more experienced teacher, and suggest that they might want to talk to the class together.

You should then make plans to follow up with the teacher (a return visit or a phone appointment) so that it's clear you want to hear how things went with the intervention (the class discussion, the separate session with the ringleaders, if it's clear who they are) and how they're going now for your child.

If you don't receive the response you want from the teacher, go to the principal. Make it clear that you see this as a serious issue and that you intend to stay involved. If your child is being teased or bullied partly on account of a disability, make it clear that you regard this as especially serious and possibly illegal. We've tended to use the word *teasing* rather than *bullying* when talking about younger children, but persistent teasing and targeting one child easily cross the line into bullying, and you may find that if you use that word, teachers and school administrators will take the problem more seriously.

Talking to the Parents

Should you, ever and under any circumstances, consider calling up another parent to say, "Can't you make your daughter stop tormenting my son?" Certainly, if you're ever going to do such a thing, it would be in the elementary years. Once your child gets to middle school, it's probably out of the question. If you decide to do this, tread carefully. You may make an enemy. The more you know about the other parent, the better, and the more contact you've had in the past, the better. Ideally, you want to present this issue as important, but potentially just a bump in the road in the long careers of your children as they attend school together.

Remember that you are placing other parents in the uncomfortable position of hearing something negative about their child. Try, as much as possible (this will be rather difficult), not to make it sound as if you think the other child is a horror, a monster, and a lower form of life.

Offer a specific solution: "Rachel probably doesn't realize it, but Lisa feels really bad about not being able to read yet. If Rachel could understand her feelings better, I'm sure she wouldn't tease her about it." Also, be polite in suggesting options: "I'm afraid that if Rachel pulls Lisa's hair on the school bus once more, they're going to ask Rachel to stop taking the bus, and I would really like it if we could put our heads together and talk to the girls and find a way to stop that from happening."

We have heard only a few positive stories of the parent-calling-other-parents-to-complain variety, and a lot of nasty ones. You shouldn't have to resort to this, and we hope you never do, but there have been a number of successful (and highly public) lawsuits in recent years in which children were bullied, teased unmercifully, or sexually harassed in public schools, and their families sued those schools for failing to protect them and won large judgments. The teacher—or certainly the principal—will be aware of this nightmare scenario, which should make it much more likely that your highly reasonable and civil request will be taken seriously. If it isn't, and if things are very bad, you might then have to talk to a lawyer.

For more information on bullying, see pages 200–202 in this chapter.

The Cool and the Uncool

By first grade among the girls, and by fourth or fifth grade among the boys, the question of who is cool starts to become an issue. Quirky kids, by and large, are not cool. And just because they aren't teasing your daughter doesn't mean that the cool girls are including her at the lunch table, where everyone wears the trendiest clothes. And although you can, to some extent, help fight your child's battles when it comes to teasing, at least in elementary school, there are no parents on earth who have ever succeeded in making the cool girls open up another place at the lunch table, no matter how many pieces of trendy clothing they buy for their child. And the problem is, as it becomes more important to be cool, more children begin to worry that uncoolness may be catching, like cooties.

In Megan's class, it became clearer that her development was well behind that of the others. The sixth-grade girls especially, who were trying to be more independent, made her life miserable, and she became an outcast. At that time, she started acting out. She actually kicked a boy when he accidentally knocked a shell off her desk and it broke. She continued her spaced-out episodes of looking out the window and missing what was going on in class. We knew that our family needed help.

By fifth grade, the boys are getting to a point where there are cool kids. Cool guys are smart and funny and socially savvy, and they sit together at lunch—and Gabriel doesn't notice any of this yet. His friend Ken is also not cool, but he's more aware and more with it. Ken is cool enough to know that Gabriel is the weirdest kid in the class, so he's not going to hang around with Gabriel in school, even though they're friends outside.

For some children, and not all of them quirky, all of this is heartbreaking—although they are not being teased, they also are not being included. There is not much that a parent can do about it directly, except listen when your child wants to talk, offer comfort and reinforcement, and promise that this, too, shall pass.

Friendships

There are some less direct things you can do, strategies aimed at helping your child find a peer group, social contacts, and friends, thereby freeing him or her, to some extent, from the strictly limited social dynamics of the classroom.

For both boys and girls, a single good friendship can change the world. Going through elementary school is much easier if you have a best friend. If the right one comes along for your child, that can be a blessing. Cherish that best friend, who may also be a little quirky. Help them find time to be together so that the feeling of really being friends, with mutual experiences and in-jokes, grows and expands. If a best friend isn't available at school, and if your child doesn't seem to be part of a wider circle of friendly peers, it is probably worthwhile helping your child look elsewhere for friends and companions.

> I was happy with my daughter's dinosaur obsession. I became an expert on dinosaurs because she knew so much. We would go to the library and get books and I would read them to her, and she really seemed to absorb it all, retain it. Right now, Pokémon is Lisa's obsession. Her father and I had bought her Pokémon cards, and she went out with the neighbors and traded every one of her good cards for really crappy cards. I said to her dad, "If it helps her get along with other kids, I'm happy." Pokémon seems to work for both boys and girls, whereas when she was obsessed with dinosaurs, it was hard to talk to other girls. Now she has a couple of good girlfriends at school.

- *Think seriously about community activities,* such as Boy Scouts, Girl Scouts, religious groups, or bowling leagues, especially for the older elementary school child. A somewhat more structured setting may make it easier for a quirky kid to interact with peers. It will give him a wider circle of kids at school with whom he has something in common. We recently read about a mother who organized a Cub Scout pack specifically for boys with autism spectrum disorder (ASD), attention-deficit/hyperactivity disorder (ADHD), and other developmental issues, tailoring meetings and activities to their needs and interests.

- *Look at school-based after-school activities.* For younger children, this will probably mean the school-based after-school program, if one exists and if your child seems to enjoy going. Going to an after-school program, even a couple of days a week, can give a child the chance to interact with a slightly different mix of kids, some older and some younger. It will broaden social horizons within the school and may help a child learn to play more comfortably.
- *As your child gets older, look at extracurricular activities,* such as band, orchestra, or chorus, if the school offers them. A child with musical skills can easily make this into an important peer group, and, once again, it will mean children in other classes and other grades who say "hi" in the hallway or stop to ask what they're supposed to practice that evening.
- *Consider enrichment classes.* A child with a splinter skill may find peers and friends in a special program or an after-school enrichment class such as math groups, computer classes, and art schools.

When your child finds an out-of-school friend, make it work. Get to know that child's parents, figure out the logistics of getting them together every now and then, and think about carpooling to and from their activity. Keep in mind, though, as you're looking for extra activities, that the elementary years are often the years most crowded by therapy appointments and other special supports, some of which, after all, are aimed at helping your child develop social skills. Ask yourself, which is more important right now, occupational therapy or math group? Keep in mind that these children grow and change. The mix that's right for now may not be right a year from now.

> Before John found baseball, he liked playing with younger kids. They didn't challenge him socially, and they would help him catch up with things he hadn't done earlier, like playing with the train set or building with blocks, which he never did when he was supposed to!

> Abby had a little girl in our old neighborhood who was 3 years younger, and they would ride bikes together and play dolls together, and the younger kid was flattered that here was this big girl who wanted to spend time with her.

Some children will find their friends—or even their soul mates—at therapy appointments. It may be that in a pragmatic language group, your child will encounter another child who is a soul mate and they will recognize each other with joy.

> Caitlin has not had many friends but now has a friend through her
> social skills group who also has autism. They text each other, and
> I have to say, texting is a wonderful thing for a child who misses
> nonverbal cues. She only has to deal with the words, and the two of
> them share interests, so it has worked very well.

If a child needs social contact beyond what school seems to be offering, consider the possibility of a virtual buddy or texting partner. Many quirky kids learn to type and use computers fairly early. Some find it easier to text or email, without the pressure of having to decipher the social cues of body language and tone of voice. Email lists are available for children with certain specific diagnoses (eg, autism spectrum disorder, learning disabilities), and it can be both a pleasure and a comfort for children to email back and forth with others whose experience matches their own.

If you decide to go this route, remember that quirky children, like all children, need very strict guidelines about social media and, because they tend to be more socially naive, may be at special risk. A parent should make sure that the virtual buddy is genuine—is, in fact, a child—and probably should make contact (email is fine) with the child's parents. If last names and addresses are to be exchanged, it should be by the parents. Basic rules for a child are as follows: **Never give out your address or your last name on the internet. Never arrange to meet someone over the internet. Never post your picture on the internet.**

Of course, your extended family, if they are in the area, may be a source of companionship. Many kids accept cousins, a little older or a little younger or a little quirky, with a sort of tribal inclusion that doesn't necessarily apply outside the family. If your child has been in contact with cousins or aunts and uncles not so much older, they may continue to serve as playmates and a special peer group.

Remember that many quirky children find that they enjoy spending time with children younger than themselves. When it comes to connecting with kids in their own grade, the single most important step that many quirky children take toward friendship is to find an interest, or even an obsession, that is socially acceptable among children of that age. A 9-year-old boy obsessed with baseball and sports statistics or a 7-year-old girl who cares about Pokémon more than anything else are children whose obsessions may work for them socially and may help them appear not so different from many of their peers. Whatever the cards and collectibles are for your child's age group, whatever the collective fads, think about encouraging your child to participate.

Birthday Parties

It's inevitable that many kids in your child's class will have birthday parties. As your child ages, depending on her social skills and social milieu, she may have to face the heartbreak of not being invited. But while she's young, you are more likely to have to face the heartbreak—or at least the severe stress—of her *being* invited and having to go and behave. Certainly, some children don't like birthday parties at all—we know one boy whose mother always just says "no"—but many of them want to go, even if the party poses a social challenge.

> As my son gets older, he's better able to say, "Wait, that's not something I want to do," but you don't always know. He was invited to one birthday party, and he really wanted to go because he liked the kid, and it turned out it was a laser-tag birthday party. It was really loud, really dark, really scary—and he'll never do that again. If it's a pool party, he's not going to go because he hates water, or he'll just come at the end for the cake. We have to allow him the choice and help explain when he doesn't want to go.

Certain aspects of children's birthday parties are rather ritualized. You can help your child prepare for those, from the blowing-out-the-candles-and-singing moment to the good-bye and thank-you-I-had-a-very-nice-time, which needs to be nudged along by parental prompting for a good 9 out of 10 children. But it can be hard to predict the games, the activities, even the entertainment. That is why many parents of quirky children end up being the ones hanging around at the party, offering to help and planning to stick it out just in case the bowling, or Murray the Magician, or the treasure hunt somehow goes awry.

Keep your own child's birthday parties small when she is young. Invite grandparents, siblings, a favorite babysitter, a couple of playmates. The experience of being the center of attention is overwhelming for many quirky kids, and the social responsibilities that devolve on the host—saying the occasional thank-you, not winning all the prizes, not biting anyone—can just be too demanding. As your child moves along in school, however, you may find yourself in a situation where inviting the whole class is obligatory, or at least all the boys or all the girls. You should consider some kind of short and highly ritualized party outside the home if there is a venue that your child finds comfortable and pleasant: a pizza party, a party at the science museum, a party in a theme or fast-food restaurant, or a party at one of those activity zones.

Most children nowadays seem to be so conditioned to these parties that they arrive knowing exactly what to do, eager to see the IMAX movie or the dancing rat, depending on the place. They depart feeling they have gotten exactly what they came for, and you don't have to deal with the question of whether you somehow gave a weird party because your kid is, well, weird. You also maintain a certain amount of family privacy by keeping the party out of the home and eliminating the possibility that a child might, for example, discover the personal hygiene sticker charts on your upstairs bathroom wall or the doll collection in a house where all the children are boys. Hosting a party out of the house may be much easier for many quirky children than having to entertain in their homes and watch other children handle their possessions.

Social Life for a Middle Schooler

For many, the middle school years are the most troubled, the years when your body's changes can race ahead of your social readiness or lag behind everyone else's development. They're years of self-consciousness and self-doubt, and many kids take refuge in conformity, in blending in with the pack and being one with the crowd. A quirky child's issues may mirror the experiences of more typically developing kids, but often with extra intensity as the issues of social hierarchy become more intense.

> **Junior high school was hell. Megan's one friend moved away, and that was a tragedy for Megan. Also, the other girls in her sphere at school were into pop music and culture and talking about boys and clothes, and they would say mean things to her. At this point, we tried a girls' social-skills group.**

Where your child is in school during these years really matters. Middle school grades are grouped differently in different systems. We know, of course, that many people don't have much choice: the town has one junior high, and that's that. Still, we hope that even if your choices are limited, thinking this through and preparing for your child's experience will help.

Generally speaking, quirky kids are much better off in a separate middle school or in a kindergarten through eighth grade setting. They are unlikely to benefit socially from being with true high school students (although there may be some quirky kids for whom the availability of advanced math, advanced music, or advanced art classes is an advantage). Because they may already be a little behind their middle school peers, they could appear hopelessly slow and young in a world full of 16-, 17-, and 18-year-olds. If your school system puts seventh and eighth graders in the high school, you need to find out what special arrangements are made to guide and protect the younger children.

Eating lunch in a high school cafeteria or hanging out in high school hallways is probably going to be a challenge. Could a child eat lunch and then go to the library? Is there a counselor's office if someone needs to talk? Can a kid who is becoming anxious go to the nurse?

When middle school is part of elementary school, some quirky children find a certain relief from the social pressures of puberty because they are in a place full of younger children who just aren't there yet. Sometimes in kinder-garten-through-eighth grade setups, parents feel that the last two grades are tacked on. The building is not really adequate for their needs, and most of the teachers are oriented toward the early grades. However, this arrangement offers the comforts of familiarity during some pretty confusing years.

A separate middle school for grades 7 and 8 only (or for grades 6, 7, and 8 or occasionally for grades 7, 8, and 9) can work well socially for some quirky kids. These schools offer children an opportunity to go through these awk-ward years without constant side-by-side comparisons to true adolescents (comfortably on the other side of puberty) or to young children (innocent, not self-conscious, and generally cute). Middle schools also attract teachers who find this an interesting age, delight in what middle school minds can produce, and sympathize with the emotional and social currents these kids navigate. Because quirky kids are often more comfortable with adults than with people their own age, teachers offer both intellectual growth and emotional support.

Some quirky kids need to be with other quirky children in a more therapeutic environment. Usually, they are the kids for whom major learning issues or major mental health issues are getting in the way. They may need some kind of special placement, often with the goal of returning to the regular high school. And although this placement decision is rarely made for social reasons, a separate school can be a real social refuge for a very quirky child, offering a context in which the child is not an outlier and providing, with luck, a social matrix of friends and acquaintances.

Whatever your middle school arrangement, you will probably have limited access to information about your child's social life during these years. You will probably perceive certain truths about how your child's social life is going from his or her general emotional state. And then, of course, there will be the obvious clues of whether you meet any friends, become aware of weekend invi-tations, and perceive a general sense of activity. If your child seems isolated, depressed, or angry and confused, these are years when a relationship with a therapist or counselor can make an enormous difference.

The Differences Between Boys and Girls

Some educators strongly believe that during these years, the differences between boys and girls are so extreme that they are almost two different species, from an educational point of view as well as from a social perspective. These educators argue that the needs of boys and girls are so different during this period that you cannot serve the girls properly without shortchanging the boys and vice versa. Although we don't want to make any claim as global as that, we say, with caution, that for any given quirky child who does not seem to be flourishing in a regular middle school or for whom middle school looms as an enormous social challenge, you might want to consider whether an all-boys or all-girls school would provide a better environment. The schools do remove some of the social pressures that middle school kids experience. At some all-girl schools, there is much less pressure about how to dress and about looks in general. At an all-boys school, the embarrassment of having a voice that suddenly shifts registers may be much easier to live down.

Bullying

In middle school, the kids get meaner and sharper, and pressure to be like everyone else gets stronger and stronger. Any eccentricity or difference can make a child vulnerable to teasing and bullying: wearing an assisted-hearing device, going to the school nurse several times a day to take medications, or walking with any kind of odd gait. Of course, no one should make the mistake of thinking that bullying happens because the target is quirky. Bullies target whomever they can. There are plenty of cases of children being picked on for no obvious reason or because they happened to be physically small or were unlucky enough to be assigned a locker next to the bully.

Systematic bullying on the basis of disability, race, sexual identity, or national origin constitutes discrimination, and is illegal, as well as immoral and pernicious. Quirky kids who are children of color are at higher risk, as are children in these other categories that have historically been targets of racism, discrimination, and bullying, which can amount to persecution—and that have not always been appropriately addressed by school systems. There is, we hope, increasing awareness of the prevalence of subtle and not-so-subtle racism in our society, and about the importance of the conversations that all parents need to be having with their children. Parents of these kids who are at higher risk know all too well that they are going to have to be vigilant and make sure that the schools are appropriately vigilant and protective.

Bullying is increasingly being recognized as more than a minor social problem in schools. Schools need to protect their students. All schools and all teachers have a responsibility here, and parents need to make sure that they live up to it. Children need to know who in the school they can safely turn to for protection if they are feeling bullied or unsafe in any way. Children should be taught strategies to defend themselves, bullies should be punished promptly, and the whole school should cultivate an attitude of mutual respect and safety. We have had to refer children for counseling because of bad experiences they had at school with bullies, attempted to get school bus arrangements changed because our patients were afraid to ride the buses with bullies, and talked to teachers and principals in attempts to protect children who were scared to go to school. Sometimes these efforts simply have not worked, despite a willing school administration, and sometimes, in all honesty, the school administration has not been all that willing.

As we mentioned earlier, several lawsuits have been won on behalf of children whose schools failed to protect them when they were bullied. Schools are taking notice of these results. Psychologists and educators also have developed a number of protocols and curricula aimed at equipping children to deal more effectively with bullies and to protect themselves. These include at least one curriculum aimed specifically at children with ASD and several programs designed for working with schools to counteract bullying. To date, there is not a lot of evidence about whether these programs work for most children, but some important points need to be emphasized:

- Some programs teach children to reply with a smart comeback when they are teased. This is by and large not a great idea for most quirky kids, who are less likely to be able to gauge the effect of what they say.
- Carol Gray, author of *Gray's Guide to Bullying*, advises kids with ASD to memorize one sentence and say it well: "I need you to stop. I don't like that; stop it." Anyone with a child who has one of these diagnoses might want to examine Gray's full program, but the notion of one simple sentence as a response to bullying might work for many quirky kids of all types.

- All antibullying programs rely on the child's finding backup. Whatever the child says to the bully on the spot, he or she then has to be able to go to an adult and get help promptly. The school cannot have a "kids will be kids" or even a "boys will be boys" attitude toward bullying. The school needs to step up; the child needs to be protected; and the bully needs to face prompt consequences.

Being the target of bullying can be crippling for a quirky child, and the middle school years may be the most vulnerable. In addition to making a child unhappy, bullying can interfere with nascent social development during these complicated years, leaving the child hurt and stunted in connecting with other people.

You need to pressure the school, and by all means ask your pediatrician or your child's therapist to help you. And if that doesn't work, you should consider legal action. In addition, think about whether, in your child's best interests, you might want to change schools. Yes, in a certain sense, it's running away, and, yes, in a certain sense, "the bad guys" win, but it can also be an incredible escape and liberation for your child.

Some families of quirky kids do cite bullying as one of the factors that pushed them out of their schools. Homeschooling does not have to involve a multiyear commitment. You aren't necessarily promising to teach the child at home right through high school. But for the child who needs urgently to escape a middle school situation in which he is being tortured, and for the family with no satisfactory school options available, homeschooling can be a respite and a chance to relax, take stock, and recover.

We haven't focused on cyberbullying in middle school, but, clearly, decisions about when to let a child have a smartphone and how closely to supervise social media activity do come up for many families in the middle school years, and will be heavily influenced by whatever seems to be the norm in your child's class. We offer the general advice that it's better to be a little behind the curve here; your child should not be one of the first in the class to be on social media. When you do decide that it's the appropriate time for a smartphone, you will need to have very clear conversations with your child about how social media interactions work and about what's okay and what's not okay; you also need to establish from the beginning that you are entitled to check the messages coming through. Cyberbullying is a huge issue for some kids, and quirky children, much as they love screens, may find the complex rules of digital social interaction difficult to figure out. Parents aren't always the best at understanding this either, but you need to keep trying and keep talking, and consider involving an older sibling or a beloved babysitter—someone closer to your child's age who can help decipher this side of life as your child takes those first steps.

The Cool and the Uncool

In middle school, quirky kids are seldom numbered among the desperately cool. The lucky ones are over on the more oblivious side during these years. Boys, especially, can often avoid the issue and remain a little more childlike a little longer. If you are lucky, your child will be in a middle school where there is an entire group of children who are simply untroubled by the cool-uncool axis. That is, they are clearly not in the running, but they are also clearly not even competing. These kids, the ones not in any hurry to take on the prerogatives of adolescence, the ones not dying to be asked to the parties to which they are not invited, can be the appropriate companions for your quirky child.

As we said in Chapter 7, there is, nowadays, a certain nascent nerd-pride movement, at least in some schools. Many kids seem to be happy to identify themselves as nerds and look out at the world from that perspective, with a certain sense of superiority. Those who self-identify as nerds are unlikely to be torturing themselves over not being cool: they may actually be proud of it. As a 13-year-old boy said to one of us in horror, "Are you kidding? I'm a nerd! Nerds don't go to school dances!"

The saddest quirky child is deeply aware of cool and uncool and longs to join the club that may never accept her as a member. This is certainly not unique to quirky children, but it can be heartbreaking to watch when a child combines the exquisite awareness of what she wants with certain traits and attributes that indelibly mark her as someone who will not get it. And so we are left with a certain paradox: The more oblivious the child, in many cases, the easier the social aspects of the middle school years may be. The more acutely socially aware the child, the more miserable she may make herself, appreciating not only her exact place in the hierarchy but also the place she wants and cannot have.

Friendships

Middle school friendships can be powerful. If your child finds the right friend, or friends, during these years, the difficult transition to adolescence and high school can be much easier. Friends during these years reinforce a child's identity and preferences and offer advice—much more valuable, and much more readily heeded, than a parent's—about every aspect of life, from popular culture to school activities.

Chrissie did make a couple of friends last year. She's especially close to one girl, who slept over for her birthday in June. They visit back and forth pretty often. They've been eating lunch together in the school cafeteria. Chrissie often takes the initiative to call her, which

I think is great. She's overcoming her fear of voicemail, she's able to leave messages that make sense now, and she's pretty happy when her calls are returned. So all in all, she's growing up into a nice, if slightly awkward, girl.

Girls tend to be more socially aware and more likely to appreciate the nuances and webs of relationships through which middle school girl culture operates. Also, girls are just plain nastier to one another than boys, with cruelties so complex and subtle that many grown men cannot understand them. Girls, even more than boys, may define themselves by their social place in the world. Boys this age often travel in a pack, with room in the pack for those who lag behind a little bit developmentally. On the other hand, a boy who does find himself excluded may become the target of physical violence, whether pushing and shoving or real fighting.

This is the time when you are hoping that some of the groundwork you laid with your child during the elementary school years—all those months and months of social skills training—will yield a more socially skilled child. How else can you support your quirky child through the minefield of middle school friendships?

- Accept that it's pretty much out of your hands. You can't just call the parent of a 12-year-old, the way you did the parent of a 6-year-old, and say, "Can Susie please come over and play with Mary?"
- More and more, a splinter skill, a special interest, or a talent may provide your child with a way to find peers, companions, and friends. If your child has something she likes to do and does well, she should spend as much time on it as possible in as social a setting as possible.
- Support your child's friendships, as they emerge. Get to know the parents of the friends. Offer the occasional evening or weekend activity—a movie, bowling, pizza—as a treat for the kids.
- Don't go overboard. You don't throw all the house rules out the window just to please a potential friend. It's normal for kids this age to push a little bit for adult privileges, but that doesn't mean you have to say yes to a request to take them to a midnight R-rated movie.
- Keep community activities in mind: scouting, church groups, sports teams, charitable organizations. Anywhere that your child plays and works with other children within a fairly set structure can be a great help.
- Encourage extracurricular activities, which are more important in middle school. Working on the school newspaper or serving on the student council can lead directly to high school activities and can give your child a circle of acquaintances beyond the homeroom class or the seventh grade.

- Social life is happening more and more on social media, even in middle school. Some quirky kids will find these interactions easier to manage than face-to-face contacts, because they won't have to worry about nonverbal cues, and they can take their time composing what they post, but others will find the complex dynamics of virtual social life bewildering, and may be crushed to realize that virtual relationships that matter to them tremendously don't actually translate into real friendships.
- Remember that sometimes you will strategize and plan, and other times your child will take over and show you the way.

One day, Megan came home from school and announced, "Every kid in my class is going to sleep-away camp this summer. I want to go, too." We were stunned. She was so dependent on us for everything and hadn't ever spent the night anywhere else. The morning she was supposed to leave, she asked us to call the camp and tell them she would come next year. She was terrified. We took her literally kicking and screaming. She cried and had a tantrum for a very long time. The following morning, she calmed down a bit and had a wonderful time. She went for four summers for a month each time. She really didn't have any friends there, but she was included in everything because that's the way of the camp.

The Approach of Adolescence

Imagine sitting outside a middle school, a building that houses only seventh and eighth graders. Observe the kids going in in the morning or coming out in the afternoon. You'll see boys who are 6 feet tall and boys who are 4 feet tall. Girls who look 25, both in their physical development and in their hair, makeup, and clothing, and girls who are almost indistinguishable from those 4-feet-tall boys. Many girls will be taller than most of the boys. A few boys will have crashed right through puberty, while many others will be in the embarrassing in-between phase of breaking voices and strange new body odors.

Their social lives will vary just as wildly. Some of those eighth-grade girls are dating high school juniors and live from dance to dance. They know more than you think about drinking and drugs, not to mention sex. Some of their classmates are still, literally, playing with dolls.

The positive aspect of all this variation is that in most middle school environments, there is room at both ends of the continuum. Everybody is going through a transition, some in fits and starts, some smoothly, some with terrifying speed, and some with agonizing slowness. Eventually, most of them will catch up at least physically, but it can be a strange, even scary, time.

Puberty

Puberty hits many quirky children like the proverbial ton of bricks. Their bodies erupt in all kinds of directions. Their emotions, maybe never under good control in the first place, take off on the hormonal roller coaster of adolescence. Explain puberty to your child in terms that make sense to him or her. Tailor your explanation to where your child is developmentally, both in understanding and in physical change. When we ask our middle school–aged patients whether they learned about puberty in school, they always say they have, but then frequently turn out to have absorbed only scattered pieces of information, much of it somewhat dubious. Go over the basics, and try to answer any questions they may have as clearly as possible. We often give out or recommend *It's Perfectly Normal*, by Robie Harris, to adolescents because it contains excellent chapters on puberty. For the child whose understanding is less advanced, she has also written *It's So Amazing!* You definitely want to have one of these books—or some other book you like—around so that your child can do some quiet private reading *after* you have had "the talk."

Puberty and Boys

If there is no father in the home and the mother feels it would be better for him to talk to a man, enlist an older relative or a male pediatrician. Tell your child frankly and clearly about wet dreams. Quirky children, who may not be in touch with their bodies, can be terrified by nocturnal emissions. He needs to know that they happen to all boys as they grow and that they aren't wrong or dirty or disgusting.

Tell him about masturbation and that it's OK, everyone does it sometimes, and you did it, too. Make it clear that it's only to be done in private, something that people do to make themselves feel good, and that this particular good feeling is a sexual feeling.

Explain personal hygiene as he reaches puberty:

- His sweat will start to smell, so he needs to be scrupulous about showering after exercise and wearing clean clothes.
- Deodorant. Toothbrushing. Shampoo.
- If he is uncircumcised, he needs to start routinely retracting his foreskin and washing under it every time he showers.

Tips for "The Talk"

- Traditionally, the adult of the same gender gives the talk, although some parents—and kids—are comfortable discussing these subjects across gender lines.
- You need to use all the terms—that means the slang and the vulgarities—that your child may hear in school to refer to pubertal changes and other physical manifestations. Your goal is for your child to understand what is happening to her own body and not to be bewildered by the conversation around her in school.
- This is not really the birds-and-bees conversation. You can provide as much information about human reproduction as you want, but the main goal is to equip your child to understand and survive the onset of puberty.
- Discuss the topic of touching—other kids or adults touching his or her body without permission or in ways he or she doesn't like—and what is considered inappropriate. Ensure that your child knows he or she should come to you if ever put into an uncomfortable position. Make it clear that you will never be angry with them for telling you something like this and that you will always protect them.

- If he's starting to be troubled by acne, take him to a doctor sooner rather than later. Acne is much more treatable now than it used to be. Untreated acne can make a kid feel really bad.

A good time to talk to your son is when you notice his body starting to change or by the time he is 13 years old, whichever comes first, or if he asks you about any of this ever. And then remind him, at regular intervals.

Puberty and Girls

If there is no mother in the home and the father feels it would be better for her to talk to a woman, enlist an older relative or a female pediatrician.

Tell her about menstruation and show her pictures so she'll understand what's happening. Tell her about the first time you got your period. We calculate loosely that daughters nowadays are beginning to menstruate about a year earlier than their mothers did, which may give you some sense of when to expect it for your daughter.

Explain to her, as clearly as possible, what she needs to do when she gets her period—at home or at school. Talk with her about how women handle their periods. Show her a sanitary napkin and a tampon. Practice with her how to use them, how to know when it's time to change them, and how to dispose of them. Emphasize that this will be her personal hygiene responsibility. For some quirky girls, the ones with sensory integration issues and awkward relationships with their own bodies, menstruation is no simple proposition. You need to start thinking about the routines and prompts that will make it easier. Talk about breast development, bras, and special sports bras for exercise.

Your daughter needs the same conversation about masturbation. Tell her it's OK, that everyone does it sometimes, that you did it, too. It's only to be done in private, something that people do to make themselves feel good, and that this particular good feeling is a sexual feeling.

Explain personal hygiene as she reaches puberty:

- Her sweat will start to smell, so she needs to be scrupulous about showering after exercise and wearing clean clothes.
- Deodorant. Toothbrushing. Shampoo.
- Emphasize regular baths or showers, especially during her period.
- Depending on hair growth and hair color, she may tell you that she wants to start shaving. Once again, this will pose particular challenges for a girl with fine motor delays or with sensory integration problems. Show her how to do it. Buy her easy-to-use razors and creams.
- If she's starting to be troubled by acne, take her to a doctor sooner rather than later. Acne is much more treatable now than it used to be. Untreated acne can make a kid feel really bad.

In terms of personal hygiene, Chrissie still needs a little push. Her skin is starting to break out, which grosses her out, so that has actually worked in our favor in terms of keeping her clean.

Talk to her when you see her body starting to change or by the time she is 12 years old, whichever comes first. Keep these conversations going. It's an ongoing process.

Dances and Dating

What about dating? What about dances? We can't say we like it, either as mothers or as pediatricians, but dating is going on in most middle school settings. The girls, at least, tend to be very aware of it. By eighth grade, there are often dances. In some schools, these are occasions for everyone to go in a pack, whereas in others, they are attended mostly by those kids who are already dating, already coupling off. Whatever the custom is in your school, you and your child are more or less stuck with it.

Encourage your child to attend school dances if she wants to and if she has friends to go with. Remind her to check with other kids about what will be worn, especially if she has trouble understanding subtle social cues. The dress code for some eighth grade dances is jeans and sweaters, and others involve what look to the maternal eye very much like cocktail dresses. Warn your child that middle school dances often don't feature a great deal of dancing. A few of the already-dating kids get out there and dance. A big group of boys stands on one side of the room, shoving one another, and a big group of girls stands on the other side of the room, talking about the boys—or about one another's cocktail dresses. Or maybe the girls dance with the girls and the boys watch them.

Trevor is naive about social situations. He is immature. His friends tend to be a year or more younger than he is. He frequently misjudges his abilities and is confused by other kids' reactions sometimes. For example, he came home from a "dance club" meeting at which the other kids laughed at him because of the way he dances. He demonstrated for me, and indeed, he dances in a peculiar way that other kids would think is weird. He still didn't get it when I explained it to him.

George is very interested in girls, and girls seem to like him. He doesn't have a girlfriend, but seven girls asked him to dance at the first dance he went to. I think this is because he stands by himself, and it's not so scary for the girls to ask a boy who is by himself. I asked his older sister if it was some kind of pity on the part of the girls, but she felt it wasn't. She felt that George is sweet and not scary or threatening.

Practicing a little dancing beforehand is generally a big favor to a quirky child. Our parental generation fortunately is not stuck with our own parents' lament: "I just can't do that rock-and-roll stuff you kids call dancing." Most of us can do it just fine, and it's an easy kind of dancing for a quirky kid to learn, because it has no rigid rules and does not require body contact. Put on some music, loosen up, and try to leave your child with the sense that it's OK to go to a dance and then not dance, but that if you try to dance, you'll be just fine.

But what about dating? Let's assume that your quirky child is not dating, at this point, but may be functioning in an environment in which other kids are coupling off. Keep your eyes and ears open, listen to what your child reports, and to what other parents are saying. If couples are obviously forming in the school, ask your child about that. Talk with your child about the fact that some kids are dating and others are not, about what dating actually means, and about his or her understanding of what is going on. If kids are clearly dating and it's on your child's mind, don't write it off. Make it clear that seventh grade is seventh grade, and for most people, serious dating occurs in high school, college, and beyond. In other words, from an adult perspective, what goes on in seventh grade is unlikely to be life-determining.

Your child may start asking questions about what your own social life was like in middle school, or about how you and your spouse or partner met. For some quirky kids, watching social patterns form among their peers, even if they aren't participating, opens up their curiosity for the first time about love and sex and relationships. Your child may also refuse to discuss the issue with you. Either way, make sure your child has access to good books and knows that the conversational door is always open.

There is always more going on in the way of sex, drugs, and alcohol in middle school than parents would like to believe. That doesn't mean that all the kids are involved or even that your child has any idea about this. But somewhere in that middle school are a couple of kids whose sexual experimentations have gone well beyond a little kissing, and they may or may not be conveying their discoveries to the group at large. Similarly, somewhere in that middle school are kids who know more about drugs and drinking than anyone thinks they do, and they may well be passing this information on. You will not find an absolutely protected school and social environment for your child, no matter how much you would like one. You need to be ready to help your child interpret, understand, and judge—and above all, stay safe.

Safety

Quirky children's poor sense of social skills, their relative immaturity, and their eagerness to be part of the group can make them vulnerable to being pushed sexually, even abused. That's one reason why the talk (discussed on pages 206–209) should always include the subject of being touched when you don't want to be. Any child in middle school who is going out to dances needs to know that kids sometimes try to push other kids into doing things they don't want to do, whether it's drinking beer behind the gym or playing strip poker. Your child needs to hear, over and over, that he or she is entitled to say no and entitled to ask an adult for help, and that you will never be angry about any of these things.

Because middle school is often a time of increasing independence, it's also worth repeating the warnings about being wary of strangers, with a special emphasis on sexual predators. An eighth-grade girl needs to know that the guy who sits next to her on the subway and asks if she goes to college in the area is bad news, however momentarily flattered she may be. She needs to know that she should get up and change her seat if he persists. To understand the potential danger, she must have some idea of what he might be after.

Parents should also keep in mind the importance of internet safety, especially because for many quirky kids, what happens online is an important part of their social lives. This will not be a new topic in your family because you have been discussing and monitoring internet use since you first allowed your child to use social media. However, it is important to keep talking and reviewing the rules of staying safe online, and that means explaining to your child what some of the dangers are. The same factors that may make that eighth-grade girl vulnerable on the subway may mean that at home, one of these kids is going to be a tempting target for an online predator. Take a look at the American Academy of Pediatrics (AAP) recommendations for media use and stay involved in their online lives (https://www.healthychildren.org/English/family-life/Media/Pages/How-to-Make-a-Family-Media-Use-Plan.aspx).

Almost all parents keep their kids under closer supervision now than when we were children. Quirky children's parents are often even more protective. Parents of quirky kids tend to know where they are at any given moment, defer independent travel and escort them back and forth, and hover more closely. As a result, these children can reach middle school age without having had a lot of practice and drill about not getting into cars with strangers, not talking to people who come up to them on the street, and not responding to the questions of the guy on the subway. You're going to have to explain all this to your child as clearly as you can and probably take him on a few experimental journeys where he takes the bus or the subway "alone," with you a few yards away, or he walks home "alone," with you trailing a block behind. Doing this probably will not be easy, and you will worry about whether your child is really ready. However, you do not want to send your child to high school with no sense of the world's dangers and no practice in navigating them. You have to walk a careful line here; you don't want your child to feel scared of everyone and everything, but you do want your child to be careful and vigilant and able to manage independently in the world, which means that your child should be able to identify a possible threat.

High School

High school is often a little easier socially than middle school. In most places, the rigid conformity of middle school relaxes. There are more possible social strata, more groups with which to identify, and a wider range of normal. Almost all adolescents struggle with issues of identity, risk-taking, achievement, substance abuse, sexuality, family relations, and self-esteem. The developmental task of every adolescent is to separate, to become an individual adult. However, being the parent from whom that separation takes place is never easy. Against this somewhat tumultuous background of change, rebellion, and self-definition, the quirks that are present in middle school or toward the end of the elementary years can be much less noticeable. Many high schools are more forgiving, more varied, or simply bigger.

However, high school is where some kids—and not just quirky kids, by any means—seem to go seriously wrong. As students get closer to adulthood, the ways in which they can hurt themselves—or others—get more dangerous, with cars and alcohol and drugs and sex coming into the picture in various ways. We need to address some of the darker fears that confront parents, which is not to say that they will be relevant for every quirky child, but it is important to acknowledge that these concerns are out there. There's the very frightening image of the child who is excluded or feels marginalized and then turns violent, and there have been school shootings and other public tragedies in which this isolation was part of the perpetrator's profile. A teenager who says, writes, tweets, or posts on social media anything that could be interpreted as a threat will probably be taken very seriously. A quirky boy whose special interests include anything to do with the military or weapons may frankly scare people, and he may be asked to undergo an evaluation. Many school districts have a professional, usually a child and adolescent psychiatrist, who can conduct threat assessments if a concern is raised. If you feel your child is increasingly withdrawn or angry or perhaps getting drawn into something that alarms you, you need to get professional help.

We aren't trying to say that the kids who have committed school shootings were necessarily quirky kids, by our definition, but rather that these relatively new and scary images have come to be associated with high school loners and outcasts, with kids who became sullen and withdrawn and often were the targets of bullying.

If you sense that anything like this may be going on, you need to get help immediately. Your child needs to see a counselor, and you need to be in close touch with the school to find out what is going on with respect to classes and social life. It's more likely, however, that your child's high school social life will be affected by more mundane factors, that your child will find a somewhat precarious footing on the rapidly shifting ground of adolescence, and that she will eventually get safely across. But it can be a pretty winding, indirect, and painful trip. Any quirky kid dealing with some extra challenges along with common everyday adolescence surely ought to at least consider the advantages of having a counselor or therapist. Plenty of people who work with the high school population believe that basically every adolescent could use such a relationship.

Friendships

Almost every high school is divided into multiple little worlds, and some exist side by side for 4 years straight, never touching. The secret to high school success is to find the right zone. For the nonathletic and chronically uncool, many watering holes are available: the math club, chess club, computer club. There's also orchestra, the debate team, or any other activity that reflects a child's true interests. And as we've said, it's generally more acceptable these days to be a geek or a nerd, and understanding computer technology can be a real social asset.

If the high school itself does not offer the right niche, think again about community and religious activities. Some children simply do better with adults, and they just might be happier in charge of ticket sales for a local theater group every weekend. But if your child is participating in an activity such as that, keep suggesting that it might be worthwhile to find a high school equivalent— someplace where tickets need to be sold—that would enable your child to connect at least a little to a group of schoolmates.

You don't have to be defined by an extracurricular activity in high school, though it can be a major help in finding like-minded peers. You can find an academic identity if you have a subject you love. Teachers have pretty good noses for this, and the girl who gets totally carried away by geometry will probably be noticed and appreciated by her teacher. Your child can find his or her niche in art or shop or any vocational courses (from auto mechanics to cooking) that the school happens to offer.

> George is exceptionally musical and plays the trombone in the school band. He has perfect pitch, which only 1 in 10,000 people in the general population has but 1 out of 20 with ASD has. His music teachers are thrilled. They've never had a kid with perfect pitch before. And George likes to play in the band. He'll practice when he is told to, but he doesn't spontaneously play on his own. He also sings beautifully but doesn't seem to realize it or care about it.

Every once in a while, a high school kid asks us to be excused from gym. Sometimes it's a kid who is getting teased or bullied, but sometimes it's someone who feels self-conscious about a changing body or is inept at games and sports. Under those circumstances, we try to refer for counseling, we discuss body-image issues, but you know what else we do? We give the kid a note to get out of sports.

It's true that exercise is important for physical health, as well as well-being and mental health, and it may be especially important for children with ADHD, many of whom are quirky kids. So certainly, some of the most self-conscious kids—the child who has obesity, the boy who is embarrassed by the breast development happening in part because of overweight—would profit most from taking gym. We talk with these families about the benefits of physical activity for physical and mental health, and we talk about limiting screen time and building in family walks and outdoor activities. But for those kids who see gym as being forced, kicking and screaming, into a setting in which people make fun of their bodies, making them attend is probably not building good habits of regular exercise. Sometimes a teenager needs a respite. Sometimes schools offer what is called *adaptive physical education*, which may be better suited to some teenagers' needs. More schools are installing exercise equipment, and some offer students a fitness option for physical education in which they can work out and measure their progress only against themselves. For the quirky child who has some athletic ability, a team sport can offer an automatic high school identity, a circle of friends, and perhaps an area in which to shine even if academics are difficult.

With a little bit of luck, all the social skills your child has acquired through the years, combined with the wider variety of social options, will give him or her a fighting chance to find a peer or peers, a friend, or a circle. Stand back and watch, try to express a counter opinion about prevailing fads and fashions ("no, you do not need to wear very tight revealing clothing that makes you self-conscious," "no, vaping is not a safe thing to do," "no, it will not make you seem cool to lie about your age and get a tattoo"), and offer whatever advice you can. Certainly, support the friendships that seem to be good ones, offer to chauffeur, pick up at the movies, and open your home for the occasional get-together or homework group effort. You are entitled to set certain limits, and with a quirky child, you should make those limits as clear and explicit as possible. Go ahead and set curfews and demand the name, address, and phone number for any place your child is going. Go ahead and say "no" to unsafe and illegal ideas (10 kids in the minivan driven by one who just got a license, heading for the shore 200 miles away on a holiday weekend). Wall yourself off with all the traditional parental lines ("If everybody else jumped off the Brooklyn Bridge . . ."). Quirky adolescents who have not always found it easy to be included can be so overjoyed to find an opportunity, a potential social slot, that they are desperate to go along with any crazy ride. Stand your ground and feel comfortable saying "no."

For many adolescents nowadays, a large part of friendship takes place by text message and social media. Be aware of the kind of activity on your child's phone: Instagram accounts that offer stories of impossibly cool adolescent lives, intense discussions of the school day via group text, or whatever the app of the moment may be. Adolescents, almost by definition, are more skillful at navigating this technology than their parents, but you need to continue to keep the conversational window open, asking to have things explained, prying a little, and setting firm limits on screen use that you've been enforcing since your child was young. Adolescents should not have their phones in their bedrooms (especially in their beds) overnight; there's a real risk that they'll be up texting, worried about missing out. They also should not have phones at the dinner table. In fact (and this does not apply only to quirky kids), this is a time when you need to be discussing cell phone manners (it's rude to check your phone when Grandpa is telling a joke, even if it's a joke you know; it's rude to text at the theater; and everyone can tell when you're sneaking a look at your phone under the table, so don't). Take a look at the AAP screen time and media use recommendations mentioned earlier. It's completely normal for adolescents to prefer interacting with their friends and peers to being stuck with their parents, so these restrictions are unlikely to be received with joy, but if you apply these rules to the whole family and stick to them, you will be helping your child get a little respite from what has become the 24/7 social cycle of high school. Similarly, you may get a break yourself from a culture in which it's the norm in many jobs to send emails all evening and weekend, if not all night long.

In fact, more generally through all the ups and downs of adolescence, you continue to exercise the prerogatives (and exorcise the anxieties) of every high school parent, including trying to keep your child safe, setting curfews, arguing about screens and phones, making rules about drinking and drugs, and just plain hanging in there. You're doing the right thing by staying in the game and keeping the conversation going.

Love and Dating, Sex, and Sexuality

Some quirky kids are going to make it all the way through high school and still not understand what all the fuss is about. Really. These girls and boys will, of course, have undergone the physical changes of puberty, which they may regard with amusement or disgust or may seem to have hardly noticed. However, they have somehow escaped a little longer than most the emotional upheavals, susceptibility to crushes and falling in love, and yearning and fantasizing that are the lot of most high school students. As a parent, you will, of course, worry a little about this, but you will probably also feel somewhat blessed and somewhat spared.

> **Megan was invited to her friend's birthday party. By this time, her friend had a boyfriend. She had started dating in tenth grade, and Megan, of course, had no interest at all in boys. So her friend spent most of the party with her boyfriend, and Megan didn't really know any of the other kids. She called her friend afterward and said, "I didn't like the way you acted at your birthday party." Her friend has never called her since, and the friendship is basically over.**

Other quirky kids are swept away and turned upside down by their first rushes of sexual attraction, sexual fantasy, and romantic emotion. These, after all, are kids who have always been inclined to obsessional thinking. They may find themselves consumed by a crush, obsessed with a romantic object to the point of constantly thinking of and fantasizing about that person. They may even end up doing something that looks rather like stalking that person. Quirky kids may overstep the line and make fools of themselves, or they may even occasionally elicit complaints or concerns about safety on the part of their adored.

Other adolescents—quirky or not—are tortured by doubts about sexual identity. Sometimes they are merely responding to the rather diffuse sexuality of these early postpubertal years, in which people often develop crushes on teachers, close friends, and singers and movie stars of both genders. Others are realizing that they are not heterosexual—or not exclusively heterosexual—which can be a complex and difficult realization for a high school kid. An adolescent struggling with issues of sexual or gender identity in a homophobic culture (we're talking high school locker rooms after all) is at risk for depression and even suicide. Such a kid needs to feel unprejudiced support and unconditional love. A quirky adolescent, who already has complex feelings about being different from other people and being outside the group, may be particularly bewildered, troubled, or depressed. In pediatrics, we've learned a lot over the past couple of decades about how to take care of gender nonconforming adolescents in a helpful and nonjudgmental way, and a good number of quirky kids fall into this category. If your child is expressing any issues around gender identity, make sure to find an adolescent medicine doctor or a clinic (major medical centers all have them) where there will be some experience and expertise.

Dating scenes vary enormously from high school to high school. There will always be a certain number of kids coupling off and going steady, but in many circles, hanging out in groups, even including couples, is common and this may be less pressured. In all high schools, formal school events, dances, and proms are held, and, of course, parties occur outside school.

We'll say it again: Wherever you are, whatever you think the school enforces, more is going on with regard to sex (and drugs and drinking) than you know or would hope to see. We live in an era in which many high school students are sexually active and with multiple partners. Whether your child is in that category or not, he or she is certainly exposed to the conversation, information, and behavior of those who are. Our job as parents is to make sure that our children gain the judgment they need to evaluate what they see and to give them the support needed to function in that environment.

If your child does begin dating, you can offer support and suggestions, but you probably are not going to be listened to. However, a willingness to do some of the driving, or an offer to treat to a special dinner or theatrical event, can help the relationship along and give you some sense of where it's going. Just as quirky kids may be at higher risk of developing those obsessive crushes, they may also be more likely to be destroyed when a high school relationship comes to its natural end. For some quirky kids who are not easily social, this ending may bring disillusionment, despair, and clinical depression.

As in middle school, the desire to be included can make high school students vulnerable to sexual exploitation. It's an awful thing to say, but you probably should be suspicious of a daughter's sudden popularity, especially if accompanied by other danger signs: mixing only with older kids, all boys and no girls calling the house, and vagueness about where she is going and what she is doing.

When it comes to social media, kids who are vulnerable and eager to be liked may be pressured into some form of sexting—sending photos of themselves, perhaps, which may then be passed around and forwarded online. Once again, you need to have these conversations with your child, and you need to play the heavy, explaining how things don't stay private on the internet, and that being pressured to send suggestive photos (or to let someone take suggestive photos of you) is in fact a form of abuse. Kids also need to understand that sending or receiving sexual photographs can compromise them legally and some of these cases have been treated as child pornography because they involved images of underage subjects.

We have heard about a number of older teens and young adults with ASD who have a fascination with child pornography. We suspect that some of these individuals are trying to come to grips with their own sexuality, yet their developmental age lags behind their chronological age, and they may find themselves more comfortable with images of children. This is extremely dangerous territory, and if you have any reason to think your adolescent or child may be looking at such websites, you need to have a serious conversation in which you explain that this behavior is illegal and dangerous. While they may be unlikely to act on any of these urges, anyone can be arrested for having child pornography on his personal laptop. There is no gray area here: child pornography is illegal. An adolescent who is bewildered by his own sexual thoughts needs to be talking with a therapist, but he also needs to understand that this set of images is absolutely off limits.

After all these negatives and fears, let's offer a word or two about the possibility of finding positive romantic relationships. Adolescence is a time of exploration, and in their romantic relationships, as well as in their friendships, quirky kids can find new opportunities to make connections, form affectionate bonds, and care for one another. Adolescent affection, attachment, and even love can be beautiful and moving and, of course, profoundly educational.

The romantic lives of many high school students are carefully shielded from parental examination. If there's going to be a conversation, you probably have to initiate it:

- Talk to your child about sex and also about love. Talk about the power of the emotion and the difficulty of fixing your affections on someone who doesn't return them.
- Use movies, TV shows, or news stories as ways to discuss these subjects. Quirky kids often have unusual takes on human relationships.
- Use books to open a dialogue. Find out how your child views the decisions made by Romeo and Juliet or any other characters who happen to wander

onto the scene. (*Romeo and Juliet* is read in many eighth and ninth grades, and it is, after all, a story of crazy, obsessive love that ultimately destroys both characters!)

- Make absolutely sure that your child understands the physiology and mechanics of sex and the meanings of all the most commonly used terms, however vulgar.

- Do not assume that your child's sexual feelings will be heterosexual. You want your child, who may be struggling with issues of sexual identity, to feel comfortable coming to you for help and support. Many people in early adolescence find themselves attracted both to those of their own sex and to those of the opposite sex. And if your child talks about same-sex or opposite-sex crushes, be positive and supportive, but don't assume that that necessarily means sexual identity is determined for life.

- You owe it to your child to make sure that he or she has a good understanding of how to prevent pregnancy and of the dangers of sexually transmitted diseases and how to prevent them. Although you can state clearly that abstinence is your preferred choice for your adolescent, the truth is, you need to talk about condoms and how important they are and how to use them.

- If you have a son, you *must* discuss with him the issue of date rape. A quirky boy who doesn't quite get other people's social signals and who pushes a girl too far is going to find himself in terrible trouble. He has to understand that he must absolutely clarify whether each additional intimacy is welcomed and must desist immediately if it is not. And as we've said, you should convey to all adolescents that they have the absolute right to set bounds on touching and other sexual activity, and that "no" should always mean "no." Since quirky kids may sometimes be targets because of their vulnerability, it is especially important to review with them what to do if they feel at all pushed.

- Talk about sex. Talk about love. Talk about taking care of people you love and about accepting it when someone doesn't love you back. Talk about relationships and what happens when they go wrong and about all the joys and satisfactions when they go right.

Alcohol and Drugs

Most of what there is to say about alcohol and drugs and the quirky adolescent could apply just as well to all adolescents.

The desperate desire to be accepted may make some not-easily-accepted kids do dumb things. Many high schools now have zero-tolerance policies in which any breach in the drug or alcohol rules can land a student in serious trouble. Make sure your child understands the rules and the danger.

For adolescents taking psychotropic medications, discussing with your doctor any possible interactions with alcohol or common street drugs is a basic issue of health and safety. Your child's doctor should be willing to talk this through with her and make it clear that the risks can be severe.

Sometimes when teenagers find that alcohol and various other drugs are available, they begin treating themselves for long-standing symptoms, without realizing what they are doing. Thus, for example, marijuana may calm the insufficiently medicated adolescent with ADHD. Be aware that adolescents may either share their prescription medications with their friends (or even sell them) or start taking their own medications in the wrong doses or on the wrong schedule to achieve a desired sensation. Some stimulants are popular recreational drugs in some circles.

Anyone who is near the edge of mental illness is at much greater risk when it comes to drug use, especially regarding hallucinogens. A single LSD (lysergic acid diethylamide) or PCP (phencyclidine) experience can precipitate a psychotic break, especially in a person whose state of mind is already tenuous. Your child may need very specific scenarios for avoiding trouble with drugs or alcohol, the kind of step-by-step instructions that you once provided for birthday parties.

Tell your child:

- Never go to a party if the parents are out of town or not at home.
- If you find yourself at such a party, call us and we will come get you, and we will not be mad at you.
- If someone offers you drugs, say "no thank you" and go somewhere else.
- If people are drunk or acting strangely, call us and we will come get you, and we will not be mad at you.

For many parents, the single greatest anxiety is about mixing drinking and driving. You need another set of explicit instructions.

Tell your child:

- Never get into a car where the driver might be drunk.
- If you are in a situation like that—however far away you are, however late at night it is, however against the rules it is for you to be there in the first place—call us and we will come and get you, and we will not be mad at you.

- If, on the other hand, you are riding with someone who is drunk—
  or drinking and driving yourself once you have a license—terrible
  consequences will follow, and you will have lost our trust.

Your job, as parents, is to help your quirky adolescent make the most of his
high school years, reminding him of your love and acceptance, cheering him
on in his achievements, and supporting him socially as best you can to help
him enjoy the pleasures of his peer group without falling prey to the dangers. It
isn't easy and it isn't always pretty, but together you can make it through.

Physical Distancing

You probably noticed that we did not make note of the circumstances in which
this book is going to print, with the demands for social distancing and infection control. Social distancing is a particular challenge, or perhaps a welcome
relief, for kids whose main difficulty is in the social realm. Every aspect of
social life, and not just for kids or quirky kids, has obviously been affected by
the need to distance ourselves from each other. During the pandemic, kids
were deprived of social contact with friends and relatives, including, and
maybe especially, their grandparents. Families got creative about virtual visits,
bedtime stories, and playdates. Optimistically, we are hoping that by the time
you read this, in-person social life is strong again, but we do want to salute
all the dedicated and exhausted parents who helped their kids through this
extraordinary time.

3

The Science, the Medical Science, and the Pseudoscience of Quirky Kids

Literary Glimpses

Hanno's gratitude to his teacher was boundless, and he abandoned himself to his guidance. The same boy who brooded over arithmetic without any hope of ever understanding it, despite all his special tutoring at school, understood everything that Herr Pfuhl said to him at the piano, understood it and made it his own—if you can be said to make your own what has always belonged to you. Edmund Pfuhl, however, seemed to him like a tall angel dressed in a brown swallowtail coat, who took him in his arms each Monday afternoon to lead him from his everyday misery into the realm of sound, where everything was gentle, sweet, consoling, and serious.

In his heart, Thomas Buddenbrook was not pleased with little Johann and how he was developing....He would fix on these very points: the dreamy softness, the weeping, the total lack of vigor and energy....He was not doing well in his subjects. He was absent too often because of illness and was totally inattentive because his thoughts would linger over some harmonic relationship or some unraveled marvel in a piece of music....Senator Buddenbrook knew nothing about such details; but he saw that his son's development, whether as a result of nature or external influences, was not, as yet, headed in the direction he would have wished....If he could have suppressed and banned the music at least—it was certainly not good for his health, absorbed all his mental energies, and made him ill-suited for the practical side of life. And that dreamy way he had about him—did it not sometimes border on simple-mindedness?

—Thomas Mann, *Buddenbrooks*, 1901

Speak sharply to Jeremy and you will bowl him over; he can't stand up to things. You'll get further being gentle with him, but I always remember that too late. He puts me in a fury. I don't see how he could let himself go the way he has. No, letting yourself go means you had to be something to start with, and Jeremy was never anything. He was born like this. He is, and always has been, pale and doughy and overweight, pear-shaped, wide-hipped. He toes out when he walks.

His hair is curly and silvery-gold, thin on top. His eyes are nearly colorless. (People have asked me if he is an albino.) There's no telling where he manages to find his clothes: baggy slacks that start just below his armpits; mole-colored cardigan strained across his stomach and buttoning only in the middle, exposing a yellowed fishnet undershirt, top and bottom, and tiny round-toed saddle oxfords. Saddle oxfords? For a man?... [Our mother] thought the sun rose and set in him. She thought he was a genius. (I myself have sometimes wondered if he isn't a little bit retarded. Some sort of selective, unclassified retardation that no medical book has yet put its finger on.) He failed math, he failed public speaking (of course), he went through eighth grade *twice* but he happened to be artistic so Mother thought he was a genius. "Some people just don't have mathematical minds," she said, and she showed us his report card—A+ in art, A in English, A+ in deportment. (What else? He had no friends, there was no one he could have whispered with in class.)

—Anne Tyler, *Celestial Navigation*, 1974

He was still leaning against the wall. He had been leaning against the wall when I came into the room, his arms folded across his chest. As I pointed he brought his arms down and pressed the palms of his hands against the wall. They were white hands, sickly white hands that had never seen the sun, so white they stood out garishly against the dull cream wall in the dim light of Jem's room.

I looked from his hands to his sand-stained pants; my eyes traveled up his thin frame to his torn denim shirt. His face was as white as his hands, but for a shadow on his jutting chin. His cheeks were thin to hollow-ness; his mouth was wide; there were shallow, almost delicate indentations at his temples, and his gray eyes were so colorless I thought he was blind. His hair was dead and thin, almost feathery on top of his head.

When I pointed to him his palms slipped slightly, leaving greasy sweat streaks on the wall, and he hooked his thumbs in his belt. A strange small spasm shook him, as if he heard fingernails scrape slate, but as I gazed at him in wonder the tension slowly drained from his face. His lips parted into a timid smile, and our neighbor's image blurred with my sudden tears.

"Hey, Boo," I said.

—Harper Lee, *To Kill a Mockingbird*, 1960

What You Should Know

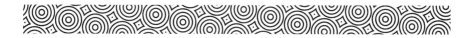

Many quirky kids manage all right at home and in school and even in the social realm, thanks to a vigilant and understanding family, a tolerant environment, a terrific school, or a good friend at the right moment. But the truth is, those children are the ones who don't carry the heaviest baggage. Their quirks are milder, perhaps less troubling to those around them, and maybe they are less rigid in how they behave. Many other children—even with wonderful families, homes, schools, and friends—still need extra help along the way. And then there are the many, many children whose life situations are more stressful, who may have to deal with a less-than-ideal school setting or a less-than-sympathetic peer group and may hit a bad emotional or developmental patch as a consequence. In other words, many quirky kids need extra help and support along the way, sometimes a little, sometimes a lot.

In Part 3, we look at the wide range of supports and interventions that parents may find themselves trying: therapies, home behavioral programs, and medications. We examine what is understood—and not understood—about these children from the standpoint of medical science. We would all like science to provide us with straightforward answers about the causes of developmental differences, but such explanations are rare. Still, research is filling in a lot of gaps in information about these children, which can make it possible to understand them better and sometimes help them more effectively.

Many less-than-scientific theories are also circulating about quirky children and the roots of developmental differences, and a lot of not so scientifically based therapies are available. Our goal is to help explain what has been tested and shown to work, and also to give you a framework for thinking about new ideas as they come along.

If you are just starting to delve into the world of therapies and medications, there may be terms and outcomes discussed in Part 3 that make you confront your biggest fears and worst-case possibilities. No one, looking at a quirky 3-year-old, wants to think in terms of years of medications and five different therapies. Not all quirky kids need medications and not all need intensive therapeutic support. However, many quirky kids go through a difficult phase at some point, and you will at least want to consider whether a therapeutic intervention or a medicine might help. You need to know what's out there.

It is certainly not your job, as a parent, to try every therapy, nutritional program, behavior-modification exercise, and new religion that may be suggested to you. It is your job, however, to look at your child and think about what could make his day-to-day life easier and more joyful—as childhood should be. This is why we have organized the chapters on therapies and medications according to problem or symptom: what's getting in the way? Whatever a child's underlying diagnosis, if the major daily problem is anxiety, you need to deal with the anxiety. For that reason, you may not want to read through these chapters from beginning to end; it may be more helpful to use them as resources and look up the specific problems that affect your child.

We watch parents wrestling with the obligation they feel to do as much as possible for their child. There are always more possibilities, another expert in another city, another therapist with a special intensive program, another blood test to look for some new trace element that someone thinks may be linked to the problem, another nutritional theory about how to modify the family diet. We don't suggest that you stop looking for alternatives that may be right for your child, but we do know you cannot go down every single path at once.

In picking and choosing the right kind of help for your child, you need to consider a few basic realities:

- What type of help your child needs depends on who he is and what his "package" is: his strengths and weaknesses and skills and problem areas.
- The help she needs will certainly vary as she grows; as she comes up against different situations and different expectations, she may need different supports, in quantity and in kind. Your goal in certain respects is to get her help early on, so that she can acquire the skills

she needs to function more smoothly when she's older. Other issues come to the fore only as children age and need to be dealt with later on.

- The type of help you get may differ depending on whom you ask. Psychiatrists tend to think in terms of psychopharmacology and starting kids on medications. Other practitioners might want to try something else first. This is not to say that one way is right and one is wrong, just to point out that, as the saying goes, "If the only tool you have is a hammer, everything looks like a nail."

- Keep an open mind about what might help; don't make blanket decisions (eg, no behavior-altering drugs, ever!) without learning what the possibilities are. The goal is to help your child, and you will help your child best by finding out as much as you can.

- You need to get over any embarrassment at having a child who goes to special therapy sessions or takes a medication. That doesn't mean this has to be everybody's business, but if your child senses that you are ashamed, she will be too.

Different children respond differently to any given kind of help. You will find out what's right for your child by knowing him well and testing everything you are told against that knowledge, against your experience, and against your common sense. You may only find out what really helps by trying it. Sometimes you may try things that are no help at all. It's important to remember that even within one relatively narrow category of therapist or specialist, people vary enormously in their skills, their personalities, their general approach, and, above all, their knowledge of quirky kids. You aren't just choosing the therapy, you're choosing the therapist. How much good your child gets out of treatment may depend as much on the fit with the therapist as on the need for the intervention.

Your best bet in almost any field is probably going to be someone who has worked with quirky children and knows the range of issues. Within any given specialty, training and experience can vary widely. You don't want your child to spend session after session with a speech therapist who focuses only on articulation issues if what he really needs is a speech and language therapist who will leave his diction alone and concentrate on helping him use language in realistic, practical ways.

Some parents speak of a eureka moment when they feel they finally met the person—the doctor, the therapist, the special education teacher—who really understood their child and their child's issues completely.

> When we met Dr. R, we could really see that he got our kids. We've met neurologists and OTs and PTs and our pediatrician, of course, but this was just a eureka moment, when we felt we've finally met someone who gets the whole picture. And we feel like he's going to see us through. We'll probably see him for years, now and again, and if things get rough, we know he's in our corner.

Keep an eye out for that one person whose understanding of your child seems to be larger, fuller, more complex, and more informed by experience. You want to stay in contact with that person. You want that person in your corner, helping you figure out how to respond to new challenges and adjusting whatever regimen you and your child have developed together.

All of this can add up to major decisions and complications in the lives of parents and quirky children, and siblings, too, for that matter. Take it on piece by piece. We realize that Part 3 contains a lot of information, and much more information is available on each individual topic. You need to regard the project of getting help and evaluating the help you get as a lifelong job, perhaps never to be definitively completed, and as a partnership with your child who will grow older and more able to participate in these choices and decisions. The goal is to help, and help means different things at different times. If your child is given a particular diagnosis, and you believe that it fits, you will certainly be able to find books for parents about that diagnosis, and you likely will be able to find parent advocacy groups and websites, many of which are listed in the resources section of this book. We don't want to suggest that this book is the ultimate resource for every diagnosis, and you certainly will want more information on the topics most directly of concern to you. But we hope the information offered here helps you think about this complex parental project, whether in the setting of a quirky kid with some specific difficulties or in the setting of a more global diagnosis.

Give yourself a break. How your child does in life is going to be a highly complex mix of the package he started with and the environment in which he grew, the help he received, the times in which he lived, and that thing called luck. You are doing your best, keeping an open mind and trying to stay in close touch with how he's doing, ready to change the mix if things are slipping. There is no one right way, and there is no sense beating yourself up about how much better everything would have been if you'd just done something differently. You do your best, and life only goes forward. The goal of therapy, medication, or any other support is not to bring your child to some guaranteed endpoint but to assist her along her own trajectory and help her function as well as possible as the person she is. And be ready for surprises—quirky kids are full of surprises.

During the 2020 global pandemic, with school closures and social distancing, a lot changed for quirky kids. Evaluations and therapies went virtual, and many special education services were similarly delivered over the internet (and still may be). We do not reference this specifically in the discussion of therapies that follows but want to acknowledge that for some children and families, this was and has been a barrier and a problem; some children have trouble engaging. The "digital divide" further increases inequities in services, and some therapists adapt to these modalities better than others. On the other hand, we have heard inspiring stories of dedicated therapists and supportive parents, and the learning curve here is steep. Some therapies can actually be delivered quite effectively on a virtual platform, which increases their availability to kids regardless of their location.

You are doing your best!

9

Therapies: Finding Help and Evaluating the Help You Find

Most quirky children encounter some difficulties in mastering expected skills at the expected time. No two children are alike—and no two children with the same label are exactly the same. One physically awkward or clumsy child may need a specialized physical education program, while the next might be reasonably well coordinated but have problems with fine motor skills such as buttoning or snapping. A third may have sensory processing disorder that affects many aspects of daily living. Almost all of these children struggle with social interactions, managing the interpersonal aspects of living with others, playing with others, and going to school with others. Call it what you will—social communication disorder, deficient theory-of-mind abilities, nonverbal learning disability, auditory-processing disorder—this aspect of development is skewed for most quirky kids, whether they are aware of it or not. Regardless of whether an individual child is aware, parents, teachers, coaches, camp counselors, and therapists—and most of all, peers—will be aware of the ways in which your child may need some help. In fact, as they grow and the social tasks expected of them become more complex (and the peer-group setting becomes less forgiving of eccentricity), many children who did not receive—or need—a diagnostic workup early in life will become the focus of increasing concern and attention.

Deciding when or whether to pursue any of the therapies that are recommended for quirky kids is quite a task. Sometimes, the developmental concerns are evident early in a child's life, prompting an early intervention (EI) referral. If you have concerns about your child's development in those early years, it's essential to obtain an assessment and to get help fast. Talk with your pediatrician and obtain a referral for EI, or you can refer yourself. In addition, ask if a more detailed assessment by a developmental specialist is warranted. There's good evidence that for children whose developmental differences are evident early in their lives, intensive early therapy—in particular, applied behavior analysis (ABA), which we discuss later in this chapter—can make a real difference. Interventions for the very young may follow one specific approach (eg, ABA) or may integrate aspects of several approaches (eg, many therapeutic preschool programs). Some families embark on intensive behavioral programs to deal with disturbing or disruptive behaviors or with noticeable delays. If families start down this path in the early years, it usually makes sense for intervention, therapy, and special support to continue—though they may change in nature—as the child grows. Often this leads to a special education evaluation as the child approaches school age, and this evaluation will, in turn, lead to a recommendation for more therapy. As children progress through elementary school, their teachers may continue to suggest new evaluations and new therapeutic possibilities, which may be profoundly helpful. But you can't follow every suggestion. It definitely helps to pause periodically and take stock, asking yourself whether new recommendations or, in fact, the familiar therapies you are already pursuing really make sense for your child, here and now.

We've said this before, but it bears repeating: Individual children change as they grow, and so do the expectations of what they will be able to do. Therefore, the help they need—or whether they need help at all—changes accordingly. The preschooler is expected to be able to sit at circle time, the second grader to play well with other children and sit at a desk for long periods, and the middle schooler to have a degree of developing executive function manifested in academics and organization. Academic expectations change, social expectations change, and so do children's individual ambitions; they may want to play a sport, play in an orchestra, dance in *The Nutcracker*, or accumulate followers on social media. "Success" with a therapeutic intervention depends on figuring out what your child wants or needs to accomplish at any given point, and finding the right kind of help. But parents can also feel overwhelmed by the sheer number of recommendations they are offered, and may worry that because none of these problems is likely to be completely cured, the therapies don't have obvious endpoints. So as a parent, you may find yourself pushing to continue a therapy even if the school feels it is no longer necessary, because you feel it is helping. The school may be guided in part by staffing or budget constraints; on the other hand, you may find yourself deciding that a certain therapy, even if it's potentially beneficial, is not worth the time and effort for your child, given all the other balls in the air.

> Every time we went for a new evaluation, the doctor would rec-
> ommend that we see someone else for yet another evaluation. It
> never seemed to end. Finally, we decided that Gabriel was doing
> reasonably well, and we all needed a break from this constant
> running around to evaluations and therapies. I don't think many of
> the therapists ever tell you that your child doesn't need to see them
> anymore. I am getting suspicious that these kids are keeping a lot
> of people in business and that, as parents, we need to take some
> control over our time and money.

There's no question that many children derive real benefits from the range of therapeutic interventions. Unfortunately, from our point of view as pediatricians, we have to face the fact that for many of these therapies, only very limited (if any) serious research-based *evidence* can be cited attesting to their effectiveness. There is research to support early intervention, ABA, speech therapy, and occupational therapy (OT), but it's very hard to extrapolate from these studies to figure out what will be helpful for any particular child with a particular quirky profile. When we suggest some form of therapy for a quirky child in our practice, we see that help is needed and we make an educated guess at where to start, but we cannot assure anyone that it will definitely have the desired effect. This is a process of trial and error, of finding the right therapy and the right therapists to address your child's particular needs and struggles. For a pediatrician, this process is not quite the same as getting a positive throat culture back from the lab, diagnosing strep throat, and telling a parent that the optimal treatment for the child is a specified dose of penicillin for a certain number of days.

The Schlep Factor

Keep the ever-present "schlep" factor in mind: How much of your time and energy is the program you are designing for your child going to require? What are the ramifications for other areas of *your* life—your job, the rest of your family, your own spare time. Many parents of young children feel they have no spare time at all, and, as mothers, we certainly understand that. The idea of selecting therapies may be daunting, but our intent is to help you think about what really matters for your child, without losing sight of the need to care for other family members and yourself. If you are thinking of signing up your child for a therapy that is offered on the day you often stay late at work or the day you usually take her brother to karate or the only day you can take an exercise class or go for a swim yourself, you should think carefully about (1) whether it's worth it and (2) whether someone else can get her there. Increasingly, many supports and therapies for quirky kids take place in schools, relieving the burden on parents to run around after school or on the weekends. This isn't the case for all kids in all schools, but progress has been made in this area since publication of the first edition of this book.

Guilt is potent for many parents, arising out of the pain they feel at watching their child struggle. It's easy to take a more is better approach to therapies, and it's a short step from there to the idea that you're doing something selfish by deciding to forgo any particular option. But more is not necessarily better. You and your child, and any other children you have, are all entitled to lives. Therapies and appointments should enhance your quirky child's life, not run him ragged. The schlep factor really adds up over time, and many parents reach a point at which they are just worn out!

How to Decide What to Do for Your Child

The following are some questions to consider as you look at possible therapies, therapists, and therapeutic regimens:

- *Does therapy target the problems that are really getting in my child's way?* Keep in mind what *you* are targeting, and what your child wants to target. What specific skills are you and your child hoping to gain, or which behaviors would you like to decrease? Does this therapy seem like the place to start?
- *How will we know if it's working?* This is a good question to ask the therapist during an initial evaluation. Ask the therapist how progress is measured, what kinds of assessments are done at the beginning, and how often the child is reassessed.
- *What if it isn't helping?* Ask yourself if you trust the therapist to let you know if it seems like the intervention isn't working or that she and your child aren't a good match.
- *What kind of commitment are we making if we start this course of therapy?* If it's a group, determine how important it is for your child to stick it out for an entire semester or year, and how it would affect the other kids in the group if she didn't.
- *How long will it take?* How much time a therapeutic intervention takes—and how intense it is—is quite variable. None of the therapies we discuss in this chapter are intended as quick fixes.
- *Is my child at the right age for this kind of therapy?* As we stated previously, there is good evidence to suggest that you can make better progress if you address some of the more troublesome behaviors, or the most significant delays, at an early age. Younger children who don't receive help may experience relatively more delays, or their behaviors may become more troublesome as time passes. For parents, it is a lot easier to cart around

toddlers, or work with them at home, than it is with older children who have more demands on their time and energy. At a certain point, an older child may balk at all this so-called help. It becomes harder to continue with a therapy, no matter how much good it's doing, if the child won't go.

The Right Program

What do we mean by a program? We mean a combination of therapies (or maybe a single therapy) tailored to your child and your child's development and needs, as well as the needs of your family and its schedules. If your child is already enrolled in a special school—for example, a school designed for kids with autism spectrum disorder (ASD)—or, in some cases, a special education program within a regular school, you may have comparatively little planning and scheduling (and schlepping!) to do. Most of these schools employ all the most likely types of therapists in addition to providing academic support. For anyone not in that situation, there's a lot of evaluating, planning, and thinking to do.

> I've always felt that if he could survive in a regular education setting, that is best because it's more like the real world. What I didn't realize was that all the extra help he needs is on my time around the edges of the day. It takes a toll—on him, on me, and on our family as a whole.

Make sure you leave your child some time to kick back and be a kid. Hanging out with you in the kitchen or running around the playground may help him as much as any therapeutic regimen. Home is, after all, where most of a young child's growth takes place. Be alert for opportunities to help your child at home.

> While I limited television drastically for my other children, I felt that Sesame Street was George's best social pragmatics intervention.

In working with our patients, the two of us have watched different children experiment with various therapies, and we have developed some biases. We aren't experts (that is to say, therapists) in any particular regimen, but neither are we ideologically committed to any one approach. Still, although we hope you finish this chapter with a better understanding of the kinds of help available, as well as the jargon that may be used to describe it, we also know that nothing really takes the place of checking out any interesting possibility for yourself to see if it's a good match for your child. Many of the therapies we describe are highly therapist dependent—find the right person and you're golden—and that is going to require your judgment, your willingness to trust your impressions, and the help you can get from other parents in the vicinity who know your local players.

> Once we found the right person to help us, we felt so much better. The therapist who helped Abby the most was a woman who was both an occupational therapist and a psychologist. She just got it from the start and seemed to know exactly what we needed to do to help her. It was a giant relief. In many ways, it was just the beginning, but it took a long time to find her, so in that way, it felt like the end. It has made an enormous difference.

What Behaviors or Concerns Can Be Addressed by Different Therapies?

Matching behaviors or concerns with potentially helpful therapies is a challenge. In this subsection, we consider some of the specific concerns parents of quirky kids have and the therapies that may address them (Table 9.1). Be aware that there is plenty of overlap; one child's OT may be remarkably similar to another child's physical therapy (PT).

Table 9.1. Targeting Therapy to Your Child's Needs

BEHAVIORS OR CONCERNS	THERAPIES
Her speech isn't developing normally. He can't carry on a conversation.	Speech and language therapy, including pragmatics
My child just isn't with it. He doesn't make eye contact. He always seems off in his own world. She doesn't play with toys in a normal way. She just hangs on to that DustBuster. He doesn't connect with other kids his age. He's always off by himself.	Applied behavior analysis (gold standard for kids with autism spectrum disorder [ASD]), play therapy for the younger child, pragmatic language therapy for the older child
My son isn't walking yet. My daughter falls off of benches. She just can't seem to hold herself up.	Physical therapy

Table 9.1 (*continued*)

BEHAVIORS OR CONCERNS	THERAPIES
She can't manage a knife and fork and spills whenever she pours something. He can't get himself dressed. He can't figure out how to get his legs into his pants. He can't figure out how to do things that come naturally to other kids his age: mount a tricycle, ride a bike, pump on a swing. She's klutzy and always breaking things, such as toys, lamp switches, barrettes.	Occupational therapy
His feet never leave the ground. He's scared of stairs, curbs, swings, and slides. She has a meltdown when something unexpected happens: a sneeze or sudden laugh, a touch. He misjudges the quality of objects—how heavy the pitcher is, how much pressure to use on the pencil. He can't erase without putting a hole in the paper.	Sensory integration treatment
She pulls out her hair and eyelashes. He's washing his hands 99 times a day.	Cognitive behavioral therapy, medication management
His behavior is driving us crazy! We can't take her anywhere, and life at home is a nightmare. All the babysitters have quit.	Applied behavior analysis, cognitive behavioral therapy for older children
She is completely disorganized. He can't see the forest for the trees. Homework is a nightmare. School projects are hell.	Occupational therapy, pragmatic language therapy, individual academic support, executive function programs
He is becoming depressed and more anxious as he gets older. She's much more aware of how different she is, and she feels really bad about it.	Child psychiatry or psychology, friendship groups, social skills groups

Many experiences in day-to-day life can be highly therapeutic. The right piano teacher, the right karate class, the right new school may help your child with some of the issues mentioned in Table 9.1. As children grow up, they are more likely to put time and effort and energy into activities they love. Your best strategy may be to help them find those activities and support their participation. A martial arts program, a butterfly club, a robotics club, or a Dungeons & Dragons group might be just the ticket to engage a child in his special interests while fostering social skills.

What Choices Do We Have?

Children whose problems show up early in childhood usually will take part in some amount of speech and language therapy and OT, most likely through an EI program. Children with a diagnosis of ASD will likely be referred for ABA, the evidence-based program in which parents and therapists respond to every aspect of the child's behavior, positively reinforcing desirable behaviors. Many young children are exposed to some aspects of this and other techniques in integrated preschool settings. Behavioral therapists work with kids in school and at home, where parents need support with challenging behaviors. Whether or not other forms of therapy are suggested depends on your child's unique combination of abilities, issues, and, well, quirks. Resources at the end of this book help you learn more about each of these branches of therapy.

Many of these therapeutic programs expect the child's parents to be active partners and to keep the therapy going at home (well, maybe not swimming with dolphins or therapeutic horseback riding). You should expect to be invited to participate in most of the exercises and activities. When you do, you can form your own opinion of whether it's useful and learn strategies for home to make it more effective. Some of these therapies, such as ABA, entail shaping not only the parents' behavior but also the behavior of everyone who comes into contact with your child, so you must think carefully about the type of commitment you are willing and able to make.

Applied Behavior Analysis

For toddlers and preschoolers who receive a diagnosis of ASD, ABA is the gold standard therapeutic intervention to address behavioral challenges; it combines many elements of other recommended therapies for quirky kids with the same emphasis on language, social skills, and a reduction in undesirable behaviors, like aggression or self-harm. Applied behavior analysis is integrated into many aspects of a child's daily life, with intense, often one-on-one and face-to-face interventions.

A certified therapist observes and analyzes a child's behaviors. He or she collects voluminous amounts of data to determine the function an unwanted behavior serves. For example, does a child tantrum or scream because it relieves anxiety, or to avoid having to do some activity that frightens him, or because something in the environment such as loud noises or bright lights make him uncomfortable? Once the behavior is understood, the therapist gets to work with the child to extinguish the behavior through a series of trials, using positive reinforcers (eg, praise, stickers) to promote the desired alternative behaviors (eg, sitting quietly during circle time). Fortunately, negative reinforcers are no longer used. The therapist collects data continually to document progress, which is immensely satisfying for parents.

Applied behavior analysis is intensive and requires a substantial commitment on the part of the child, the family, and the therapist. Sometimes less intense forms of ABA can be used successfully to treat problematic behaviors in much more functional quirky kids. The principles of ABA are used in Pivotal Response Therapy (PRT), a play-based therapy program used to elicit positive behaviors, self-motivation, and initiation of social interactions. A typical ABA or PRT program today may involve 25 hours per week and can take some creativity on the part of the family to put together.

> When Trevor was 2 years old, he had no language at all. When he did start to talk, he had echolalic speech and repeated what people said to him. He reversed his pronouns, and he had odd behaviors like waving backward. At about age 3, we had him evaluated by a behavioral intervention group in California, and we started an ABA-type program with an emphasis on his social skills and fine motor skills. We did things such as pretend birthday parties to help him learn the "script" he would need to use at a real party. We also hired students to help us work with him.

Although many major cities have certified ABA therapists or organizations with a staff of certified therapists, they may be harder to find in small towns or rural areas. You want the best possible person working with your child, so it's worth doing some digging or extra traveling early on to get on the right track.

Other Behavioral Approaches

Other behavioral approaches include Floortime and TEACCH (Treatment and Education of Autistic and Communication related handicapped CHildren). The Floortime approach, developed by child psychiatrist Stanley Greenspan, is a good example of an approach to enhancing development without dividing tasks into areas such as speech or motor or sensory. Greenspan's theory is that a close emotional connection with a parent or another important person in the child's sphere will promote optimal development. Rather than addressing the child's deficiencies, this approach is more likely to build on areas of strength. It requires parents and close associates in your child's daily life to spend 20 or 30 minutes on the floor, at least once a day, playing with the child, gradually challenging the child during play to learn from and build on the variations and changes the partner introduces. Many quirky toddlers and preschoolers have a limited imagination and play skills. The kind of playfulness we expect from children just isn't there. Letting go of your expectations and following your child's lead isn't as easy as it sounds. As the attachment deepens (the theory goes), the child's skills develop.

The TEACCH program, based in North Carolina, is directed at teachers and offers a structured approach for the classroom in which a set schedule is combined with clearly defined areas consisting of different activities and individualized visual reminders. Home-based programs are also available and use the same approach.

Therapeutic School-Based Programs and Approaches

Many communities now offer therapeutic nursery or school programs that incorporate many of the philosophies promoted as beneficial for quirky kids, and, again, they also emphasize language, social skills, and functional abilities. Although each of these programs is different, they have many similarities. Your child's options will be based largely on where you live and on which programs are established in your area.

Speech and Language Therapy

Speech and language pathologists are the friends and supporters of quirky kids, and most will perform a speech evaluation for delayed onset of speech or for atypical development of speech and language. Speech and language therapists can be credentialed in a variety of ways—from a bachelor's degree to a master's degree and on to a doctoral degree. These therapists are trained to work with many different populations, including kids or adults with head injuries or strokes that have affected their speech; kids with oral-motor problems such as feeding or swallowing difficulties and cleft lips or palates; and kids who are slow to acquire language or whose language is not intelligible.

For the very young child with absent or unusual speech development, a hearing test and a speech and language evaluation are critical. Sometimes the child is just a late bloomer, but when something more is going on, a good speech and language therapist will notice behaviors that you may not notice and make suggestions for further evaluation. The earlier the delay is detected and understood, the better. If your child cannot cooperate for an evaluation, that is useful information too. Speech therapy for the preverbal child can start at 15 to 18 months of age, if not earlier. Many quirky kids receive years of speech therapy for slow onset of speech, articulation difficulties, and general communication problems. Fortunately, most kids find it fun.

> We started speech therapy for Charlie when he was about 18 months old. The speech therapist from early intervention came to our home twice a week, and Charlie attended a playgroup at the early intervention center that included a few different kinds of therapists. He loved the extra attention, and he seemed to know that this was going to help him talk. The therapist got right down on the floor with him, right in his face (after he knew her well enough to tolerate that) and worked hard at getting him to produce sounds. He learned where the different sounds are made in his mouth and throat. I remember him saying "frog" and holding his throat as he made the hard "g" sound. She brought toys that he loved and used them to help get the words out. Now that I have learned so much about the things that help these kids, I see that she was using lots of strategies at the same time.

Increasingly, EI programs and preschools are using sign language for nonverbal kids who may be very frustrated by their inability to express themselves with words. The Picture-Exchange Communication System is another strategy, in which small cards with photos of daily activities are posted, and the child can pick a card to indicate a wish, something to eat, or a desire to go outside or play with a specific toy. This is communication, even if it does not involve words.

Pragmatic Language Therapy

Speech therapists with additional training in the pragmatics of language are most likely to be of help to the older quirky child who has trouble communicating and/or may have been given a diagnosis of social communication disorder. Part of what we are calling quirkiness often involves difficulties with the pragmatics of language—that is, with understanding the dynamics of conversation beyond the ability to say words and form sentences. Problems with language pragmatics may mean that kids have trouble with the following:

- Starting or stopping a conversation
- Following up a comment with a related comment, rather than starting a new conversation about a personal interest, which is off-putting to a conversational partner
- Asking appropriate questions of a new acquaintance
- Knowing when the information he or she is trying to convey is getting across and when it is not
- Understanding that conversational style or tone of voice should change according to the audience; people don't talk to a police officer the same way they talk to their best buddy
- Reading the body language or cues of the person across from them and understanding when the person is interested and when he or she is losing interest

For typical kids, the ability to understand another's point of view develops at about age 4 years. This is the theory-of-mind concept: You can appreciate that another person has a different experience from yours, sees things differently, may know things you don't know, and may not know things that you do know. Many quirky kids can't do this or can't do it as well as other kids their age, and it wreaks havoc with their conversational skills.

This is where *pragmatic language groups*, sometimes called *friendship groups* or *social-skills groups*, come in. The point is to get a small group of kids together with a speech therapist who teaches them the mechanics of conversation, such as making eye contact, assessing the listener's level of interest, communicating your own attention to another speaker. Each session involves a topic or a place to start that is chosen by the therapist, who then helps the kids navigate conversationally. This therapy can involve frequent redirecting, gentle reminders about paying attention or reducing interruptions, and role-playing videos that the kids watch and then comment upon. For the younger elementary school children, there may be cooperative games or activities in which the kids are instructed to talk with one another in order to finish the game or project.

In second grade, Sam started a friendship group at a local university with supervision from a professor of speech and language therapy and some graduate students. The group was all boys, and they all needed some help with their social and conversational skills. They did exercises and games geared toward understanding facial expressions and nonverbal body language. They did role-plays, which they later watched on video and loved! Then they would dissect their own and one another's behavior, with a lot of assistance from the group leaders. Some days they played cooperative games—again, with a lot of help where they were required to talk to one another to reach a common goal. Sam found it challenging at times, but I think it helped him to see the perspective of another person. We used the strategies at home a lot, over dinner especially, to help him get the social rules of conversation that seem to come more easily to other kids.

Does It Work?

There is a growing body of evidence that group social skills interventions can yield improvements in social communications and reduce children's tendency to focus only on special interests and repetitive behaviors. We suggest that you discuss the potential benefits with the consultant who really knows your child, as well as observe a group session and trust your own knowledge of your child and sense of her needs in deciding whether it's worth a try. Checking in with your child's classroom teacher can also help you assess whether a pragmatics group is helpful. Teachers observe kids interacting with one another more than do most parents and are in a good position to let you know if they see any improvements in social skills.

Physical Therapy and Adaptive Physical Education

Muscle weakness or low muscle tone, motor clumsiness, and poor coordination are quite prevalent among quirky kids, who can be rather klutzy. Physical therapy and OT are often recommended to address these troubles. Parents are likely to notice delayed walking, poor balance or instability, low muscle tone or weakness, poor fine motor skills for eating, writing, or dressing, and poor ball-playing skills. Physical therapy for the youngest kids is geared toward improving function through enhanced strength and balance, as well as improving coordination through enhanced ball skills, obstacle courses, and the like. Most young children love PT and the equipment in the rooms. Strong data support the efficacy of PT.

Physical therapists can be found in all EI programs, most hospitals, and most public schools. Also, independent groups of PTs working together with other kinds of therapists are sprouting up in many communities. Most school-based PTs have some experience with the quirky-child population and the approaches that are most likely to be successful. Talking to a therapist about your child and the issues you most want addressed is worthwhile, and observing one or two sessions can help you determine whether your child and the PT are well matched.

The PT was David's first therapist, and we were referred to her because he was motor-delayed. He couldn't roll over or sit up. He started to see her when he was about 9 months old, and that relationship lasted a long time. It was through his PT that we figured out many of his other issues, and that his motor delay wasn't an isolated thing. Fortunately, he loved going to see her, and it definitely helped him. He continued it for a long time, and now he attends a special education school where there are PTs on the staff.

John was really uncoordinated as a small child. He had a lot of difficulty with the most basic things, like learning to go up and down the stairs. His PT explained the combination of strength, coordination, and motor planning that is required to do something that seems so simple. He worked on strength and balance with her, walking on the balance beam, practicing going up and down the stairs, and worked with other kids with similar issues. He enjoyed it, though he was exhausted when it was over. As he got older, he worked more on ball skills and eye-hand coordination and developed confidence in those skills.

As kids grow, the options for PT broaden in some communities. Many quirky kids develop basic motor skills but still have difficulty with the coordination and communication necessary for team sports or playground games. Continued individual or group work with a PT is necessary for some of these kids, but a number of other activities also can foster improved coordination, confidence, and strength. Families whose children take martial arts classes such as karate or taekwondo swear by them as activities that have helped in all three of these areas. A growing number of gymnasium-based programs, staffed by special educators, are available for kids who can benefit from some good old-fashioned physical activity with cooperative gross motor games followed by small-group processing sessions with a counselor. These programs address both motor and social skills in each session.

Some schools offer *adaptive physical education programs* for kids with physical handicaps or more severe coordination problems, which can be complicated by perceptual difficulties. Adaptive physical education is not available in all schools, but it is worth knowing about because the gym teacher may be willing to team up with an OT or a PT to create such a program. Chances are good that a number of kids in any given school could benefit from an adaptive physical education program.

Occupational Therapy

Occupational therapy is the treatment most likely to be recommended for a quirky child. It is a huge and growing field with many areas of specialization. Some OTs specialize in the small muscles of the hand, in feeding and swallowing disorders (some focus particularly on picky eaters), or in visual and perceptual differences, and a growing number are obtaining certification in sensory integration (SI) treatment. As with PTs, OTs can have a bachelor's degree, a master's degree, or a doctorate. A number of OT assistants are also working in this field. Occupational therapists can be found in virtually all EI programs and most schools and hospitals, and an increasing number are working in large private organizations with all the equipment in one place.

> We saw a highly recommended OT for 2 years for John. We were told she knows her stuff, and she was trained in SI, which is a big part of what he has, but she spent a tremendous amount of John's time on his fine motor skills. They did mazes; he had to hold the pencil and try not to bump into the edge of the line. Now he works with a different OT who is much livelier and helps him work on stuff that really impacts his daily life—keyboarding, cello playing. In retrospect, I think the earlier OT experience was a complete and total waste of time. He didn't complain about it; I just don't think it made that much difference.

Younger kids may be seen by OTs as part of their EI evaluation or may be referred specifically to OT because of feeding difficulties, generally low tone, or an inability to use both hands together in a coordinated fashion. Toddlers or preschoolers with developmental delays in fine motor skills, unusual reactions to textures (eg, Play-Doh or certain foods), extreme irritability or whininess, or difficulty following directions, as well as quirky kids who are preoccupied with unusual objects that prevent interactions with toys or other people are all good candidates for OT. School-aged kids with attentional, organizational, or fine motor deficits also may benefit from working with an OT.

> Charlie's OT visits his preschool class periodically to observe and educate the staff. When his preschool teacher was worried about his behavior and not paying attention at story time, his OT noticed that he was flopping all over the place because it is hard for him to maintain his posture if he has nothing to lean back on. As soon as he was moved to a place where he could lean against the wall, his

attention improved and he was less disruptive. When he refused to participate in activities that the other kids loved, his OT helped us to see that he was overwhelmed by the happy chaos all around him and that his difficulty with things like cutting and drawing made it easier for him to observe rather than participate. Occupational therapists have an eye for this sort of thing. It worries me that, without her perspective, Charlie would have been seen as a behavior problem, when the solution was so simple. Ultimately, it was the insight of his OT that helped us realize that Charlie was in the wrong preschool setting. We moved him to another school where there was more structure and many more adults to help kids with transitions and play skills, and he has absolutely thrived.

Occupational therapists are terrific at helping kids, families, and schools make (sometimes quite simple) modifications that can help with day-to-day functioning. A particular kind of chair may help a child maintain his posture in class. Simple tools can attach to a pencil or pen and make writing easier for a child. For some kids, the mechanics of writing are just too much, and OTs can set them up with technology and software programs and teach keyboarding skills. For kids who need strategies for following directions, OTs teach them how to break things down into small, discrete steps.

Does It Work?

Many quirky kids are referred for OT at some point. In our experience, most parents whose kids receive OT believe it is helping, and a growing body of evidence supports the effectiveness of a range of different interventions. But keep in mind that a great deal has to do with defining your child's wants or needs and finding a therapist who can develop a helpful program. Part of the picture is a warm and supportive relationship with an adult who understands the child's difficulties interacting with the world around him. Occupational therapy helps him develop a vocabulary to describe those difficulties and strategies to cope. This can be an enormous comfort to kids struggling with these issues, and many keep coming back for more.

Sensory Integration Treatment

One form of OT that comes up for many quirky kids is sensory integration treatment. *Sensory integration* (SI) refers to the ability of the nervous system to integrate incoming information with the senses and act on it. Most of us can appreciate a child's struggle with her sense of vision, hearing, taste, and smell, but it may be more difficult to observe the subtleties of touch in its various components, balance and movement, body position. Each of these more subtle senses is addressed in SI evaluation and treatment.

Many quirky kids have difficulty integrating sensory input from their environments, and some parents are relieved to have an explanation and a strategy. For some kids, these sensory issues are the biggest problems they face, and *sensory processing disorder* is the *main* diagnosis or the one that best explains a child's unusual behaviors.

> Jack was about 6 years old when we first heard the term *SI dysfunction*, and it made so much sense to us. He had been such a difficult baby, screaming and arching and barely sleeping, and he developed horrendous tantrums as he got older. We knew we were good parents, and this had to be something about the way he was wired. Finding a professional who understood him was a great relief, and now he is receiving SI therapy, and he loves it. We have new strategies to help him at home, and we just understand it better.

Sensory integration evaluations should be conducted by occupational or physical therapists with training in SI. With a certified therapist, there will at least be some consistency in the approach, which will enable you to make a more meaningful assessment of whether or not it is helpful. A typical SI program lasts from 6 months to a couple of years, with frequent assessments throughout the treatment, though some families have used an on-again off-again approach over the years with reasonable results.

> When Gabriel started his EI program, the OT suggested that we try to improve his sense of his body in space and to help him overcome some of his hypersensitivity to sensation. He had to have the tags cut out of all his clothes and couldn't stand the seam on his socks. As he got older, he saw another OT certified in SI, and she worked with him on things like gravitational insecurity—the fact that he didn't like to have his feet off the ground. They worked with various types of swings, and he developed more strength and coordination and less anxiety about these things. I can't really put my finger on it, but it did seem to help him, and he is pretty coordinated now.

Psychotherapy

Growing up quirky can be pretty rough, and it is our belief that most kids will need some mental health intervention at one point or another. Anxiety, depression, obsessive-compulsive disorder, and tics are common and, if untreated, are additional obstacles to growth and development. As we have said, a relationship with a caring psychologist (PhD), social worker (licensed mental health counselor [LMHC] or licensed clinical social worker [LCSW]), or psychiatrist (MD, especially if you think medication might be necessary) over the years can be immensely comforting for quirky kids and their families. Different families need different kinds of help. Treatment ranges from play therapy for the youngest child to individual talk therapy to family therapy to group therapy. Some child psychologists run social-skills groups much like the pragmatic therapy groups described earlier.

Individual Talk Therapy

Children come to talk therapy for many different reasons and finding a therapist who is a good fit can help a child in a wide range of ways. Talk therapy can help children develop insight, recognize patterns in their own emotions and behavior, and give them a place to review their emotions and experiences. Depending on their communications skills—or difficulties—some quirky kids may seem less likely to be able to engage successfully one-on-one with a counselor or therapist. Because of these children's typically poor interpersonal skills and lack of insight, this is a reasonable question. Supporters of this type of therapy argue that much is to be gained for the socially awkward child and that, in a good therapeutic relationship, a child should experience a positive social interaction with a caring adult. Challenging for the therapist as well as for the child, talk therapy has the potential to help a child learn to identify feelings and the facial expressions and tone of voice that may accompany them. An empathic attachment with a therapist fosters improved communication and the development of empathy itself. A therapist may start out by acting as a translator for the child, giving her clues to understand the actions of people in her world. Parents whose children have developed good relationships with therapists invariably tell us that it takes a long time for the kids to get the hang of it but that talk therapy can be a great help for the kids and for their exhausted parents.

> David has a therapist at school whom he sees weekly. It took a while for him to understand the point of it, but he now looks forward to it, and it helps us as a family that he has another trusting adult to talk to. He is developing a vocabulary for describing his feelings and experiences that will help him make it through adolescence.

Individual therapy with a child psychiatrist is actually a rare event these days; most therapists are social workers, psychologists, or guidance counselors.

You probably will want to see a child psychiatrist if your child needs medications to manage his symptoms (developmental-behavioral pediatricians and psychiatric nurse-practitioners also have expertise in prescribing these medications). Although some child psychiatrists are knowledgeable about quirky kids and may even have a particular interest in what makes them tick, their time is generally too expensive for most families to be able to hire one for ongoing therapy. Many child psychiatrists function as consultants to other mental health professionals, especially regarding medications. Pediatricians can perform this function, but we generally consult with our psychiatric colleagues as well. They understand the subtleties of psychiatric medicines the way pediatricians understand antibiotics.

Group Therapy

Highly structured psychotherapy groups are sometimes recommended for quirky kids to help them address individual and interpersonal goals, as well as to teach them about forming and negotiating relationships with others and how to follow rules and directions. These groups usually take the form of social-skills groups or friendship groups aimed at kids who are learning about body language and social cues, understanding the perspectives of others, and communicating their confusion or lack of understanding in an acceptable way. Some psychology practices offer relaxation groups, growing-up groups, or groups in which kids work on "social stories" together. Sessions can even take the form of going out for a meal together or some other social activity.

Whether a group experience works for a particular child depends on a number of factors:

- Is your child motivated and interested or at least willing to go along with you if you believe it's indicated?
- Does the therapist have experience with this population of kids and agree that your child is a good candidate?
- Has the therapist thoughtfully chosen a group of kids who can work together?

The group itself is also critical. Kids referred for these kinds of groups are, by definition, experiencing difficulty socially. They might be excessively shy and uncommunicative or boisterous and loud. For some, their attention issues or nervous habits get in the way or are distracting or disturbing to the other kids. Check it out for a few weeks. Some of these group therapy rooms have facilities for parents to sit and watch through a one-way mirror. Ask your son or daughter if the group is enjoyable, and ask the therapist how it's going. Again, this is a significant time commitment, and it's better to cut your losses if you conclude that group therapy isn't going to help.

Cognitive Behavioral Therapy

Cognitive behavioral therapy (CBT) is an effective form of treatment with a strong evidence base, and it is especially likely to be useful for children with anxiety symptoms, including social anxiety, phobias, and obsessive compulsive disorder (marked by compulsive thoughts and ritualized behaviors). Psychologists or social workers can receive special certification in CBT. Cognitive behavioral therapy focuses on specific goals, such as reducing (or replacing) an undesirable behavior (an obsession or a habit, such as picking at one's skin or pulling out hair repeatedly). It tends to work best with kids who can be taught to negotiate and parents who are willing partners in helping a child work toward a given goal. Once a behavior is targeted and its frequency measured, you and your child work together with the therapist to decide how the behavior should change. Cognitive behavioral therapy is not the type of therapy in which a child's feelings are examined in detail or the therapist reaches back into history looking for motivations or causes. In CBT, *not* a lot of time or energy is spent determining why the behavior exists. Rather, the goal is to eliminate it, reduce it to a more reasonable level, or replace it with something else altogether.

The next step is choosing a reinforcer for the desired behavioral change, a small treat or token that rewards the child for each success. Of course, your child gets first dibs on this. What can work well are treats such as baseball cards or time to play an electronic game, some reasonably small guaranteed pleasure that means something to your child. This is the basic framework of the CBT approach. It can be a terrific plan for some quirky kids, but not all have the capacity to negotiate the goals or have enough control over their undesirable behaviors that they can actually reduce them or replace them with alternative behaviors, whatever the incentive.

Behavioral psychologists are also known for teaching kids to manage their anxiety, using techniques like relaxation, guided imagery, a competing behavior that prevents the anxiety-driven one (for example, you can't pull out your hair if you're squeezing a ball in your pocket), role-playing, and humor. Lots of kids respond to these strategies, and most parents prefer to start with these techniques rather than moving right to medications. Cognitive behavioral therapy has been particularly successful for people with phobias, which are forms of anxiety. Quirky kids may suffer with phobias, which are a form of anxiety: a fear of blood draws at the pediatrician's office, elevators, airplanes, crowds, animals, or Halloween costumes. Many parents respond to these phobias by trying to protect their child by avoiding situations that may involve elevators, costumes, or animals, but CBT uses a strategy in which the child is gradually exposed to the feared stimulus, teaching that nothing catastrophic will happen, while practicing coping skills.

Activities in the Community and at Home

Many activities for kids have the potential to be therapeutic. A caring and sensitive Little League coach can make a world of difference to a quirky child. At times, you may need to talk about your child's particular quirks with an adult who is supervising an activity in which she is participating. Many adults who work with children on a regular basis are going to figure things out on their own. Over time, many parents develop a kind of sixth sense about these issues: whom to tell, what to tell, and how to get the child the support he needs.

> Sam is intensely musical, but his techniques for learning and playing music are not at all standard-issue. His first teacher was pretty rigid and simply did not get him, and could only see his odd behaviors as defiance or hostility. This year, we are working with someone new, who is less rigid and more accepting of Sam's stuff, but I can see that she, too, is confused and bewildered that Sam is such a struggle to work with. I talked to her more openly about what a struggle life in general is for him, and it seemed to help the two of them relax and enjoy each other.

All families involved in any of the therapies or activities described in this chapter learn to incorporate some of these interventions in their day-to-day family life. Families may find themselves using organizational charts or dry-erase boards to keep a child on track; sticking simple pictures on the refrigerator to help a preverbal child with communication; using pragmatic language techniques at the dinner table; engaging in the type of rough-and-tumble play that the child enjoys at PT. Most therapists actively encourage parents to augment these programs at home.

A couple of programs specifically lend themselves to the home environment. Carol Gray, an educator, developed Social Stories and comic strip conversations to address the particular areas of difficulty for most quirky kids: understanding the rules of social behavior and the perspectives of others. Although originally designed for use in the school and used heavily by speech and language pathologists, these techniques are easily learned by parents and kids alike. Kits are available to help you get started.

A Social Story is a simple story written by an adult who knows the child well. Stories are written according to a formula in which certain rules are followed, and the stories are then reviewed with the child. Social stories have the capacity to help parents and other adults understand a child's perspective and special areas of difficulty, as well as increase the child's awareness of the social world.

Comic strip conversations are joint projects in which an adult and a child create a simple comic strip involving characters that have bubbles (for thoughts or words) coming out of their heads. These comic strips can help a child process an event that she may have found disturbing or plan for an event in the future at which certain behaviors are expected (such as a birthday party or wedding). They are used to help the child understand the perspective of others; for example, what someone says is not the same as what that person may be thinking, especially when sarcasm is used. Sarcasm is one of the hardest concepts for quirky kids to grasp. Drawing a comic strip and working with your child to fill in the blanks provides a good opportunity to explain what comes naturally to you but not so naturally to him.

Stanley Greenspan's Floortime technique, discussed earlier, lends itself to the home environment. Many families swear by it for helping to bring a child out of his shell. You've got little to lose and a lot to gain by making these activities part of your family life.

Putting It Together

Many parents may find it easy to read down the list of problems and indications and think, yes, indeed, she needs help with her fine motor coordination, her social skills, and of course, the SI stuff; she definitely needs to see a counselor. You won't possibly be able to do all the things that are out there, and you won't be able to spend all your home time following therapeutic regimens either. You're going to have to pick and choose. Follow your instincts and pay close attention to how your child is doing.

Not all "problems" need to be solved. If your daughter never learns to ride a bike or hates the sand at the beach, so be it. If your son types all his assignments because he never mastered legible handwriting, fine. (He'll make a great doctor!) The world is much more tolerant of these idiosyncrasies in adults. There is no expectation that all adults like soccer or science fiction movies, no requirement that they all have neat handwriting or perfect table manners. What we all want for our children is that they be happy with themselves and live the best lives they possibly can.

Be sure your child doesn't have so many appointments that there is no time to play with siblings or kids in the neighborhood or visit cousins or grandparents. Learning the basics of hanging out at home can be challenging for quirky kids, especially those with excess physical energy and those who engage in their special interests to an extreme degree. Create quiet time hanging out with your family, whether it's reading or doing crossword puzzles on Sundays, playing word games or board games or doing projects together, or watching movies on Friday nights. These activities are good for all families but can easily get lost in the hectic pace of life for families with working parents and quirky kids. Make it a priority. You will see improvement in your child's ability to relax and enjoy the company of others, although this can be a slow and gradual process; progress occurs over time, and you have to fit that time into your life.

10

Medications and the Quirky Child: Drugs, Doses, and Daily Routines

Medications cannot eliminate a child's underlying quirks, and that is generally not anyone's goal. Often, medications are recommended for children who are unable to make use of other interventions designed to help them. The hope is usually to dial down the particular symptom—the anxiety, the inattention, the depression, the impulsiveness—that gets in the way, so that the child can take full advantage of other supports and therapies. Parents almost uniformly struggle with the decision to medicate a child; this is not an easy call for anyone. For some parents, the suggestion that a child might benefit from a medication indicates that something is *really* wrong. Understandably, that can be scary.

We have encountered parents whose first reaction to the idea of medication was an unequivocal refusal; it's not uncommon for parents to announce that they have vowed never to give their child medications of this kind. It's also not uncommon for parents to report that other members of the extended family—grandparents or aunts and uncles—have very strong negative feelings about "putting kids on drugs." Some people believe that doctors are collaborating with pharmaceutical companies to sell more product by putting more kids on medications. Other people are concerned about the social justice aspects of who gets diagnosed and who receives treatment with medications (inequities show up in different and sometimes contradictory ways; children of color may be less likely to be diagnosed early with neurodevelopmental issues, but parents may worry that some teachers are too likely to request medication when a child of color behaves rambunctiously in class). Our goal here is not to convince you that medications are necessary—now or ever—for your child, but we strongly suggest keeping an open mind while we take you through some of the logic and some of the evidence regarding use of medications in children who are struggling.

Medication is not usually a first resort for children with neurodevelopmental differences or behavioral problems; always start with environmental modifications and the therapies discussed in Chapter 9 to help build your child's skills and help the family cope. However, for children with severe attention-deficit/hyperactivity disorder (ADHD) or mood instability, medications are considered first-line treatments. We believe that many neurodevelopmental disorders are biologically based; thus, it makes sense that for some children—and for some periods of their lives—medications that act on the brain and the central nervous system may be useful.

Uses for Commonly Prescribed Medications

The medications prescribed most commonly for quirky kids are those used to treat ADHD, behavioral dysregulation (as in oppositional or out-of-control behavior), anxiety, obsessions and compulsions, tic disorders, phobias, sleep disturbances, and in older children, mood disorders, especially depression. These medications include a range of categories, such as stimulants, antidepressants, and antianxiety drugs, but it's important to acknowledge that there can be a great deal of crossover; some children end up on antidepressants to address anxiety symptoms or sleep problems.

We do not go into detail about specific medications and their indications for two reasons: (1) doing so requires a highly detailed knowledge of the individual child, and (2) the medications and their indications are a moving target, constantly changing; you want to talk this through with someone who knows your child well and is fully up to date on the medications, formulations, dosages, and side effects at the moment of prescribing.

It has been our experience that a trial of medications is suggested at some point for more than half of the children about whom we are talking. In part, this reflects the general increase in the use of these medications in children (almost every classroom and every group at camp now includes a child or two who takes medicine for a behavioral or an emotional issue), but it also reflects the fact that many of the kids we're writing about go through some pretty hard times, and that even with full family support and lots of therapy, many families at some point are faced with a situation in which they feel their children need something more. There is a growing body of short- and long-term research studies demonstrating the effectiveness and safety of medications for some of these disorders, perhaps especially ADHD. This chapter is an attempt to make sense of the questions that typically come up, explain the current wisdom of the professionals who usually prescribe medications for behavioral and mental health issues, and review some of the data regarding use of these medications in quirky kids, including their benefits and side effects.

Occasionally, the suggestion to consider medication arises early in the child's life or early in the diagnostic evaluation. More commonly, it occurs as the child enters the school-age years, when academic and social demands are greater, when conformity to some notion of normal is expected, and when the child and family are feeling the stresses more acutely. The early childhood years, when parents can keep their children close to home, even if that means carting them around to different appointments and evaluations, are a bit of a honeymoon period for most families, though it may seem so only in retrospect. Medications that help children manage in school may also have beneficial effects on family interactions.

Kids exhibit stress in different ways, but the most notable feature of a child's distress—anxiety, obsessiveness, moodiness, irritability, attentional difficulties—will be the target of the suggested medications, which are offered in the spirit of helping children and families through difficult times and often to help children function and succeed in the school setting, which becomes such an important part of their world. Parents should make these decisions after due consideration and discussion and keep in mind that these are not necessarily long-term commitments; some children may need a medication to help them through a rough patch, and there's always the opportunity to reevaluate.

When Should My Child Use Medication?

No parent is ever eager to see a child start taking psychotropic medications, but some parents feel strongly that they will do anything to avoid this. They need to try all other possible approaches, perhaps nontraditional therapies or a change in schools or school programs.

Medications should only be used as a last resort. I worry that medication will make my son into a zombie, and he has a very nice disposition. He's very affectionate and loving, and despite everything, he's a happy kid.

Trevor has never been on any medications, and meds have never been suggested for him by any of the doctors he has seen. We're both happy about this, but we suspect that medications may be in his future for his anxiety, which is his biggest area of difficulty and will probably get worse.

Depending on how serious a particular child's problems, symptoms, and behaviors may be, putting off medications and trying other changes in the child's life may be the best strategy at a given point in time. Sometimes you find the right school, and the stress lessens notably. Sometimes your child takes a developmental step or makes a friend, and things get easier. Families often revisit the question at a different age, a different developmental stage, or a time of new and different challenges. No decision is set in stone. Similarly, a decision to start treatment with medication is not a lifetime commitment. You need to look at what is most helpful for your own child at this particular time.

> When Caitlin was about 6, we tried a course of an antidepressant also used to treat anxiety in kids on the recommendation of her doctor. We had already changed her school environment, hired a full-time aide, and involved her in a lot of different therapies, and she still needed something to help with her rigidity and her phobias. It helped her tremendously. It freed her up verbally and with communication. She stayed on it for 1½ years and then tapered off.

Most of the time, if someone who knows your child well is recommending medications, it suggests that the child is experiencing significant stress, that the activities of normal everyday life are just too demanding or distressing. As we said earlier, almost all parents initially resist the idea of using a medication to alter their children's behavior and would prefer to try any number of nonmedical therapies first. We're not telling you that drug treatment is inevitable. However, you may reach a place at which you feel that your child's problem is just too great, and you find yourself willing to try anything that might help. When a medication does indeed help, even parents who were initially opposed may begin to feel that it is essential, and that withholding medications is actually cruel.

> In the fifth grade, George became very anxious and depressed. By the third week of school, he had pulled out all his eyelashes and had a giant bald spot on the top of his head. He said things like, "I think my school would be better off without me," and "I think I should go away and live in a box with the homeless people." I knew this was very serious and couldn't stand to see him suffering. I quickly got him to a psychiatrist, who prescribed medications.

We have learned a few rules of thumb from working with families as they go through this process:

- *Trust your professional.* Be sure that you trust the medical professional making the recommendation. Because medications need to be prescribed by a physician or nurse practitioner (according to the rules in your state), finding someone you like and trust is imperative. General pediatricians should have a trusted child psychiatrist, a developmental-behavioral pediatrician, or a psychiatric nurse practitioner to whom families can be referred for detailed discussions about the use of medications. This person should understand the potential benefits of the drugs, have experience in prescribing them and in following children receiving treatment with these medicines, and be committed to communicating with you about these issues.

- *Seek out an expert.* Some communities have a few experts—developmental-behavioral pediatricians, child psychiatrists, pediatric neurologists—who practice in the world of quirky kids. These physicians see hundreds of families and have tremendous experience in prescribing medications. Usually, there is a long waiting list to see such people, but it's often well worth the wait. The emergence of telemedicine and video visits resulting from the 2020 pandemic has opened options for families to see experts who may be farther away, and some quirky kids may actually be more comfortable with this option. Having a long-term partner in the professional world who knows your child well is a terrific asset. As your child progresses through different developmental and educational stages, if the question of medications comes up, such decisions are easily made with the assistance of a consultant who knows your child well. In addition, such a person should be able to answer questions about the downside of treating with a particular medicine and the ramifications of not treating with a medicine at all.

- *Use caution.* Be wary of specific suggestions for medications made by people who don't have the responsibility of prescribing these drugs and tracking their effects. Be wary as well of those who condemn all use of medications in all children, whether they are your family members or people in your community.

- *Flexibility is key.* You need to stay flexible, and you need a medical partner who's flexible and truly helpful. The prescribing clinician must be open minded and attentive to the experience of your child and family, ready to try different dosages or juggle medications a little until a good result is achieved. Not all children react alike to a given medicine or a given dosage. This is even more true for quirky kids, with their different neural wiring. You need a prescribing partner with the ability to listen with care and compassion, to accept that a particular medication may not have been exactly right for a particular child, that the adverse effects are overwhelming, or that the target symptoms are not being touched. These skills distinguish truly seasoned and objective practitioners from those who are familiar with only a limited repertoire of therapies or are limited by their own agendas. No one should ever make you feel that it's your child's fault if the medicine isn't right—or your fault because you won't admit to an improvement that isn't there!

- *Give it time.* We are far more tolerant of a change in an antibiotic when the first one didn't work for an ear infection. The average family has little experience with psychotropic medications, which makes the process of finding the right drug or the right combination much more stressful. The prescribing clinician must work as a partner with the child and family. This means not just listening at appointments but also being available for short consultations and questions when the need arises, which may be at unexpected times. Many of these specialized practitioners are overscheduled and excessively busy; some will have special call-in hours or online portals to make it easier to ask questions. Be sure to ask your prescribing clinician about how you can get in touch if you have a question or problem.

It took us a while to get it right. With the kids on medicines, questions come up all the time, and one of us wants a quick conversation with their doctor. He had a system for questions and that was reassuring to us, to know that we could get our questions answered.

When your child is being treated with medications, you need a way to get your questions answered if you think there is a problem or a side effect. Ask the prescribing clinician how to call or send a message with questions, and when you do leave that message, make sure you describe the level of urgency. With all calls of this nature, call again if you don't receive a timely response.

A course of drug treatment has helped many kids through particularly rough patches at school or at home. Clearly, children with disabling symptoms can benefit somewhat more from other therapies (eg, occupational therapy, speech and language therapy, social-skills training) when their problems—anxiety, inattention, moodiness, or obsessiveness—are reduced or eliminated with the use of medications.

This chapter on medications is not intended to take the place of a consultation with an appropriate prescribing clinician. What is up-to-date at the time of writing may well have changed by the time you read this information. Do not, under any circumstances, change your child's medication, dosage, or schedule before talking with your physician. Do not ever, under any circumstances, give your child a medication that has been prescribed for someone else. Every child is different, every case is different, and information and recommendations are constantly changing. Use this book for background information, to inform yourself about what you want to discuss with the physician or nurse practitioner who actually knows your child. Be aware that there is no substitute for proper evaluation by an experienced clinician who understands the issues particular to *your* child.

A Good Diagnostic Assessment

A good diagnostic assessment means better treatment. Maybe you didn't want a diagnosis at first, maybe you resisted the idea of a label, but, generally, if it's time to think about medications, it's important to know which overall diagnostic category best fits your child. The team involved in the care of your child needs to be aware of any previous evaluations, and you and the team need to agree on the best diagnostic category.

In addition, it is helpful to agree on which symptom or symptoms, and for which settings, you're targeting with the medication: Is social anxiety at school making it difficult for him to leave the house? Is staying on task with after-school homework a real nightmare? We do children a great service when we perform thorough evaluations and create appropriate classifications of their overall combinations of symptoms or behaviors. However, we should point out that many different symptoms are treated with the same drugs. In particular, the atypical antipsychotics are the most commonly used class of medications for kids with autism spectrum disorder (ASD). The selective serotonin reuptake inhibitors (SSRIs) are also used a great deal.

No medication will correct the underlying neurobiology of quirky kids, but there is a lot of experience with medicines that have been used to treat some of the symptoms these children are likely to manifest. Many families can tolerate a given behavior or mood up to a point. When it escalates to a degree that it interferes with the child's or the family's daily functioning, it is no longer a nuisance but a symptom warranting directed treatment. The targeted symptom should be kept in mind at all times, because it is your most valuable index for assessing whether a medication is helping or not.

When Sam's moods and reactivity started causing chaos in the whole family and his tantrums were affecting his two brothers, we felt at a loss. We had tried so hard to help him with therapy and various groups as well as with lots of support and compassion. His child psychiatrist started him on medications, and things became much smoother at home. It's not perfect, but it's a lot better.

What Are We Treating?

Generally, medications are suggested for treating extreme versions of some of the behaviors, symptoms, and feelings we've been discussing in this book. Parents and professionals who have experience with quirky kids describe their rigidity, social difficulties, obsessive tendencies, attention issues, anxiety, irritability, reactivity, and moodiness tending toward depression, especially as they approach adolescence and become more aware of their differences. Some children may engage in self-injurious behavior, such as picking at their skin or head-banging, symptoms that have a considerable effect on parents and teachers and can lead to medical complications. Many of these behaviors have been successfully addressed with medications when other approaches have failed.

Can Medications Help With Learning Problems?

Learning disabilities and learning differences cannot be directly targeted by medications, but children may be able to focus better and use effective learning strategies when their overwhelming anxiety or obsessive tendencies are under better control or when their attention deficits are at least modified. In fact, many children with severe attentional issues feel that medication makes a tremendous difference in their ability to cope with school. This may be one reason that school personnel sometimes seem eager for their students to be treated with medications.

Doesn't It Seem Wrong to Medicate a Child for Not Fitting In?

Many people are troubled by the idea that children who somehow fail to fit in with their surroundings end up medicated, as if the goal were to drug children into some kind of social homogeneity and conformity. Bear in mind, though, that we are not talking about the mildly eccentric child in an intolerant world. We're talking about kids who truly can't function in school because they're so anxious or rigid, so unable to concentrate, or so troubled by physical restlessness or tics. If you have made reasonable attempts to tailor your child's environments to his strengths and weaknesses, and something is still getting in the way of his learning and development and joie de vivre, it is not immoral or cowardly to consider medication. As pediatricians, we know there's no guarantee that medications will work. We certainly have heard the stories in which particular kids don't do well on particular medications, but we feel the publicity may be out of proportion considering the number of children who are helped by medication and grateful for the help. Still, we have included comments by parents whose children have had mixed or negative reactions to specific medications to emphasize that kids need careful watching, and that a medical regimen should be seen as a work in progress.

Some parents are also deeply disturbed by the idea that their child's personality will somehow be coming from the medicine bottle. Our experience, however, is that when children who have been severely affected by one or more of these symptoms undergo a successful medication trial, what parents report is not in any way a personality change. Rather, parents describe finally being able to observe—and enjoy—their child's true personality, the personality that they have always known was there but that has been obscured or pushed aside, at least for a while, by the obsessions, depression, anxiety, or hyperactivity.

What Does It Mean for a Medication To Be Approved?

When we say that a certain medication is approved for use in someone with a particular diagnosis or that it is approved for use in children older than a certain age, we mean that the US Food and Drug Administration (FDA) has examined evidence from a considerable body of research and given an official stamp of approval. The FDA looks at risks and side effects as well as whether there is real evidence that the drug treats the particular symptom or disease. The approval process is long and intense, so official FDA approval is an indication that these medications have a good safety profile for use in kids.

On the other hand, if a drug is not approved for use in children, that probably means it has not been fully studied in this age group, not that it has been tested and found to be dangerous. In fact, physicians frequently prescribe medications for symptoms other than the approved indications. We are also allowed to prescribe outside the approved age ranges. There are many situations in which that becomes necessary when you take care of children, because many important drugs are tested first in adults, so there may be a reason to try a newer seizure drug or antidepressant that has not been tested in children. This is called *off-label* prescribing. We should point out that many of the medications we discuss have not yet been approved for use in children, though they are frequently prescribed, and, therefore, there is a good amount of clinical experience with them.

The trials necessary to test a drug in children are expensive and complex, and sometimes drug companies don't pursue them. The FDA also monitors safety and side effects and may change guidelines. A great deal of attention has been paid to the question of whether antidepressant medications carry a risk of suicidal thoughts and behavior, especially early in treatment. As of 2004, the FDA specifically required a *black box* warning on these medications regarding the danger to young adults. This issue is important to discuss with your child's prescriber. The highest risk period appears to be very early in the course of treatment, so close watching and assessment of mood is critical. Although this is a frightening issue, for parents as well as for providers, untreated depression in itself is both damaging and also can be life-threatening; the risk of suicide is higher in untreated depression.

Target Symptoms: What Can We Treat With Medications?

No list of psychiatric medications is completely up-to-date or all-inclusive, and new medications and new data come out all the time. Our goal here is to give you some general information that may be useful in your conversations with your child's developmental-behavioral pediatrician, psychiatrist, or psychiatric nurse practitioner, as well as to give you a general sense of when and how medications may—or may not—be useful as your child grows, changes, and develops. This is not an exhaustive list of every medication or combination of medications that may be recommended or prescribed for an individual, and it does not take the place of talking with your child's doctor about which medications make the most sense for your child.

This following section is organized by symptoms. Look up the symptoms that concern you, and you will see the medication options. We discuss some general classes of drugs, but we don't get into much detail because the landscape is constantly changing. There's a great deal of information here, and some of it may seem scary. We don't think you need to read it straight through, as if everything applies to your child. Almost every psychiatric drug has at least rare serious adverse effects. A list of medications is not where any parent starts with a quirky child, but if this is where you've arrived, then knowledge is power.

Target Symptom: Anxiety

The single symptom most likely in any child with one of the quirky-kid diagnoses is anxiety, which can take many forms. In younger children, this can be confusing. Restlessness is quite common in young kids and is sometimes interpreted as anxiety. Many quirky children are described as worriers, but some have more specific anxiety syndromes such as social phobia or obsessive or perseverative thinking. Some kids exhibit true panic reactions. Younger children with anxiety are generally able to get along in the safety of their families without medications. Parents often unwittingly accommodate their child's fears by gradually changing their routines to avoid situations that might bring on anxiety or worsen it. Older children often use such avoidant strategies on their own, and, eventually, they realize how restricted their lives have become.

> We learned to avoid any animals, especially unpredictable puppies, windy days, loud noises or crowds, water, or sand. We couldn't attend any movies or concerts, go outside if it was breezy, or go to

the beach. No dinners in restaurants, especially kid-friendly ones. We disconnected the doorbell and stopped grinding our coffee. We felt like we were in prison.

Making some adjustments because of a child's reactions is completely reasonable (no need to drag the child who hates crowds and loud noises to the circus), but the kind of extreme limitation in this family isn't practical over the long run, and doesn't really make sense because the child is going to have to live in the world, and the world does have doorbells. We probably would advise some cognitive behavioral therapy (CBT) as a place to start; it's often successful with phobias around animals, but if that isn't enough to dial down their daughter's anxiety, the parents might find themselves considering medication.

As children grow up, it becomes more and more difficult for their families to continue shielding them from whatever triggers their anxiety. In addition, older children often develop social anxiety as they realize they are different from their peers. Many children and adolescents do really well with CBT and the various techniques they can learn to manage their anxiety. However, some kids really struggle, and, like many adults (anxiety disorders are the most common mental health problems in adults), some need to think about a medication trial. For some children, who are living with nearly constant anxiety, a daily medication will be necessary, while others may find that they need to take an occasional dose when something particularly difficult or stressful is coming up. This is similar to adults' needing medication before getting on a plane or performing on stage.

Antianxiety medications have been used a long time in adults and children with primary anxiety disorders and also when anxiety is a feature of another overall problem such as depression. When medications work, people describe being able to go about the business of living again, without intrusive worries interfering with their pleasure, sleep, or ability to concentrate.

Antianxiety drugs, sometimes called anxiolytics, fall into several classes. Most commonly used are the antidepressants and benzodiazepines. Each class of drugs has a spectrum of strengths and side effects, and within each class, drugs have different effectiveness profiles and side effects; this is why you want a knowledgeable prescribing practitioner who will be able to discuss these with you.

Antidepressants

Antidepressants are frequently recommended for children and adolescents with anxiety with or without an accompanying feature of depression or obsessive disorders, and are often prescribed for quirky kids. The SSRIs (such as Prozac and Zoloft) are the most commonly prescribed in children and adolescents, followed by the serotonin/norepinephrine reuptake inhibitors as second-line agents if SSRIs are not tolerated or effective. These medicines work by making more neurotransmitter available to the central nervous system. They are useful in treating anxiety in adults, and their use in childhood anxiety has increased dramatically in recent years. As we previously noted, there is concern about the possibility that some children and young adults experience suicidal thoughts early in treatment with the SSRI class of medications, and this is critical to discuss with the prescribing clinician. Some of the SSRIs interact with other medications. The prescribing clinician should be aware of all medicines your child is taking, including supplements, complementary and alternative treatments, and over-the-counter medications. For these reasons, the prescribing clinician needs to obtain a thorough history of your child, his symptoms, and the family history. For example, does your child have great difficulty falling asleep at night? Are there dramatic mood swings? If there is a component of depression, was its onset gradual or sudden? The answers to these questions and others may help guide the choice of a specific antidepressant.

Antidepressants have to be taken for several weeks before they are fully effective. And when a child stops taking an antidepressant, the medication should be tapered gradually under medical supervision to avoid uncomfortable side effects that can occur if the treatment is stopped suddenly.

We have worked with families for whom antidepressants were not especially helpful or who needed to discontinue the drugs because of side effects. Other families found the drugs immensely beneficial. Effective medical treatment for the sometimes disabling anxiety that afflicts quirky kids can make a great difference in their lives. Once again, many children experience improvement over time and are able to stop taking medications. Others can learn to reduce their anxiety with CBT, which has a strong evidence base, or with mind-body techniques such as relaxation, though they may be able to learn how only when their anxiety is temporarily alleviated by means of a medical intervention.

> I was able to see Sam's "stuff" in a new light. Even though many well-meaning friends and doctors had told me to see it as a medical or biological problem, I couldn't understand that until I saw how much better he was on an antidepressant. Then I felt I could begin to accept this as biologically based, just the way he was born, rather than something my wife and I had done to him.

Benzodiazepines

These are the oldest and best-known class of antianxiety drugs; Valium has been in use since the 1960s. They are sometimes prescribed for children for periodic anxiety-provoking events, such as a sleepover that a child really wants to attend but is so anxious he can't sleep, or Halloween, which terrifies a child every year, or the annual flight to see grandparents in Florida over school vacation. Some of the names you may hear are lorazepam (Ativan) and clonazepam (Klonopin). Quirky kids are generally less likely to be treated with these medications on a daily basis. They are usually used to reduce distress related to anxiety in the short term, for example while waiting for an antidepressant to take effect, which can be weeks. Alternatively, they are used for acute periods of heightened distress or panic attacks related to a specific event or stressor, such as starting at a new school or flying on a plane. Benzodiazepines are not typically prescribed long term because people can develop a tolerance to them.

Target Symptom: Depression

Quirky kids experience depression at higher rates than children in the general population. Depression in a child can bring a whole family down, and most families look eagerly for help and advice. As a well-known developmental pediatrician said to one of us, "Parents can only be as happy as their saddest child." There is much discussion about whether depression in these kids is primary or secondary—that is, are they innately more prone to it, or is it, like anxiety, sometimes a reaction to the many other difficulties they face? What child wouldn't become depressed if he is subjected to bullying at school, if he feels that he has no friends, and if he is constantly reminded that he is different? Of course, it's worth doing everything possible to address the problems directly, and you should take up the bullying issue with the school. Still, whatever may be contributing to a child's depression, we need to acknowledge that depression is real, it's profoundly painful, and it prevents a child from taking joy in daily life; in addition, there often is a biological component such that even if you can make some environmental fixes, your child may still remain depressed. If your child has close biological relatives on either side who experienced depression or bipolar disorder, that information also should be included in the medical assessment. Bipolar disorder is a cycling mood disorder that is highly heritable and includes cycles of low and high spirits; when some people with bipolar disorder take antidepressant medication, they may respond with agitation and this sometimes leads to rethinking the diagnosis and the treatment.

Adolescence is not easy for anyone; there are lots of social and academic pressures, and nowadays this all happens in the setting of intense social media activity that parents often don't fully understand. Some studies have shown a connection between social media activity and mental health risks. A recent report indicated that social media is the most common source of stress and anxiety for teenagers. Many adolescents, quirky or not, experience symptoms of depression, and parents need to be aware of the signs, which can include irritability, social withdrawal, loss of appetite or overeating for comfort, sleeping too much or too little, loss of pleasure in their usual activities, or new academic difficulties due to concentration problems. Any comments that children or adolescents make about hopelessness, hurting themselves, wanting to die, or how everyone would be better off without them need to be taken very seriously; these children need to be assessed on an urgent basis, and not by their parents but by mental health professionals.

> When George became depressed, I longed for the days when he was oblivious to his differences. When he became more tuned in to what was going on around him, it hit him really hard. I am hoping that a short trial of medication will be enough to help him through, but I have no way of knowing if that will turn out to be true.

For the children we are addressing, supportive relationships with professionals in the mental health field can go a long way toward helping them develop insight, a fuller understanding of their problems, and strategies to cope with them. Combining other types of therapy with medication, if indicated, may be the most effective strategy, but the medication should not take the place of having a professional with whom to talk things over. In fact, taking medication makes it even more critical that there be a professional eye on how your child is responding.

The medications indicated for the treatment of depression fall into several classes, but children are most likely to be given SSRIs for the antianxiety effects.

Selective Serotonin Reuptake Inhibitors

The SSRIs, such as Prozac and Zoloft, which we just discussed in terms of their antianxiety properties, are likely to be recommended as first-line therapy for depressive symptoms in a child. They are preferred over the older classes of antidepressants because there are fewer side effects and fewer risks. They are also not nearly as dangerous when taken in overdose as some of the older anti-depressants, so they are not as scary to have around the house (where a child might accidentally take too many) or to have in the possession of someone feeling depressed (who might see them as a mechanism for suicide). Because SSRIs are indicated for treatment of anxiety and obsessive symptoms as well, they are a reasonable first choice for the quirky child who has this combination of symptoms.

Serotonin/Norepinephrine Reuptake Inhibitors

These medications, such as venlafaxine (Effexor) and duloxetine (Cymbalta) affect both serotonin and norepinephrine neurotransmitter systems. They are approved for use in adults and sometimes used off-label in children and adolescents for both anxiety and depression.

No drugs that treat depression are without side effects. Many offer slightly different profiles in terms of the symptoms they treat best. As always, it is absolutely essential to be working with a clinician whom you trust and who is available to answer questions when they arise. Depression shadows the lives of many quirky kids, at least at times, and although this is a major decision, sometimes the right medication at the right moment can really improve, or save, a child's life.

Atypical Antidepressants

A number of atypical antidepressants work on different neurotransmitter systems than the more typical antidepressants. The most commonly prescribed for kids with anxiety and/or depression are mirtazapine (Remeron) and bupropion (Wellbutrin). Mirtazapine is sometimes prescribed for children with autism spectrum disorder who struggle with anxiety, sleep difficulties, and/or eating difficulties. Bupropion, perhaps best known for smoking cessation, is used to treat anxiety and depression.

All of these antidepressants come with a black-box warning about an increased risk of suicidal thinking in adolescents and young adults. Although rare, you need to discuss this with the prescribing physician or nurse practitioner, and close monitoring early in the course of treatment is critical.

Target Symptom: Obsessive and Perseverative Thoughts and Behaviors

Many of the children we are discussing have a tendency to perseverate—to think about something over and over to the exclusion of other things—or to become obsessive in their interest in a topic. Others may have a compulsive behavior such as chewing on their clothes or picking at themselves. Just as anxiety can overlap with depression, it can also play a role in obsessional thoughts and behaviors. When quirky kids have a special interest, the interests themselves may have a peculiar quality. Some kids become incredibly knowledgeable about movie animation technology, insects and reptiles, or batteries (to choose a few kids we know) and can talk about nothing else. Although this may be charming or endearing in younger kids, it becomes less so as they grow up and is positively annoying in adults (on the other hand, plenty of adults out there—including many doctors—have an intense interest in some obscure topic and may occasionally risk boring others in social situations).

Still, parents often find that when their children are engaged in their particular interests, they are at their happiest. So we are definitely not telling you that you should medicate your child out of a special fascination or enthusiasm. Medication is only worth considering when the special interest so absorbs children that they cannot engage in the world around them, limiting their lives. As with anxiety, the first-line approach should include behavioral therapy, especially CBT. But if behavioral approaches fail to help, it may be necessary to consider medication or to try the two approaches together.

> **Our son couldn't talk to anyone about anything except the weather. All conversations revolved around the temperature, the reading on the hygrometer, the forecast, the wind speed, the barometric pressure, the likelihood of a hurricane or tornado, precipitation. At first, it was kind of cute—here was this small boy engaging everyone about the weather. Over time, we realized that he really couldn't talk about anything else and needed the conversation to be about his topic. When we stopped indulging him every single time he wanted to talk about weather, he became very anxious.**

It is worth reiterating that although many quirky kids have obsessive or perse-verative qualities as a manifestation of their anxiety and may exhibit repetitive and ritualized behaviors, they usually do not have classic obsessive-compulsive disorder. As with anxiety, if obsessional thinking is a recurring and powerful force in a given child's life, it's important for the child to undergo a full evalua-tion. We have been talking about obsessional and perseverative behaviors and thoughts as one piece of a quirky child's way of dealing with the world, but if your child is growing up in a world completely shaped by those thoughts and behaviors, the problem needs to be diagnosed and treated.

The SSRIs are the most commonly recommended medications for children with these symptoms, but sometimes other drugs such as the atypical anti-psychotics (risperidone [Risperdal], aripiprazole [Abilify], and quetiapine [Seroquel]) may be tried. As we mentioned earlier, this class of medications is now the most commonly prescribed for kids with ASD, and is FDA approved.

Chrissie's trichotillomania [twirling her hair until it came out of her scalp] was really hard to deal with, and that's when we turned to medications. We tried a variety of medicines to help with this and with her anxiety. We had tried so many strategies before that, and none of them really helped.

Target Symptom: Irritability

Irritability is a common concern in quirky kids, and it can have many implications. We've already talked about the syndrome of kids who seem uncomfortable in their own skin, about off-the-scale meltdowns and tantrums in young children (or sometimes not-so-young), about restlessness that may look like inattention, and about oppositional and hostile behavior. When we think about giving a child medication for irritability, we are not talking about episodic or occasional incidents of bad temper, but rather about a child who can't learn or can't function because of a high level of chronic irritability that gets in the way of everything else, after a thorough assessment has been done to look for environmental triggers and problems that potentially could be modified. Second, we are assuming that other possible problems have been addressed, from difficulty processing sensory input to anxiety to stomach distress to attentional issues. Less severe irritability may be managed with SSRIs, but more severe irritability—true rage attacks—may call for the use of low doses of antipsychotic medication.

Atypical Antipsychotics

Let's admit it: Antipsychotics may be the scariest word in this chapter. The antipsychotics, also called neuroleptics, are used to address many problems faced by quirky kids, from tic disorders to irritability, usually after other classes of medications have failed. The so-called atypical antipsychotics, including Risperdal, Zyprexa, Abilify, and Seroquel, are now the most commonly prescribed psychotropic medications for children and adolescents with ASD, and they are the only medications FDA approved for irritability. Originally developed for psychotic individuals, they are currently used for a number of other indications as a second- or third-line option. These newer antipsychotic medications are used with great frequency in quirky kids because they can address compulsive or obsessive behaviors, mood swings, reactivity, self-mutilating behavior or picking at oneself, and explosive or aggressive behavior.

One reason people are often scared by the term *antipsychotics* is that they remember the older antipsychotic medications, which had serious side effects, and though these side effects are less likely with the newer "atypicals," they are still a concern. Weight gain is by far the most common worry for children being treated with these medicines, but they can also cause sleeping problems and a range of other issues, and, rarely, they can cause movement disorders. Children receiving treatment with any drug from this class of medications should have a blood test once a year to assess for possible side effects.

Target Symptom: Attention-Deficit/Hyperactivity Disorder

Many quirky kids are first diagnosed with attentional problems or ADHD, and many continue to struggle with attentional issues into adulthood. It's worth repeating that many other problems can look like attentional issues; children who are unduly anxious or depressed or overwhelmed by sensory input may look like they aren't concentrating, and you want to make sure these other possibilities are considered.

For kids whose problem really is inattention, life becomes more difficult as they progress further in school and academic demands increase, along with the expectation that they sit still for long periods of time and focus on whatever subject is assigned. Many kids with attentional issues get by for a while, especially if they're academically gifted, but eventually school demands catch up with them. Other kids, especially the ones who are truly hyperactive, are perceived as behavior problems and disruptive presences in the classroom, and their parents report endless phone calls from the school and trips to pick up a child from the principal's office. Having ADHD is difficult—for the child and for the people around the child. The restless "hyper" boys often think of themselves as always in trouble, while the quiet inattentive kids (often girls) can be missed for years, going through school without ever being able to concentrate. It's clear that a subset of kids, some quirky, some not, struggle mightily with the ability to focus, to screen out distractions, to tone down some of their impulses, and above all, accomplish what they want or need to do. They are misinterpreted as being lazy, poorly motivated, or disruptive, but if you talk to them, they are often desperate to behave themselves and learn along with everybody else. We need to point out what almost everyone taking care of children will tell you: Many children and families are deeply grateful to have this problem recognized, diagnosed, and managed. And medication has a strong track record here. Decades of clear scientific evidence show that medications can help. Children with attentional issues can benefit from all kinds of additional supports and structures at home and all kinds of modifications at school. But many also function better when treated with medication.

Untreated, kids with ADHD almost invariably develop self-esteem issues (it's no fun to be the kid who's in trouble all the time) and have greater rates of school failure and substance misuse, particularly marijuana. About half of children diagnosed with attentional problems continue to experience symptoms of ADHD in adulthood, so treatment is essential and involves a real commitment to finding the right therapy for any given stage of life. The demands of adulthood can be a real challenge for individuals with ADHD, when they are expected to structure their own time, motivate themselves, make decisions, and be responsible for themselves and perhaps others. Adults with untreated ADHD have higher rates of substance misuse and traffic accidents. Those who are treated effectively may find themselves in situations in which shifting attention is actually a strength. Think of emergency department doctors, who need to constantly react to new stimuli and think on their feet. Other first responders report high rates of childhood ADHD diagnoses.

Most primary care pediatricians are well versed in the diagnosis of attentional problems, which usually involves asking parents and teachers to answer questions on a validated screening form about a child's behavior. Be sure to inform the pediatrician if your child has biological relatives with ADHD; as with anxiety and depression, there is definitely a genetic component here. It is also important to remember that although attentional issues may be one component—or the main component—of a child's quirky package, if a lot more is going on, it's always okay to seek a more thorough evaluation.

Stimulants

Stimulants have a long history of use for inattention, impulsive behavior, and distractibility, and they are effective in the great majority (at least 75%) of kids for whom they are prescribed, although the rates are somewhat lower for kids with ASD. Many parents are familiar with the most commonly prescribed medications, including methylphenidate (Ritalin) and dextroamphetamine (Adderall). In general, they are more helpful when the inattention is accompanied by hyperactivity or fidgetiness. Stimulants work through effects on the neurotransmitters dopamine and norepinephrine. The reaction is paradoxical; in a revved-up child, a stimulant calms the nervous system by increasing focus and attention. The most important side effects of stimulants include appetite suppression and sleep disturbance, so a child's growth should be monitored carefully while he is taking these medications.

Monitoring a child's reaction to the drug over the course of the day is also important. Some kids become irritable when the dose wears off, whereas others rebound or become even more moody or disorganized. Sometimes changing the medicine altogether makes the most sense; this is a process of trial and error, as with the other medications we've discussed. The first prescription may not be the last or the best, and dosages are likely to change. The maxim "start low and go slow" applies here, starting with a low dose to assess for effectiveness and side effects and gradually increasing, if necessary, to reach the desired effect. Some quirky kids seem to respond to much lower dosages of stimulants than we would expect.

Stimulants come in many different preparations, for example short acting (about 4 hours) and longer acting or sustained release over the course of a day. In addition, for kids who cannot swallow pills, there are stimulants that can be sprinkled over food and patches that gradually release the medication over time. Side effects often can be managed by a change in preparation.

A couple of caveats regarding stimulant use are worth mentioning. Stimulant use in a child with a tendency toward tics can be the catalyst that gets the tics started. About 15% of children with a diagnosis of ADHD will also have tics. Quirky kids are believed to have higher rates of tics and tic disorders like Tourette syndrome. The actual percentage is not known. Still, it is worth bearing in mind when deciding about stimulant use and when monitoring the effects of such use. Second, stimulants are controlled medications (ie, they can be misused and abused). Although the doses used to treat ADHD symptoms are not addictive, we have certainly known adolescents who diverted their stimulants (ie, selling or offering them to friends). However, untreated ADHD increases the risk of substance misuse later in adolescence. As we've said before, kids need relief from these symptoms, because being unable to focus and learn is very uncomfortable. Some older teens find relief in marijuana, which has negative impacts on the developing brain. Stimulants are highly effective in mitigating these miserable feelings, and being treated properly with a stimulant medication actually lowers the long-term risk of substance use disorder.

Nonstimulant medication

Atomoxetine (Strattera) is used as a second-line treatment for ADHD, largely in children who cannot tolerate stimulants. Because it is not a controlled substance, refills are more convenient for prescribers and families. Like stimulants, it has about a 90% response rate. As with stimulants, children with developmental disabilities tend to respond at somewhat lower rates. The alpha agonists (guanfecine, clonidine), which were originally developed to treat high blood pressure in adults, are sometimes used in children with ADHD; they may be prescribed for children who cannot tolerate stimulants or don't respond to them well, but they are also often tried in combination with stimulants and may be suggested for children with irritability, and with tics.

Target Symptom: Tic Disorders

Tic disorders occur with increased frequency in quirky kids, but provisional (less than 12 months in duration) tic disorders of childhood are quite common in kids in general, especially school-aged boys. Lots of kids go through a phase of eye blinking, throat clearing, or head turning—or something more dramatic. The hallmark of the tic disorder is that the behavior stops while the child is asleep, and provisional tic disorders tend to be completely benign and go away with time. Tourette syndrome is a diagnosis that signifies the persistent presence of motor as well as vocal tics for at least a year. Tourette syndrome does run in families. A proper diagnostic workup is especially important in this population because tics can be mistaken for nervousness (and vice versa), and the treatment options will be dictated by the correct diagnosis.

Tics do not necessarily need to be treated with medications, and, in fact, many young kids are not at all bothered by their tics, but sometimes they can really interfere with a child's life. To make things more confusing, some medications, particularly the stimulants, can trigger, or uncover, a tic disorder, though medications do not cause Tourette syndrome. A specific therapy called cognitive behavioral intervention for tics has been shown to be helpful; other behavioral therapies have not. For a child who needs medication for tics, a variety of drugs may be suggested, including some antihypertensive medications, such as clonidine (Catapres) and guanfacine (Tenex). The atypical antipsychotic drugs, the most commonly prescribed class of medications for quirky kids, may be useful here, and the first choice is usually aripiprazole (Abilify), which may also help with associated behavioral problems. It is used at a low dose when treating tics.

Other Symptoms, Other Problems, Other Medications

Other symptoms occur with higher frequency in the population of quirky children, and some of them, such as seizures, will certainly require medication. To make life more complicated, the anticonvulsant medications may also affect a child's mood and other aspects of behavior, and some of them may be suggested for children who have mood issues and don't have seizures. So there are many other categories of medication that occasionally are used to treat quirky children. Many characteristics of quirky kids do not fit neatly into the categories we've discussed in this chapter but may be amenable to medical therapy if they're so extreme that they're blighting the children's lives: their rigid natures, difficulties with transitions, anger, stereotypic motor behaviors that are not exactly tics, and sometimes bizarre social behaviors. The bottom line is this: Keep an open mind, talk with your physician about anything that's really getting in your child's way, and make sure you feel you have a trusted medical partner who is really listening to your concerns and willing to consider a range of options. You don't want to jump immediately to medication for every issue, but you don't want to rule it out either, and no decision should be seen as final or even necessarily a long-term commitment.

How Long Will I Have to Medicate My Child?

Many children take a single medication, successfully targeting a specific symptom—a tic, a high level of anxiety around starting school, a compulsive habit, difficulty sleeping, inability to focus and pay attention—and find that that medication is all they need to help them, either for a brief period or over many years. However, it's important to note that for some children, life involves multiple medications, often needing adjustment or correction as they grow. This can be challenging, but it offers some kids a chance to learn and live and function in the world on a level that would otherwise be impossible. Often, the children themselves grow to understand this.

> It took us 2 years to find the right combination of medicines to help Megan, but we felt we had to keep trying because she was so miserable and hard to live with. It had a big impact on the entire family. Megan fought the meds. She'd say things like, "You don't like me for who I am. When I'm 18, I'm not going to take them anymore. I know my rights." But when she was leaving for college a few years later, she said, "Where's my prescription? I think I need an evening dose to get my homework done." She has accepted that these meds have really helped her and knows she is more successful with them than without them.

The best news we can offer is to remind you of four comforting truths. First, the decision to move forward with a trial of medications, or even to have a child take multiple medications for a period of time, does not mean your child will need pharmaceutical support forever. Second, if you do need to try medications, the serious side effects, while worrisome, are rare. Third, many children are freed by these medications and find themselves able to thrive and experience pleasure from life when their bothersome symptoms are alleviated. Fourth, early treatment with stimulants for ADHD is associated with a reduction in adult substance misuse. When thinking about the medication options, a trusted partner in the medical profession is an important and meaningful part of your decision.

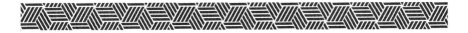

11

Medical Perspectives on the Quirky Child: Questions and Answers

As pediatricians, we find ourselves looking at quirky kids (and in fact, at all kids) through a medical lens. We see them when they're sick, and we check them when they're well, but always with a list of medical worries and what-ifs in the back of our minds. That's not necessarily the most helpful perspective when it comes to getting a kid out the door in the morning or knowing what to do when homework is agony, and we've tried in this book to recognize our limitations and to bring in educational and therapeutic expertise. In this chapter, however, we review quirkiness from the medical perspective and give you the most up-to-date science and opinions. We admit two things right off the bat: First, these scientific questions include areas of intense current research. There is a good chance that by publication, some of what we write may already be out of date. Second, when it comes to the important questions of etiologies (causes), effectiveness of therapies, and long-term prognoses, there is not always a lot of research to support definitive answers.

The risk in talking about quirkiness as a syndrome, of course, is that quirky kids are such a heterogeneous group. Some are mildly eccentric, some deeply challenged in many different ways. And then there are people who will feel that we (and perhaps that our society in general) are medicalizing or pathologizing kids whose development is not perfectly mainstream or exactly on the chart. This argument is particularly likely to be made with regard to attention-deficit/ hyperactivity disorder (ADHD), with the underlying suggestion that the problem is the environment and our expectations, not the child, despite increasing evidence that children with ADHD really are wired differently. As we said before, we've come to believe in underlying genetic, biological, or neurological differences for many of the issues included under "quirky." And we wrote this book in part because we also believe that for lots of children, these differences really can be problems, and children really struggle and can do much better with help. The science we talk about in this chapter focuses on more seriously affected children, especially those with an autism spectrum disorder (ASD) diagnosis, because they have been more widely studied and there is a growing body of evidence. Some of the questions we address may also be relevant to children with other diagnoses, or children without specific diagnoses, but we acknowledge that there is much to be learned, and that it would be a bad idea to generalize from the studies that address very specific situations.

So then, what questions do parents ask us in the office? What answers are they looking for from the medical world, from research, and from their pediatrician? Everyone has the "where-did-this-come-from?" type of questions. Parents point to other family members (or in-laws!), they think about what might have happened during pregnancy, or they worry about exposures in the atmosphere, household, or water supply. A mother may confide miserably that she drank a single glass of wine before knowing about the pregnancy, and ask if that did some damage; others worry about everything from prenatal stress to diet to infectious illnesses. And of course, many parents are aware of the controversy surrounding immunizations, and they want to know whether past immunizations may have contributed to the problem and whether future immunizations are safe.

People also want to know what kinds of information are available about the epidemiology of these conditions. Are they more common than they used to be, and do they turn up more often in some groups than in others? What do we know about the genetic factors, what do we know about the neurobiology of quirkiness?

Parents want to know about prognosis, about whether problems are likely to resolve as their child grows and develops. They want to know if all the time and care and effort they are putting into helping their child develop skills is going to result in his or her ability to manage the next stages of life: get through high school, attend college, hold a job, and live independently. Obviously, those questions change a great deal as the individual child grows and changes, but we should acknowledge that parents start worrying early and they don't stop.

Epidemiology: Are There More Quirky Kids Than Before and, if So, Why?

Whereas 40 or 50 years ago, it was a bit of an embarrassment to have a special-needs child in the family, it is openly discussed now, and there are many instances of such special children. I believe more so today than previously. Sometimes we hear of geographic clusters the way we hear of clusters of cancer cases, but I personally have not seen this, except that there are five children with autism

> in our grandson Max's class, including Max, from his small town
> in New Jersey. Among my family, friends, and in the school where I
> taught, I had no previous acquaintance with autism in any form.

Our combined experiences as pediatricians and as mothers ourselves have
certainly suggested to us that the numbers of children who fall into these
categories are increasing. Discussions with teachers and educators in all kinds
of settings reflect this same awareness. The number of children receiving
special education services has risen sharply: in Boston, it's 1 in 5 children in
the public schools, and some of these kids are definitely quirky. Schools specifically designed to meet the needs of quirky kids, with their learning profiles
or differences, are popping up in communities all over the United States as
well as in other parts of the world. While working on this book, we've found
that mentioning the topic in any social situation always yields someone in the
group who knows a quirky child and/or has a quirky child.

> We were on vacation at the beach, and I saw another child who
> reminded me of my son Max. He was flapping his hands and avoid-
> ing the water. I approached his parents, and, sure enough, he was
> "one of us"! The kids enjoyed each other in their own peculiar way,
> and I was relieved to feel that I wasn't alone.

What do we know about the incidence and epidemiology of quirky kids?
In a study published in March 2020, the Centers for Disease Control and
Prevention (CDC) reported that 1 in every 54 children meets the criteria
for ASD at age 4 years, with boys several times more likely than girls. The
American Academy of Pediatrics (AAP) recommends screening for all children at ages 18 and 24 months to assess risk and expedite referral for evaluation and services known to improve outcomes, with the goal that all children
with a diagnosis of ASD undergo a specialty evaluation before 3 years of age
(https://www.healthychildren.org/English/health-issues/conditions/Autism/
Pages/How-Doctors-Screen-for-Autism.aspx).

A lot of attention has focused on the question of whether there is an epidemic
of ASD in the United States and around the world. Certainly, increasing
numbers of kids carry the *diagnoses* of these disorders. Does that mean there
are actually more kids being born and growing up with the problems, or
does it suggest that we've gotten better at assigning the diagnoses? No one
really knows the extent to which the numbers are truly up and how much of
the increase is an artifact of how and whom we diagnose. Kids around the
edges are now more likely to receive a diagnosis than they were in the past, in

part because of increased awareness, and in part because school services for children who need help are sometimes contingent on these diagnoses. Think about what happens when a new diagnostic term is coined. The term *sensory processing disorder* is relatively new, and yet many people recognize themselves—or their kids—in its criteria. Before such a term existed, many of those people had no name for their preferences, peculiarities, or unusual behaviors.

At the same time that the numbers of kids with ASD have been climbing, the numbers of children diagnosed with intellectual disability (what was once called mental retardation, a term that is no longer used) have been decreasing. Could this represent a shift in the terminology used to diagnose kids with developmental delays, with language and learning problems? The change may reflect in part a better understanding of what's really going on with these children and in part how the label is perceived. Even if a child's IQ places him squarely in the intellectual disability range, another diagnosis may also fit the facts or account for the delays, and this other diagnosis may be easier for parents to accept.

There's controversy among researchers about what is behind the rise in ASD diagnoses. Most people would agree that some of the increases we've seen are directly related to these terminology shifts, but that doesn't exclude the possibility that more quirky kids are also being born. From an epidemiological point of view, there is a lot of work to be done investigating these questions.

We do think that children who once would have carried no diagnosis at all, or would have carried another diagnosis altogether, are now being diagnosed as having neurodevelopmental disorders, such as ASD or ADHD. But we also think that the phenomenon we're describing—the combination of developmental variations and interpersonal eccentricities we're calling quirkiness—is becoming more common. We think it's more than just increasing skill at recognizing certain diagnoses. We think there are more children around with these traits than there used to be.

Etiology: What Do We Actually Understand About the Causes of Quirkiness?

It's one of every parent's first questions: "Where did this come from?" Most of the time, there simply isn't any easy answer. Yes, in our office settings, we ask questions about family history, and often there is a relative with a similar picture, which suggests a genetic component to what is going on, though it doesn't offer any definitive explanations. Nowadays, kids who have more severe symptoms are referred to geneticists and often are re-referred every couple of years, in the hope that a new test may provide some answers.

> We often wonder where this came from in our kids. Yes, we have some funny relatives on both sides, but is that really it? We don't think about it as much as we used to, but whenever there is a new crisis, we wonder, "What did we do to deserve this?"

> My pregnancy with Chrissie was very stressful because of my career. I was working very hard, and the company was in financial trouble. I wonder about increased stress hormones in my pregnancy being a factor in Chrissie's diagnosis.

Let's just say, that at certain points, many parents have nagging questions about why their child is struggling in this way, and there is not always a clear answer about neurodevelopmental issues or about medical problems. Being a parent is a hard job. Being the parent of a child with difficulties, challenges, or serious problems is a harder job, and for all the dedication, energy, and love that parents bring to it, there are going to be some darker moments. The question of where the problem came from can sometimes serve as a focus for the doubt, sadness, and resentment. These feelings don't mean that you don't love your child; they may mean that you recognize the complexity of the assignment that life has dealt you and your child, and there are moments when that can seem overwhelming. Don't be too hard on yourself when these feelings come up, but if they are really weighing on you, or they won't go away, think about getting some additional support for yourself: a parent support group, a therapist, or a much-needed break.

We've become so much more demanding in what we expect children to do. We want preschoolers to sit still and work on the alphabet so they can learn to read in kindergarten, and we expect everyone to play nicely together in the sandbox. When a child has trouble meeting these expectations, we pin on a label. Some would argue that once upon a time, boys were restless in school and got into fights on the playground and nobody sent them to be evaluated (this line of argument brings to mind *The Adventures of Tom Sawyer*).

> I grew up in Wisconsin, where a boy like [my son] Jack would have ended up working on a dairy farm, caring for the animals, and finding a life for himself that wasn't all that different from lots of other young men there. But we are raising him in suburban Boston, where the expectations for academic performance and behavior are just too much for him. Everyone here is supposed to be good at everything.

A Long List of Theories: How Have People Tried to Explain Neurodevelopmental Variation?

Here are some of the more respectable hypotheses that have been put forward to explain neurodevelopmental variation (remember, none of this is either/or; no one single explanation covers all the children we're talking about, and probably all of these factors sometimes play roles in the incredibly complex processes of human development):

- **Genetics.** These differences in development and behavior reflect subtle differences in wiring in the brain. That implies a possible genetic origin, which we discuss in more detail later in this chapter. It's been suggested that maybe we're seeing more quirky kids because people who were once less likely to have children are now reproducing; maybe the increasing numbers of older parents play a role. Some evidence suggests that when fathers are much older than mothers, the risks are higher.
- **Prenatal development.** Maybe something happens during fetal development, perhaps because of some infection or exposure that affects the mother.
- **Environmental effect.** Maybe toxins in the environment are affecting babies' brains. It is well established that certain toxins, for example alcohol, mercury, and lead, can cause damage to the developing brain (alcohol is by far the most common exposure).
- **Technology.** Assisted reproductive technologies (ART) such as in vitro fertilization may be playing a role. Children conceived using ART are twice as likely to be diagnosed with ASD, perhaps because of prematurity or the effect of multiple gestation, both of which are independently associated with an increased risk.

- **Awareness.** We know there have always been quirky kids among us, but we may notice them more now because we notice *everything* more. The *DSM-5* diagnoses have been expanded to include a wider range of children with less extreme symptoms, and we've gotten better at diagnosing children who at one time might not even have been referred for evaluation.

From our perspective at this moment in time, there is more specific scientific evidence to back up the genetic roots of many kinds of quirkiness than there is to support the other theories of causation. When we say there are genetic causes, that does not mean that we know exactly which gene or genes are responsible for any given pattern or how these highly complex patterns of inheritance work. Currently, we are only able to identify genetic causes in 10% to 15% of children with ASD. However, there is clearly a high degree of genetic susceptibility to at least some of these disorders, based on data from family studies and twin studies.

In a 2015 analysis that looked at 13 studies, together consisting of more than 6,000 pairs of twins, there was overall almost perfect concordance for identical twins—that is, when one twin had ASD, the other twin almost always had it as well. For fraternal twins, on the other hand, the concordance was only 53%. In other words, these findings strongly suggest that there is a family predisposition (after all, half of the nonidentical twins also matched) and that the syndrome has a specific genetic cause (because the genetically identical twins were almost perfectly matched). We also know that if parents have one child with ASD, there is a significantly higher risk (as high as 14%) of having another child with ASD; if they have more than one child with ASD, the risk for subsequent children rises to about 1 in 3.

But genetics would certainly not explain why ASD might be on the increase, and although there is definitely a genetic component to at least some of the quirkiness we see, and certain families are clearly more affected than others, genetics cannot be the whole story. Genes and environment interact. It's possible, for example, that genetic heritage makes some developing brains more vulnerable than others, so that when there's an insult—an infection, a toxin, a particular problem in either the fetal or early childhood environment—the vulnerable brains are more likely to be affected, more likely to be damaged.

Many parents believe there must be some other force at work. Something is damaging children, hurting their brains, changing their lives forever. Along with the increased numbers of affected families, there has been an enormous increase in attention to possible etiologies that are largely outside the scope of traditional medical science. People have looked to dietary intolerance or allergies, environmental toxins, and perhaps most prominently to childhood immunizations as possible culprits.

As pediatricians, we are not big believers in most of these theories, and we are certainly big believers in immunization, which, of all the many putative causes, has been thoroughly investigated and clearly is not linked to ASD. Vaccines save lives—thousands and even millions of children's lives—and the question of a possible link to ASD has been exhaustively investigated and thoroughly discredited. We discuss this in more detail on pages 290–292. If you are in any doubt, we urge you to consult the AAP recommendations and evidence summary and its website for parents (www.healthychildren.org/vaccinestudies), as well as obtain information and recommendations from the CDC and the World Health Organization. Make sure your own child is fully vaccinated and protected against infectious diseases. Environmentally, there is certainly more to be learned about exposures, and, indeed, some evidence indicates that high exposure to certain pesticides and to air pollution may be linked to ASD, perhaps as a trigger in those more vulnerable brains.

When it comes to "treatments" developed to address these theoretical causes of a child's difficulties, there is little real evidence to support them, and some can actually be dangerous. Regarding the rest, some parents believe they have made a difference, and as long as they do not cost too much or interfere with other, more evidence-based treatments, these are decisions that families need to make for themselves. Still, we try hard not to send the parents of our patients down paths that will lead them to complex, expensive, and labor-intensive regimens with no research backing them. We know that a certain number of the parents we see pursue these paths and perhaps will write us off as hopelessly mainstream. However, we have no intention of telling parents to abandon anything that seems to be working. We want to make sure that our patients are immunized. Vaccine hesitancy has now been tied to outbreaks of completely preventable childhood diseases, especially measles, which can actually result in damage to the brain, as well as meningitis and even tetanus.

Many children with ASD have food allergies or intolerances, and some people have suggested that differences in digestion and diet may actually play an etiologic role for some quirky kids, and that diets can be used to treat their symptoms; however, research has not supported this. Dietary adjustments may be helpful for the many quirky kids who have gastrointestinal problems, including constipation, diarrhea, and gastroesophageal reflux (sometimes called acid reflux), each of which can lead to distress and behavioral difficulties in kids who may not be able to express where or how severe their discomfort is. More than half of these kids have a history of such difficulties as infants; they were colicky, their formula was changed, or a breast-feeding mother was put on a special diet. In addition, high rates of lactose intolerance, or difficulty digesting cow's milk, have been observed in this group of patients. The growth and nutrition programs at academic medical centers have numerous quirky kids with restricted food intake, causing a variety of symptoms, and these programs provide support and education to kids and parents.

What is the difference between an *allergy* and an *intolerance* to a particular food or substance? This terminology can be confusing. A true *allergy* is a diagnosis made on the basis of blood or skin tests that can document a response by the immune system to a given food. An *intolerance* refers to a particular reaction when a food is ingested, such as a rash, vomiting or diarrhea, or a change in behavior, that is *not* associated with an abnormal blood test result or skin test result.

There has been a lot of discussion about whether a specialized diet is an effective treatment for ASD, in particular whether a gluten-free diet is indicated. While there may be anecdotal evidence that a certain child's symptoms improved with the elimination of gluten from her diet, there is no solid scientific evidence to support a gluten-free diet as a treatment for ASD. Like any child, a quirky child could also have celiac disease, and testing for celiac disease is relatively straightforward. A child with celiac disease should absolutely be on a gluten-free diet.

There is also nonceliac gluten sensitivity, in which an individual who does not have celiac disease is still sensitive to gluten exposure. This is a more difficult diagnosis to make, and many parents have experimented with removing gluten from their child's diet to see whether it helps. Our advice is to carefully consider whether it's worth the effort to keep a child on a special diet, when there is so much else to do to support your quirky child; you want to be sure you are really seeing results by taking pasta or dairy out of your child's diet (given that many children go through phases of only eating mac and cheese).

Many parents we've interviewed discussed their children's unusual food preferences, food aversions, and restrictive eating patterns, which can lead to growth disturbances, vitamin and mineral deficiencies, as well as anemia. For some, the unusual eating habits constitute part of the restrictive or repetitive behaviors that are required to make a diagnosis of ASD in the first place. Avoidant-Restrictive Food Intake Disorder is a newer diagnostic category into which a number of quirky kids fall. This is a very difficult issue for parents, and you may well want some help. Meeting with a nutritionist—ideally one who has some experience with quirky kids—and talking it over with an occupational therapist who knows your child can help you sort out the underlying difficulties and identify strategies that might help.

Childhood Immunizations

There has been a significant amount of publicity and concern surrounding the issue of childhood immunizations, particularly the MMR (measles-mumps-rubella) vaccine. You can find first-person accounts on the internet by parents who feel their children were absolutely healthy until a certain shot was administered and then they deteriorated dramatically. Entire organizations, with publications, conferences, and publicity campaigns, are dedicated to spreading the word that vaccines cause autism.

We are pediatricians; we administer vaccines, and we know they do not cause autism. Intense and rigorous research, involving large numbers of study participants, has explored this question, which is why we're comfortable saying vaccines do not cause autism.

The MMR vaccine is generally administered for the first time between 12 and 15 months of age and then again as a booster shot between the ages of 4 and 6 years. A link to autism was first proposed by a researcher who suggested that the MMR vaccine triggers an inflammatory condition of the intestines, causing the gut to become leaky, or more permeable to toxins, which can then gain access to the brain and cause damage. His original paper, published in 1998, ignited a fiery debate that is still very much alive.

One problem is that the age at which a child receives the first MMR—12 to 15 months—is right around the time that many parents start noticing developmental concerns. This is the age, between 1 and 2 years, when children make huge strides in their development, particularly with emerging speech, and differences become more apparent. Many developmental problems do become evident around the time of the MMR vaccination, but that doesn't mean we're talking cause and effect.

The original study has been retracted by *The Lancet,* the journal that published it, because it was judged to constitute scientific fraud; investigators found that results were falsified, and the author had a financial interest in the outcome he claimed to have shown in his study. Because of his dishonest, irresponsible, and misleading behavior surrounding this issue, he was removed from the

British medical register, so he can no longer practice medicine. In addition, a number of large epidemiological studies in several countries have looked closely at the posited link between the MMR vaccine and developmental disorders and have failed to find one. In study after study, young children were just as likely to be diagnosed with autism in the time right before the vaccination as in the time right after, and they were just as likely to be diagnosed with autism if they did or did not receive the shot.

The National Academy of Medicine (formerly the Institute of Medicine), the CDC, and the AAP have all issued policy statements regarding the absence of data proving any association. But that original and now retracted paper generated such alarm that parents across the world began to decline vaccines, which, in turn, has led to outbreaks of measles, mumps, and rubella, and deaths of unprotected children. Measles is a very serious disease, and because it is so much less common than it was 50 years ago, we have little memory of the illness and its significant effects, which can include intellectual disability, blindness, and seizures. Mumps, the viral infection most familiar because of the swelling of the parotid glands of the face, also causes orchitis (inflammation of the testicles), which can result in sterility in boys. Rubella is best known for the congenital syndrome in which the offspring of a mother who contracted the illness in pregnancy is born with cataracts, heart defects, and intellectual disability. To see any of these dangerous—and completely preventable—diseases threatening children again is alarming to us as pediatricians.

Yet, the misinformation about vaccines continues to crop up, often scaring parents. Thimerosal is a preservative that contains mercury, and has been used in certain vaccines since the 1930s, but in the 1980s and 1990s, as the number of vaccines recommended in childhood increased, concerns were raised about the cumulative dose to which a child was exposed. Although extensive study has not demonstrated any ill effects of exposure to thimerosal, the AAP and the US Public Health Service asked vaccine manufacturers to remove thimerosal from all childhood vaccines in 1999. Some multidose vials of flu vaccine, which has to be formulated anew every year, and which is given both to children and adults, contain minute amounts of thimerosal. Concerned parents can also ask for thimerosal-free vaccine.

For those who distrust vaccines, none of these specifics may be convincing. They will find another vaccine to blame, because they start from the assumption that vaccines are dangerous. During our training, we watched children suffer from *Haemophilus influenzae* type B (Hib) infections, including sepsis, meningitis, and life-threatening infections of the epiglottis. We saw them die or live with complete devastation of their brains and bodies. We know why we give babies Hib vaccines, and we never want to see a case of Hib meningitis again. We don't want our patients to experience the high fever, irritability, and encephalitis that can accompany measles. We don't want to take care of any baby born with congenital rubella, see a child paralyzed by polio, or watch an adolescent's liver destroyed by chronic hepatitis B. We are encouraged by the large number of studies that have looked so closely at the MMR and other vaccines and found no associations with autism. Still, we understand why many people in the autism community are frustrated that these studies continue to be repeated, when there are so many other possible causes that have not been examined. Of the many potential reasons why there seem to be more quirky kids now than in the past, the possibility of a vaccine link has been exhaustively examined—and no such link has been found.

After considering all these possible ideas, where do we end up in terms of understanding the etiology of ASD, which is the most studied of all the diagnoses? There is no one overarching theory of etiology, just as there may be no one satisfying explanation of why this happened to your child in the way that it did. There are theories and speculations and interesting ideas, as well as mounting evidence that more severely affected children are more likely to have an underlying genetic explanation. There are environmental correlations and links to issues of pregnancy and fetal development. There is certainly reassuring evidence about vaccination, and the MMR vaccine in particular. But to date, there are not many of the answers that parents or pediatricians seek.

What Can Science Tell Us About the Neurobiological Foundation of Quirkiness?

Brain Differences

Evidence from basic research clearly shows that brain development in quirky kids is different in a number of respects, but not in a way that is likely to be seen on a computed tomographic (CT) scan or a magnetic resonance image (MRI) of the brain. Some children undergo these studies, but the results are almost always normal. However, children with ASD do tend to have slightly larger brains overall.

The key concepts of early brain development are actually quite straightforward. We define some terms in the process of explaining the ideas about what goes haywire in early brain development for quirky kids. In the first couple of years, the brain is most *plastic*, most able to be shaped by life experiences. *Dendrites*, the long, spindlelike fingers that attach brain cells to one another and enable them to communicate with one another, are relatively sparse at birth but proliferate during the early months and years and become more numerous at this point in development than at any other point in life. The neural circuits of the brain become more efficient over time, as a child's life experience fosters the *pruning down* of the number of these dendritic connections in the brain. Once this pruning has taken place, children are more able to focus on the matter at hand and tune out extraneous information or sensations. Furthermore, the brain activity centers for language shift at this point from the cerebellum, in the back of the head, to the cerebral cortex, in the front of the brain. The stage is set for learning and communication.

For children with ASD, this process seems to go awry, which may account for the sense from many parents that "everything was fine until he was about 18 months old." Without the normal pruning, there remain a huge number of connections in the brain that serve to keep the gates open for sensory experience that can be overwhelming and lead to an apparent arrest or regression of normal development. Between 18 and 19 months of age, a typical child becomes more mature in *associative memory*—that is, in memory that involves associations among all the senses—and applies emotional meaning to experience. This is a critical period for the developing child in terms of emotional connections to the world around her and the development of language. Without emotional context, skills such as language that have been gained before this period may actually be lost.

This information is useful because it lends credence to the neurological foundation of the delays and behaviors we see in these kids. On the other hand, a typical CT scan or MRI of the brain will not reveal any of these differences, as they are too subtle and require more sophisticated technology to uncover. Furthermore, the fact that there *are* brain differences doesn't yet help much with regard to interventions.

Chemical Differences

Many families are told at one time or another that the chemistry of their child's brain is different or that something is missing. Although this isn't the whole story, it isn't completely off the mark. The study of neurotransmitters, the substances that enable brain cells to talk to one another, is valuable. A number of major neurotransmitter systems have been identified as involved, and some well-done studies suggest that the concentrations of various neurotransmitters in the brains of children with ASD or ADHD may sometimes be different from the concentrations in typically developing children.

What Do We Do With This Information?

Has this type of research changed our practice or that of our colleagues in the field? It has certainly changed our understanding of these diagnoses as *biologically based*. Sometimes, by working backward, we can wager a guess about which neurotransmitter system is most likely to be involved when a behavior or symptom presents itself. Psychiatrists and psychopharmacologists are the most likely medical professionals to think this way. They work to understand the biological basis of these disorders, and pharmacological treatments are often based on their understanding of neurotransmitter systems. However, even though pharmacological treatments may be based on best guesses regarding neurotransmitter problems, they and the rest of us have a long way to go before we understand the role that neurotransmitters play and how to use the information to treat children more effectively.

Evaluation: How Your Child's Primary Care Provider Will Address Your Concerns

As pediatricians, we and our primary care colleagues are usually the first medical professionals to whom parents turn when they have developmental concerns. We are responsible for checking things out thoroughly, for making sure that whatever is going on is a developmental variation and not some other problem or disease. Although we rarely make a diagnosis of an underlying organic or metabolic disorder, parents need and deserve this kind of attention and information.

> When our son was in his infancy, with his failure to thrive and his developmental delay, his pediatrician was thinking much more about medical syndromes. He had an MRI—we wondered if he could have a brain tumor. We wondered if he might have celiac disease or cystic fibrosis because he didn't gain weight. Ruling these out was a relief on one hand, but it also increased my anxiety. It was almost as if, if it was a medical thing, it wasn't my responsibility; there was a piece of me that just wanted him to have a little medical thing. Developmental problems are much more complicated, and there's no quick fix.

There is a general consensus that an organic etiology is more likely for those disorders associated with lower cognitive function. In other words, the more severely delayed the child's development, the more important it is to look for an underlying explanation. It is now recommended that children with ASD see a geneticist for an evaluation and testing to look closely at chromosomal changes that are known to be associated with autism. All children with ASD should be tested for the Fragile X gene, the most common genetic cause of autism.

Medical History

When it comes to developmental problems, we ask a lot of questions about the medical history of the families of both parents and about the circumstances surrounding conception, gestation, and birth of the child. Some of these questions can really weigh parents down, as they can feel a sense of accusation. But every child's health and development are the product of complex combinations of genetic factors, prenatal influences, and environment, and teasing out some of the specifics is not meant as an accusation. We are trying to understand because we care about your child, and about future children; we're not trying to assign blame. Any professional evaluating your child, from your child's primary care provider to a developmental-behavioral pediatrician to a neuropsychologist, is likely to ask some of the same questions about your child's history. It can get tedious to answer repetitive questions, but it's the way we are trained, to elicit the history ourselves, not depend on the questions that our colleagues have asked. Yes, we do read each other's notes, but sometimes new history has been learned since that last interview.

- **Family history.** Is there a family history of developmental delays, intellectual disability, or ASD? Sometimes parents don't know the answers to these questions but go on a fact-finding mission with their families of origin. Keep in mind that the diagnostic labels change over time. With careful questioning, we often find someone on one side or the other who may mirror or echo a developmental difference.
- **Prenatal problems.** Were there problems before birth? There is increasing interest among researchers regarding whether prenatal factors might play a role. Does the mother have a number of miscarriages in her history? Is there a history of assisted conception such as in vitro fertilization (known to be associated with increased numbers of anatomic anomalies and now being studied with regard to developmental variations)? Were there complications or infections (especially rubella) during pregnancy? Is there a large age difference between the parents (some data suggest that when fathers are much older than mothers, the likelihood of ASD increases).
- **Perinatal events.** What events occurred around birth? Was the child born preterm or at full term? Were there complications at delivery? Was the infant deprived of oxygen for any length of time? Did he spend any time in the neonatal intensive care unit, needing oxygen, or even a ventilator? For how long? Were there any serious illnesses such as meningitis or encephalitis in the early months that required antibiotics?

- **Developmental history.** How has the child developed so far? Has her physical growth been normal? Were there motor or speech delays? Did she seem fine until a certain age at which her development arrested or regressed? Are her eating habits peculiar or different in some way? If age appropriate, is she toilet trained? What developmental concerns are most apparent now? What kind of temperament does the child have, and how does it fit with the temperaments of her parents? How does she express affection? Does she crave or avoid physical contact?
- **Current functioning.** How is a child functioning in his present setting? Are there difficulties with learning or attention? Does he engage with you in joint attention—pointing at something to interest you in it or looking at something to which you are drawing his attention? Does he make sustained eye contact? Does he respond when his name is called? How are his play skills? Is he able to transition easily from one activity to another or does he get stuck? How does he handle frustration? Is he explosive or otherwise difficult to manage at home? How do other children respond to him? Does he have friends in his community? What do his teachers say about him? Does he have any unusual skills, such as reading at a high level, telling time, a photographic memory, or perfect pitch? Does he have a hyperfocused interest in something, such as shapes, spinning objects, or insects?
- **Parental concerns.** Are you as the parents concerned about a possible medical problem? Parents often have specific worries related to an aspect of their child's behavior or development or perhaps related to something in the family history. On more than one occasion, parents have told us they are specifically concerned about bipolar disorder, depression, schizophrenia, obsessive-compulsive disorder, or a seizure disorder because of an affected relative.

We have had many conversations of this type with families worried about their children's development, and our antennae are up for possible developmental issues. What is of concern to one parent may be of no concern whatsoever to the other. In addition, parents have different expectations for their child's development. The same child may be viewed entirely differently depending on his parents. We need to be mindful of this and read between the lines to some extent. In retrospect, many parents tell us, they were concerned long before we picked up on their worries. We find ourselves wondering whether we were obtuse, or whether the parents realized only in retrospect that there were signs that something was amiss or at least not quite right.

Physical Examination

After the medical history is obtained, the next step is a careful examination of the child. With young children, this can be done quickly, although a terrified child or one who is sensitive to touch will not appreciate it. Before the child is even touched, careful observation of his behavior in the exam room can provide a fair amount of information in a short time. What are we thinking about and looking for when meeting a child?

- Does the child move easily from the waiting area to the examination area? Is she able to separate from her parent or caregiver when appropriate?
- Does the child make eye contact with us when we enter the room? Does she respond to her name being called?
- Can she tolerate being weighed on a scale, and having her head and body measured without becoming too upset?
- Is he interested in or curious about the equipment or toys in the office?
- Does he point with his index finger to draw your attention to something?
- Will she follow your gaze when you point at something?
- Does she use language? Is it functional? Does she echo what others in the room are saying?
- Does he use scripted speech—that is, recite lines from books or movies that, albeit somewhat relevant, aren't his own words?
- What is his prosody (the character of the voice and the fluency) like? Does he talk like a "little professor"?
- What about the child's level of physical energy? Is she still, constantly moving, or sitting all curled up in her mother's lap?
- Does she have any stereotyped movements, tics, or nervous habits that may be more likely to present themselves in the stressful environment of a doctor's office?
- Does he seem overly anxious?

A pediatrician with an interest in these issues and the time for proper observation will take notice of unusual behaviors or development. A second look may be necessary, or perhaps one visit will be spent entirely in observation and you'll make a new appointment for the physical examination. In any case, if you have concerns, make an appointment within a couple of months for a second look.

What are the specific aspects of a physical examination to which we pay particular attention when we are considering developmental questions?

- **Dysmorphic features.** Does the child have an unusual appearance? Are his eyes or ears different in any way? How large is his head? (One-quarter of the children diagnosed with ASD have large heads, that is, their head circumference is greater than that of 95% of children their age.) Large heads also tend to run in families, so don't be surprised if the doctor wants to measure your heads as well. Children with dysmorphic features are more likely to have an underlying genetic syndrome. Fragile X syndrome is an example:

This is an abnormality of the X chromosome, affecting mostly boys. It is a known genetic cause of ASD, especially in boys, although girls can also be affected. These children sometimes have large heads and large ears.

- **Skin lesions.** Some of the neurocutaneous syndromes—specifically, tuberous sclerosis or neurofibromatosis—can first appear as developmental differences due to small lesions or tumors in the brain. The associated skin lesions have a characteristic appearance (café au lait spots or ash leaf spots), though sometimes a special lamp, called a Wood's lamp, is required to see them clearly. These syndromes are serious but rare. A small number of kids turn out to have one of the neurocutaneous syndromes.

- **Abdominal examination.** Does the child have an enlarged liver or spleen? Enlargements in these abdominal organs are associated with certain rare metabolic disorders in which a missing enzyme can lead to buildup of a metabolite in the abdominal organs as well as in the brain, sometimes affecting behavior and development.

- **Careful neurological examination.** Not the easiest thing to do with an uncooperative toddler, a neurological examination can uncover subtle weakness or low muscle tone, poor coordination, and poor fine motor control. In addition to checking the reflexes, we usually ask a child to draw something with a marker or pencil to observe the manner in which he holds and uses the writing instrument. Depending on the child's age, we may ask him to stand on one foot to assess balance or close his eyes to determine whether he can maintain his posture without the visual input. These sorts of maneuvers will sometimes expose the subtle neurological weakness or poor coordination that is frequently seen in these children.

What Is the Optimal Management as My Child Grows?

While there is no simple blood test that will lead to a diagnosis for a quirky child, questionnaires and lists of possible behaviors are used by specialists to figure out what is going on. They interview parents to detail the child's developmental history and perform a careful behavioral assessment of the child. In addition, some commonly used medical tests often assist in figuring out what is going on with a quirky child.

Any child with a speech delay should undergo a hearing test. It should be repeated in a few months if the child's speech doesn't improve. Although very few children are actually deaf, a child may not have adequate hearing to pick up human speech, and a hearing device may help enormously. Some children may have fluid buildup behind the ear drum, which makes hearing difficult, and they may need tiny tubes inserted into the eardrums to reduce the fluid and improve hearing.

All children, and especially those with developmental delays, should be tested for lead poisoning. These simple tests should be part of the evaluation of any child with a suspected delay, and in fact are included in basic well child care for all children. A speech and language evaluation is indicated for any child with a clear delay in speech, particularly if there are other concerning aspects of development. Because certain chromosomal abnormalities are identified with ASD, a chromosomal analysis may be useful, especially if there is unexplained intellectual disability in other family members.

Referral to a geneticist for specialized genetic testing, including a Fragile X evaluation and a chromosomal microarray (both simple blood tests), is indicated for all children with a diagnosis of ASD. A geneticist is likely to perform a chromosomal blood test to look for gene mutations that could explain a child's presentation, and the findings may help with determining recurrence risks in future children. As mentioned earlier, the Fragile X gene is the most common genetic cause of ASD and is often associated with some physical features that may not be apparent until a child is about 3 years of age. That is relevant for genetic counseling because many families have already decided to have another child at that point. Prenatal testing for Fragile X is available, but the actual outcome for an individual child is nearly impossible to predict.

If an underlying disorder is suspected on the basis of the child's history, the family history, or the physical examination, certain targeted laboratory tests are indicated. For children who experience severe regression when they have a minor viral illness, a search for a metabolic disease is indicated. Kids whose parents describe cyclic periods of abnormal behavior may undergo electroencephalography (EEG) to look for a seizure disorder.

Although there is an increased incidence of seizures—particularly a rare kind called *complex partial seizures*—in older children with ASD, one neurological disorder associated with seizures is worth special mention: Landau-Kleffner syndrome. This rare syndrome can show up as developmental delays or developmental regression in a slightly older child. The diagnosis is made according to a specific pattern on the EEG, and about 25% of affected children will respond dramatically to treatment with seizure medications or steroids.

Although we support the targeted medical evaluation, most of the quirky kids we see are unlikely to have a clear medical explanation for their developmental differences. Still, a medical evaluation may help set a parent's mind at ease, may rule out some scary possibilities, and may be important for genetic counseling and planning for future children.

Genetic Implications: What About My Future Children?

The search for an etiology often ends without an answer, just as the deep basic questions about epidemiology have no clear answer. *Most* quirky kids do not have an underlying syndrome, a congenital infection, or a chromosomal abnormality. The first question many parents ask after "Why?" is "Will it happen again?" No one can tell you exactly. Other than the Fragile X syndrome, which we have discussed as a genetic cause of ASD, no diagnosis can be made on a prenatal genetic test for any of the quirky-kid diagnoses. But we do know that there is a genetic component. Based on empiric observation over time, the recurrence risk of ASD in a second child when the first child has ASD without a specific genetic explanation ranges from 6% to 14%. The risk is slightly higher if your first child is a girl. For families in which more than one child is affected, a subsequent child is 35% more likely to have ASD as well.

Does this change your mind about having another child? These are intensely personal decisions. There is no question that raising a quirky child involves heartache, but the prospects may look worse when the child is very young and all you have are unanswered questions about the future. If you have time, wait it out a bit before making such a lifelong decision. By all means, consult with a geneticist. A lot of progress has been made in the years since this book was first published, and many families have genetic information now that wasn't available 10 years ago. Geneticists will offer advice based on a family's genetic history in addition to chromosomal analyses. When a careful analysis of both families is complete, a geneticist or genetic counselor is in a better position to offer more specific risks for recurrence based on each family's history.

Associated Conditions: Are There Medical Problems to Expect as My Child Grows?

As you help your child deal with the implications of the diagnosis, be sure to keep the lines of communication open with your child's pediatric primary care provider. Our job in primary care does not end just because a medical etiology for the quirks has been considered and ruled out. Many questions remain, and a number of associated conditions may need attention in the years ahead, though it is impossible to predict which ones might affect a given quirky child. Once again, parents should look to the family history. If a cousin, an uncle, a brother, or a sister has a seizure disorder, that will increase the likelihood of seizures in your child. If there are family members with depression or obsessive-compulsive disorder or Tourette syndrome, these, too, may be more likely to become a part of your child's picture.

Seizures are probably the single most common medical condition associated with these disorders—specifically with ASD. About 20% of kids with ASD will have seizures, and they usually do not appear until adolescence. *Partial complex seizures* are the most common type and are not always immediately obvious as seizures to observers. Partial complex seizures usually present with facial grimacing and twisting, sometimes with staring or drooling or lip smacking, and they are sometimes confused with strokes because they can make the face look strange. These seizures are treatable with medications.

Some quirky kids don't grow well because of their peculiar dietary habits or because, once again, they seem to be wired differently. Many have constipation and many are slow to become toilet trained. They may have more trouble managing their allergies or following any other medical regimen that's prescribed. You and your child will benefit from a close relationship with a primary care provider who understands the whole package. And for children who struggle with restrictive eating, severe constipation, or acid reflux, a pediatric gastroenterologist and feeding team will be a helpful addition to the child's care over time.

Of course, quirky kids will experience the usual ear infections and strep throats, stomach viruses and drippy noses. You want those problems treated by someone familiar with your child's patterns and preferences, someone who understands, for example, that it's hard for your child to swallow medicine or that she can't cope with wiping a runny nose and needs antihistamines.

> Our doctor has told his staff that if I come in, I need to be brought right to an exam room. He is lovely with my kids and always asks me, "How are you?" I can't always answer that, or sometimes I don't want to, but I really appreciate that he seems to understand the trials of my life with my kids.

Most quirky kids are rather healthy, but it helps to have an ally who knows your child over time. Make sure your child's provider understands what your challenges are. Today's pediatricians and pediatric nurse practitioners all have experience with quirky kids, and are much more informed than even 10 years ago.

> We have a wonderful pediatrician whom we cannot praise enough. In the early years of our son's life, he was a learner along with us. His staff knows that we simply cannot wait for the usual time in the waiting room when Ben is sick. He is too restless and becomes agitated. He asks us to call in advance so his staff can set up a room, and then he sees us as promptly as possible. This is so kind and understanding, so generous, and it makes a huge difference. Our son likes going to the doctor and thinks of him as his friend.

PART

Looking Ahead

Quirky Characters

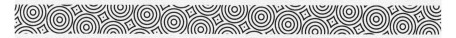

Among the many people, fictional and real, about whom it has been suggested that they have (or had) autism spectrum disorder:

Dilbert

Professor Henry Higgins

Sherlock Holmes

Mr. Spock

Jane Austen

Emily Dickinson

Thomas Edison

Albert Einstein

Glenn Gould

Alfred Hitchcock

Wolfgang Amadeus Mozart

Isaac Newton

Henry David Thoreau

Andy Warhol

Bill Gates

Dan Aykroyd

What You Should Know

> I worry about my daughter's future. Will she ever find someone to be
> with, of either gender? How would that person live with her? What
> if he or she also has a disorder? Should she ever have a baby? With
> the increased risk that she would have a special-needs child, I really
> don't think she could manage. I am not sure she could manage with
> a typical child. But of course, these aren't my decisions; they're hers.
> I think there is a place for her in the science world, and she will
> probably be able to live independently, but other aspects of life, I
> just don't know. She will need more support than a typical young
> adult, that's for sure.

Once quirky children have graduated from high school, they are
in certain respects no longer children. Eighteen-year-olds have to
be allowed a certain adult status, however nervous it makes us as
parents. In fact, many quirky kids with greater challenges may be in
high school until they are 22. Your child always remains your child
in a certain sense, though, and you go on watching closely, hoping
for the best, and vicariously experiencing both triumphs and tragedies. For the parents of a quirky child—bound together by having
traveled a more difficult, more unusual, and often more roundabout
road—the tendency is often to hover a little more closely and keep
on smoothing the way.

That is not necessarily a bad thing. Yes, you have to learn to hold
back a little, as your child grows into an adult. All parents do. Most
likely, the high school years have already started teaching you that
lesson. You probably will have progressively less say over many
details of how your child chooses to live. There's still no getting
around it: Quirky kids can have different issues or different time-
tables. Some of them aren't adults yet, despite their chronological
ages, and some struggle with the demands of adult life or are not
completely functional adults. Keep in mind that we are all learning

a lot about high school, college, and adulthood as these children grow. And a lot has been learned in the years since the first edition of this book came out, as many quirky kids have come of age and are functioning in the world in a wide variety of ways.

We don't want to patronize or offend those parents who are beginning to suspect that their children's entire futures will be circumscribed and even blighted by the adult versions of their quirks. Neither would it be fair to paint too bleak a picture, because many quirky children either will learn to accommodate to their differences and look less odd against the wider range of choices available to adults, or will actually find more or less triumphant ways of making their special traits work to their advantage as their lives unfold. These children grow up in so many different ways. It can be difficult, looking at them when they're young, to predict how things will develop and change.

We know you're in this for the long haul, and in Part 4, we talk a little bit about perspectives on quirky adulthood. We can't cover all the many situations that may arise, but we do offer some thought about how quirkiness fits (or doesn't fit) into various corners of adult life, some realistic looks at the accommodations that sometimes have to be made, and some hopeful stories and happy endings.

Brian's outlook is so much brighter than we ever imagined in his elementary school years. There were a lot of bleak times, when we thought he needed a residential program, when we worried that his options were severely limited. He's had a lot of help, but he has surprised all of us, even his psychiatrist. This summer he has a job ghostwriting proposals and doing spreadsheets. This is the same boy who couldn't get a sentence on a page until he was in fifth grade. It's just amazing what kids can outgrow.

12

Adolescence and Adulthood: Quirky Kids Grow Up

Adult life poses certain specific challenges, which, for some quirky kids, are especially difficult and, for some, frankly impossible. For some quirky adults, it may be particularly problematic to meet some of the basic expectations of adult life:

- Live independently and care for themselves
- Hold jobs and support themselves
- Maintain the human relationships needed to make them happy

All these are tall orders, and not just for quirky adults; they are the stuff of lifetime goals and internal struggles for many people. However, adult life offers considerably more scope for quirkiness than the rigid everybody-needs-to-be-good-at-everything sociology of childhood.

Quirky adults can shape their own worlds to fit themselves, choosing niches and platforms and stages from an almost infinite array of possibilities. Your job with your quirky child was at times to bend and rearrange his school so that his life fit better. Her job as an adult is to choose the right work, arrange her home, and set up a social life, creating the world that fits her best and in which she functions most happily and fully. Differentiating between the kids who are eccentric but still pretty functional and those who really struggle has been a balance throughout this book, and that's true in this chapter as well. When we say quirky adults, we could mean anything from someone with a genius IQ who cannot balance a checkbook to someone whose paralyzing anxieties and rigidity make it impossible to hold a job. We talk about general concerns that arise for just about everyone and don't presume to tell you where your kid is going.

What Happens After High School?

College is not for everybody. Kids, quirky or not, for whom academics are either uninteresting or incredibly difficult and who have interests or talents leading them in another direction should wave their friends and classmates off to college, and you should help them figure out what type of training or apprenticeship will be the best next step. There are vocational-training opportunities and entry-level jobs. If you're lucky, you started thinking about this before the last year of high school, and your child has had a chance to find out whether she really does love working in a garden supply store as much as she thought she would. In more academically oriented families, parents may have difficulty with a child's decision not to attend college or to delay attending, but remind yourself that everything can take a little longer with a quirky child.

Because many quirky children will at least want to try going to college, which may raise special issues around living away from home, we dive into those questions in some detail, but want to emphasize that this is not the only path.

Help your child look into other possibilities. A kid who is good with his hands, who has a knack for working with machines, or computers, or dough, or puppies, may be able to find a job that will pay him while he learns. Or there may be a particular certification to work toward or a course to take at a community college or a specialized academy.

Vocational Training Opportunities

Kids who attended vocational high schools, and those who extended their high school years, may already have had the chance to develop skills in their chosen fields and to serve internships and apprenticeships. Many community colleges offer certificate programs in vocational areas including preparing kids for fields as diverse as cosmetology and barber certification, veterinary technician assistant, floral arrangement, plumbing, electrical work, HVAC licenses, and many jobs in the medical field. These fields require a wide range of skills; some will require passing academic written tests, but others will rely much more on practical and technical knowledge. Many people who come out of such training programs end up working in medical centers, libraries, museums, post offices, animal care facilities, and the National Park Service. This tremendous range of possibilities means that parents can help a young adult think through them and look for a good match, and can also help research the training and certification requirements that may in themselves be daunting or difficult to decipher.

State disability agencies can provide funding support for young adults for technical or vocational training. Many states have vocational service agencies where a sheltered internship program provides support for an individual with a disability who is learning occupational skills and may actually provide specific help with workplace social expectations as well. If your son or daughter has had a good experience with vocational training or with an internship placement, you might consider offering to meet with a key person to discuss next steps. Community agencies and advocacy groups may also provide coaches—sometimes described as vocational coaches, or life coaches—who can work with young adults on an ongoing basis, helping them process the inevitable complexities of entering the workplace.

Don't forget about the importance of family, friends, and special contacts. Many young adults get their first jobs in a family store or some other business where a relative or a neighbor can keep a friendly eye on things.

College: Where to Attend

College isn't for everybody right away, either. Quirky kids tend to lag behind their chronological ages. Some kids stay in high school until they're 22 because it's written into their individualized education plan. Even when they graduate, they may not be ready for a full-time college experience, let alone for living away from home. Your child can stay home and attend a local school as a commuter or day student or enroll in school part time at a community college or an extension school; doing so offers an opportunity to try out college-level academics while living in a familiar situation, with all familiar supports. Anyone who starts out this way—or who starts out assuming that she isn't going to college at all—has the option of changing directions later on and going to college when she feels ready and eager for it.

> George did make it through college as a music major. He was close to home and I went to see him frequently. He also got a driver's license and had some independence. He has struggled in the work environment for a variety of reasons, so it's still very much a work in progress.

Many parents send their quirky kids to a college within an hour's drive, so they can visit regularly and welcome their child back home on weekends. That leaves parents more clued in to what's going on in their child's life than an occasional email asking for money or those unsatisfactory phone calls late at night from college student children who sound a little bit distracted.

College is a rich intellectual and social opportunity, but it is also a high-pressure environment. Parents need to recognize the high pressure and think realistically about their child's history, vulnerabilities, and the supports that need to be in place. A growing number of colleges have programs that cater to this population of kids who need extra academic and social support to thrive in college; if you think this might be your child, talk to a guidance counselor and to other parents, and do some research.

Your child is off to college. Now there is the question of finding a psychotherapist or counselor. By this age most quirky kids have some insight into what makes life difficult for them, and the social demands of a college campus can be dizzying, and not only for the quirky. You want to find out what the student health service offers. If it doesn't seem to have too much going on from a mental health point of view, you probably want to ask about outside referrals. If your child has been seeing a psychotherapist for some time, that person may be able to refer you to someone for the college years—the right person in the right place at the right time.

Another advantage of doing a certain amount of self-exploration in high school is that, with any luck at all, your child will develop a much greater degree of self-awareness, a stronger sense of emotional balance, and a heightened awareness of danger signals that something may be going wrong, such as increased anxiety, obsessive thoughts, or depressive moods. Having said this, many kids of all types find the first semester of college daunting and end up needing some counseling and support; a certain number of kids of all types also end up taking breaks and not going straight through to graduate in 4 years. If you can set your child up with a therapist who already knows her quirks and her history, this is more likely to work out. Some kids, quirky or not, realize fairly early in the first year of college that they aren't ready—for the academics, the social life, the being away from home—and decide to leave. This is not a failure; it is a change in plan. College will always be there.

Any child planning to go away to college right after high school ought to have been away from home before that for at least a couple of weeks. Parents of quirky kids sometimes tend to hold them close, but if a child can't go to math camp for 14 days the summer after her junior year of high school, that child probably isn't ready to move to another city and live in a dormitory.

College is a challenging time for everyone. A certain number of kids just go off the deep end, in one direction or another. Sometimes it's too much partying, experimenting with drugs or alcohol, or academic crashing and burning; sometimes it's eating disorders, destructive relationships, or withdrawal and depression. Many others seem to manage okay, but find themselves troubled by doubts and insecurities, academic, social, or both. Colleges vary in the level of support and supervision they provide, though many schools have been working hard to improve their mental health services. Consider the size of the school and its level of intensity. More fragile students do better in a smaller school where adults know them, watch them, and can help them if they're in trouble. Despite their best efforts, most big universities and state schools are rather anonymous places. That includes the Ivy League schools and many other prestigious seats of higher learning. At these institutions, supervision and support are likely to mean a dorm proctor or an adviser, often a graduate student with no professional training in counseling or psychology, and an academic adviser, who, in some cases, may provide a required signature on a study plan or a drop/add petition and not much more. And although more help is usually available from trained counselors, clergy, and doctors if you ask for it, the truth remains, at many big schools, a student can get into deep trouble of one kind or another before anyone in authority notices.

Many high schools encourage academically successful seniors to apply to the most prestigious colleges and universities, at least as "reaches." And the entire competitive ethos around college applications may encourage kids to try their luck and find out whether they can score the plum acceptances. Still, a kid who gets accepted by a big and prestigious university but is not quite up to dealing with this level of anonymity and fend-for-yourself spirit may be better off turning it down to go someplace smaller and more personalized, even if this means breaking a sacred family tradition. Alternatively, it may mean that for a student to function successfully at that big school, parents have to take even more responsibility and make sure that all the supports and help—both inside and outside the school—are in place.

Whether the school is big or small, parents need to keep track of what is going on, and remember that if the situation begins to go awry, no one's grade point average or dream of graduate school in engineering is worth a breakdown. As pediatricians, we have these discussions with many families, whether the kids are quirky or not, but as you probably already realize, if you have a college-bound quirky child, the experience is going to be more difficult and more intense for children who have struggled with standard expectations at earlier ages.

Dormitory Living and Other Arrangements

College may also mean living in close quarters with others. Some adolescents who may be academically ready are definitely not able to cope with dormitory life. When it comes to college living arrangements, think hard about what will work and what will be a problem. Many schools are willing to arrange a single room for a student who has special issues.

> The first year, Megan had a roommate. On parents' weekend in
> October, Megan and her roommate came to meet us, arm in arm, and
> I teared up, because this had never happened before. But it didn't
> last. By March, the roommate had moved out. We never got the
> whole story, but it had to do with the fact that the roommate had a
> boyfriend and he was spending time in their room, and this led to
> a lot of conflict. Other girls in the dorm sided with the roommate,
> and Megan lost friends and ended up living on her own. We didn't
> even know this had happened until she came home for the summer.
> She told us that it was none of our business but said, "Could you tell
> when you met her that she was evil?" That was her black-and-white
> way of explaining it to us.

Certainly, all colleges are making more accommodations for students with
learning differences and disabilities. Special programs or special adjustments
in the program or special arrangements for taking tests or for handing in
assignments are increasingly available, and a student who needs to take
exams in a quiet room alone or type all essay exams on a computer is likely
to be easily accommodated. You should make sure that the relevant office at
your child's college (eg, the office of learning disabilities, student support, or
academic affairs) is provided with complete information about your child's
learning needs.

> His college has a special education coordinator. She is there to help
> kids with accommodations they may need, but the kids have to go
> to her to get any help. She doesn't go looking for them. When we
> took our son for the first time, we went to meet her. I told her about
> his learning profile and anxiety, and she knew what we were talking
> about. When he did poorly on a physics test, he went to see her and
> took the next test untimed and did much better.

The most important thing about college, from the quirky person's point of
view (and indeed for all students), is that it is a golden opportunity to figure
yourself out according to your interests and preferences. High school may be a
bigger and more varied world than middle school, but college is a much bigger,
more interesting, and even more tolerant universe. Do you want to hang out
with the Trekkies who congregate every evening before dinner to watch *Star
Trek* reruns? Do you belong in the science center library that stays open until 2
in the morning?

College is a time for trying out new intellectual and personal interests and identities, and it can be a very forgiving place in which to experiment. Many quirky kids come into their own in college, with the social peculiarities and rigid hierarchies of high school long ago and far away. College has social pressures too, and whether it's the hubbub of a giant dining hall, the complex rules of fraternity and sorority culture, or the need to work on group projects that many colleges require, there are plenty of social situations that can be pretty tough for many kids, and especially complex for the quirky. It's probably also worth mentioning again the hot topic of sexual assaults on college campuses; students need to understand absolutely the rules about sexual consent, and also the arrangements in place to keep them safe on campus.

Embracing Their Identity

One important theme in your child's engagement with the somewhat daunting responsibilities of adult life will be his sense of himself, including his understanding of all that we have been calling quirkiness. Does your child see herself as belonging to a particular diagnostic category? A person living with ASD, attention-deficit/hyperactivity disorder, obsessive-compulsive disorder, or all three? If so, that can make for a different sense of identity than might evolve in a kid whose understanding of herself is that she is a math genius who gets anxious sometimes and has to take some medicine for it.

We are not saying that these are two different ways of describing the same person, but rather that each person formulates a sense of self based in part on how he interprets his quirks and challenges. One tempting syndrome affecting many medical students is the tendency to diagnose themselves with any syndrome they read about. In writing and researching this book, we realized that we have, at various times, sensory processing disorder, attentional difficulties, autistic features, and obsessional thought patterns. A young adult who has carried several diagnoses in her life may be particularly susceptible to this "medical student syndrome" and may be constantly constructing and reconstructing herself according to different combinations of mental and developmental disorders.

How quirky young adults formulate their ideas of self—identity, level of success, happiness in the world—depends on many things. There will always be a family context, a cultural context, a social context. We all know people who consider themselves failures despite multiple successes in life and people who consider themselves successes on the basis of making it from day to day. Some define themselves to one extent or another by their quirks—whether that means identifying with one particular diagnosis and forming a social circle from its support group or just limiting their social lives to some category of people with whom they have a great deal in common. Others resolutely refuse to define themselves in this way, insisting, perhaps, that it's the rest of the world that's weird.

Some young adults choose to identify themselves with specific communities, sometimes linked by a common diagnosis, and rely on support groups composed of others with similar wiring. Others may decide to reject the diagnosis completely in adulthood—call it denial or call it free choice—and construct their identities in other ways. As a parent, you should be sensitive to the kind of experimentation that goes on in these years of self-discovery and self-definition and, to the extent possible (with safety always in mind), let your child set the terms for how you talk to him and about him (and that can include gender and preferred pronoun), and attempt to forge together a new and somewhat different bond, one adult to another.

Living Independently

The parents of quirky children often worry tremendously about whether their children will be able to live independently and take care of themselves as adults. It is certainly true that there are individuals who take much longer to achieve any kind of independent life or whose independence, when it comes, may require regular support from nearby family members. Others may need special arrangements such as a supervised living situation or a group home. And those who are living on their own, as well as those who are not, may continue to need the support of a variety of professionals, from an occupational therapist to a psychiatrist. If this is what your child needs when the time comes, you will be out there looking for the best options, protecting and assisting the adult as you have protected and assisted the child. Many people also choose to live at home for all or part of their adult lives, and this choice does not necessarily reflect an inability to manage in the world. How many of us have adult siblings still living with their parents?

Sometimes parents worry that their young adult is refusing the adventure of adulthood or taking refuge online from the complexities of navigating the real world. We know some families of quirky young and not-so-young adults who are living with their parents and essentially refusing to be engaged in employment or a social life outside the home. With social media exploding in recent years, many young adults, not necessarily quirky, spend countless hours online. Motivating an adult child to reengage in the outside world can be a particularly heartbreaking challenge for parents, and they may welcome the support from therapists or other specialists who have known this young adult as a child and helped at other points along the way.

> My son is now in his late twenties, living in a group home, and has
> created a life for himself, with a job and a few friends with whom he
> shares his interest in sports. He can't manage on his own, though,
> and we worry as we age about how to be sure he is cared for and
> whether that is the responsibility of our other children. He's a pretty
> happy guy, though incredibly anxious. He often says he misses being
> a kid because the demands of adult life are hard.

For the great majority of quirky young adults, however, there will indeed be
that challenge of learning how to take care of themselves. Every detail of adult
life, from paying the rent to cooking, can pose a challenge to someone who
looks at the world from a different angle, whose motor skills never caught up,
and who struggles to understand the "hidden curriculum," those unspoken
rules that operate at work and in life more generally.

Some quirky kids, as they achieve adulthood and independence, take the
opportunity to cast off certain conventions or behaviors that have never made
sense to them. These can be anything from maintaining a clean apartment to
shaving every day. They may live in chaos and squalor, or in rigidly neat and
ordered environments in which nothing is ever allowed to be out of place.
Without family members or college roommates dictating a slightly more
conventional setup, some quirky young adults take the opportunity to finally
indulge their preferences to the extreme.

You can help your young adult get ready to take care of herself in much the
same way you once helped her get ready to go to a birthday party. Break down
the tasks of independent adult living and make sure she understands them.

- **Food.** Every quirky adult (well, every adult, if you ask us) should know how
  to prepare a few basic items and, most important, know how to buy, store,
  and prepare the things he really likes to eat and drink regularly. They should
  know how to scramble an egg, construct their favorite kind of sandwiches,
  make coffee, and prepare two or three of their favorite easy dinners. If this
  is truly not possible for your young adult, you may want to consider group
  living in a supportive environment.
- **Money.** Make sure your young adult knows how money is transferred and
  stored (checks, cash, debit cards, credit cards) and make sure she has some
  sense of relative sums. Explain how different bills are paid—the rent with
  a check left in the landlord's mailbox or possibly paid online, the phone
  bill paid online, and so on. If she is going to have access to a credit line,
  either through credit cards or a bank account cash reserve, make sure she
  understands that these debts accumulate interest at high rates.

- **Social Security.** Many adults with ASD qualify for Social Security income on the basis of their disabilities or their inability to make a living wage. This is worth looking into, as expenses related to supporting a quirky adult can be formidable.
- **Medical care.** Determine how your young adult will obtain health insurance. There's no one easy answer to this (although anyone with a severe disability of any kind ought to be eligible for any of several programs), but it's not something that can safely be left up to most young adults because the medical insurance world is a maze of confusing options. As of this writing, all young adults may stay on their parents' health insurance plan until age 26. Some insurance companies allow parents to apply for ongoing insurance for an adult child with a disability. And some young adults will qualify for public health insurance plans based on income.
- **Special medical care.** Does your child know whom to call if her problems act up? If her medication stops working or starts to produce strange side effects? Be sure she's connected in all ways she needs to be, but shift some of the responsibility for making and keeping appointments to her, if she's ready.
- **Maintenance.** Whom does your child call when the toilet won't flush, the stove burner won't light, or the water heater starts to leak? Many of us can remember calling our parents! Be available for consultations, but also make sure your child has a little basic grounding in changing a lightbulb or tightening a loose screw.
- **Logistics of daily life.** Opening a bank account, registering to vote, or renewing a driver's license can be hard to figure out the first time around. Once again, quirky kids and the adults they become often have a harder time figuring out even the things that come naturally to other people. The more you can help them break life down into manageable tasks and then get through those tasks, the easier it will be for them to keep safe, functional, and well connected.

It's generally a parent's job to provide a place of refuge if all this independence gets to be too much for your adult child. Most parents who have children, quirky or not, see this as part of the deal: *If you need to, you can come home and start again.* Many quirky people spend some part of their adult lives at home with their parents, and if you find yourself in that situation, you will quickly realize that it raises some difficult questions, maybe some you've been thinking about and wrestling with for a long time. If your quirky child is not completely able to live independently and take care of himself, who is going to be responsible for whatever care and support are necessary when you are no longer able to do it? Is this going to devolve on your child's sibling or siblings? Do you need to make special financial arrangements, set up a trust fund or a special annuity account? Do you need to write a will that leaves the house and money to one child, the one you think needs it most? If so, have you discussed it with the other family members? We feel the need to raise this issue once more—certainly not any parent's favorite long-term fantasy for a child—in the context of the quirky young adult's experiments in independent living.

Give your quirky child some space to figure out independence and adult life. You may be troubled, sad, or mildly disgusted at the arrangements he makes for himself, at the state of his kitchen or bathroom, his junk-food dependence, or the rag he calls a bathrobe. For the most part, keep quiet about these things (this could all be true with a nonquirky child as well, and we would give the same advice). Yes, you need to be there as a backup and resource and refuge, and you're certainly entitled to your opinion. But when your child starts to live independently as an adult, give her some space. Stand back a little, which can be harder for parents who know their children often have a more difficult time coping. But independence is independence. As long as nothing seems to be unsafe about the situation, you need to let your child make these attempts and explorations.

Holding a Job

Chrissie would like to do design work or something where she doesn't have to be around people too much. I don't think she'd be happy in the back office of a bank feeding data into a computer, but she also isn't going to be a public relations maven. Anything that requires a lot of quick changes during the day, such as journalism, won't be her strong suit.

There are many eccentric adults out there, some working in jobs that they have chosen to fit their kinks or that allow them full-time access to their obsessions—from feeding animals at the zoo to scheduling trains to splitting subatomic particles. Others work at more generic jobs, such as office jobs and civil service jobs, but they are unmistakably different from most of their colleagues in one way or another. In fact, some employers find quirky adults excellent employees: They follow the rules, arrive on time, are singularly focused, and don't get bogged down in office gossip. Some choose jobs that require no social skills, thus finally escaping the repeated ordeal of trying to figure out what other people are all about. Others pursue an all-consuming interest to the very top of academia, or Silicon Valley. Still others are creating art or playing music. That doesn't mean that any of these paths were necessarily straight or easy.

Quirky people, throughout life, may be subjected to teasing, bullying, and outright discrimination. This can happen in school, but it can certainly happen in the workplace as well. Discrimination on the basis of a disability is illegal, as is discrimination on the basis of race, sex, sexual identity, religion, or national origin—but that doesn't mean that these problems don't exist in many workplaces. Quirky young adults who are people of color are at especially high risk, as are those in the lesbian, gay, bisexual, transgender, queer, intersex, asexual (LGBTQIA) community and those coming from immigrant backgrounds. Parents may have to stay involved in helping their young adult understand what discrimination is, and figure out how to report and follow up on problems that are making the workplace difficult, uncomfortable, or unsafe. A vocational coach, especially one who is connected to an advocacy organization, should be able to guide your family here, and along with you as parents, reiterate to your child that this is illegal and unacceptable. The conversations you have been having with your child all through school about understanding differences, about bullying, and about racism are not going to stop when your child enters the workplace.

Many quirky young adults cycle through a number of jobs, sometimes very disappointed when things don't work out. Some do much better in a supportive work environment, structured for people who have difficulties functioning in a more typical workplace. Some can't manage a full-time job, but part-time work can be meaningful and satisfying.

What this means is important: Most quirky kids grow up to be quirky adults who find ways to function and to contribute to society. Most find places in the world. You need to help your child find that place and, above all, not fix your own and your child's ambitions too firmly on any one particular professional destiny. She has to choose, and you have to be proud of her, not disappointed, once she's chosen.

Some quirky children grow to achieve as much as anyone; they start companies, make discoveries, write symphonies, or win Nobel Prizes. Most of them, however, just like most of the rest of us, will live reasonably decent lives and do their best. So make suggestions, but let your child take the lead and show you where she wants to go.

Relationships

Marriage and children are Chrissie's dream, but I don't know if she'll be able to handle it. What I really worry about is her loving spirit being taken advantage of.

We all want our children, as adults, to find the interpersonal connections and important relationships that lead to happiness and even love. We don't want them to be alone and we hope they will be surrounded by people who appreciate them, understand them, value them, take care of them, and love them. In other words, what we most want for them is that which has been most challenging all along: meaningful social relationships with people who treat them well. We don't have the ability to make that happen (and neither do the parents of nonquirky children). It's up to the adults themselves and to chance and fate and circumstance.

Many of the points we've made about puberty and sexuality apply here as well. It's very important to keep having those conversations with your grown-up child about safety, about respecting other people's boundaries, and about treating people well. There are dedicated dating platforms for people with ASD, and lots of books, websites, and videos to help the quirky navigate this side of life. One important issue in this population is gender identity; a disproportionate number of quirky kids are not comfortable with the gender they were assigned at birth. They are more likely to find themselves in the LGBTQIA community, with all its different possible self-definitions. Some will be gender nonconforming, nonbinary; others may define themselves as asexual. Your job as a parent, here as elsewhere, is to love and understand your child as he (or she or they) most wants to be understood and appreciated.

Some quirky children always get along better with adults than with children their own ages. Once they are adults themselves and no longer have to deal with children at all, social life can become easier. Their colleagues and social contacts are much less likely to tease or bully them, although they may perceive them as odd, eccentric, or weird. Adult life is full of alternative places to meet and greet. By choosing their venues carefully, most adults can find at least sporadic opportunities to assort themselves with like-minded folks.

Probably the most hopeful and useful advice you can give quirky adults is to do exactly that: Find your own special peer group, the club or clubs of which you are a member. The internet has made it much easier for small groups of people with rarefied interests to find one another and connect. Certainly, there are quirky adults who live their realest, truest lives during the time they spend at particular kinds of conventions—from historical reenactments to fantasy game sessions. Some of these individuals have complete alter egos, characters they assume—down to the attitudes, accent, and costume—when they are outside their own often humdrum daily lives and able to associate with their true friends.

Is any of this comforting to a parent who fears that, in a basic sense, this quirky child—now quirky adult—will always be alone, will never establish a long-term relationship, find a mate, or build a truly secure base of home and family? We have no way to answer this question. Thus, taking our place in a rich tradition of people with no firm answers, we can offer only a little philosophy.

Some really quirky adults do find long-term relationships, astonishingly good fits. Of course, there are also many not-at-all-quirky adults who never find the long-term relationships they earnestly and endlessly seek. And there are many adults, quirky and not, who are not seeking a single permanent long-term relationship but have other ways of living their lives and establishing their place in the world. It's more important to think in terms of the many relationships that keep most people connected in the world and look at strategies for finding them if you happen to be a little eccentric. Quirky adults, as we previously said, often need to search out a peer group, not necessarily as a way of finding that one special someone but as a way of finding a setting in which they are not seen as odd.

Remember that your quirky child who has grown into a quirky young adult may not define romantic success in the same way that you do. Don't set yourself up for disappointment by projecting your wishes and imagining a Hollywood ending for a child whose whole life has been anything but. If your young adult is actually yearning for some kind of connection and finding it elusive, then by all means try to help, but be sure the yearning is not your own.

Many adults find connections and contacts through religious groups or community groups or through volunteering. The more ways you can help your young adult link up with other people, the more likely it is that those people may include friends, companions, and even perhaps something more.

Some of the quirky children we love grow up to be relatively solitary and definitely quirky adults. Others find ways to make their quirks work for them and draw friends, admirers, and even disciples. You can't predict an adult's social future by watching a child on the playground or even on the high school dance floor. Though some adult lives are sad and disappointing, others are remarkably happy, and many are downright quirky.

I have managed to live a whole lifetime—I'm 71—and somehow, I could never learn things. I didn't learn to drive until I was 45 years old. But I am an artist, the greatest artist in the world. I had to teach myself how to draw and how to paint. I can teach anyone to draw like an old master. I give talks a lot about art.

A Final Word

The world would be a poorer, plainer place without the quirky. Without the quirky children, who extend the range of normal in the schoolroom, in the pediatrician's office, or on the playground. Without the quirky adults, who remind us that not all lives are alike or predictable or easily explained. The world would be a duller and more monochrome place without the artists and musicians and writers who have seen and heard and felt a little differently from the rest. And the world would be a less-understood place without the scientists and visionaries who have seen around corners with their unusual eyes and thought through walls with their differently wired brains. We honor the different drummer among adults when we hear the beats as creativity or even as conviction and principle.

Children, on the other hand, live in a more conformist and regulated world. Despite a great deal of romantic twaddle about the freedom and innocence of childhood, the truth is that many children's lives are strictly regulated, and no major deviations from the norm are tolerated. A child can't wake up one morning and say, "That's it. I'm through forever with math, with riding those dumb buses, with pretending I like the great outdoors." But adults can easily make such arrangements for themselves.

Quirky children, as you know, can be frustrating, inspiring, puzzling, delightful, devastating, and highly entertaining. Our goal in writing this book was to offer some practical help and some general philosophy about doing the always hard and always different parental job with these children, and to do that, at least in part, from this standpoint: The world needs its quirky children, its quirky adults, its quirky minds, and its quirky sensibilities. For all the challenges they face, quirky people enlarge and enhance life for us all.

Resources

Although this list is by no means exhaustive, we have found these resources most useful, both for us as pediatricians and for the parents of children in our care. Older kids and young adults have given positive feedback as well. These days, most resources are web-based, although there are still some great books that we recommend here.

General Resources

The American Academy of Pediatrics HealthyChildren.org website is an excellent resource for parents, families, and educators working with children of any age from newborns to young adults. Featuring evidence-based guidelines and information, HealthyChildren.org is an excellent place to start for more information.

www.HealthyChildren.org

The American Academy of Child and Adolescent Psychiatry Family Resources website is useful for parents of children with any emotional, mental health, or behavioral disorders. There are resources for families for all of the diagnoses we have discussed in this book.

https://www.aacap.org/AACAP/Families_and_Youth/Family_Resources/
Home.aspx

The Centers for Disease Control and Prevention "Learn the Signs. Act Early." website provides developmental tracking tools for parents.

https://www.cdc.gov/ncbddd/actearly/index.html

ep Magazine provides practical advice, emotional support, and the most up-to-date educational information for families of children and adults with any sort of developmental difference.

www.ep-magazine.com

Specific Resources

Here are some resources that address some specific issues common among quirky kids.

Anxiety

Pincus DB. *Growing Up Brave: Expert Strategies for Helping Your Child Overcome Fear, Stress, and Anxiety.* Little, Brown and Co; 2012

Autism

American Academy of Pediatrics. *Autism Spectrum Disorder: What Every Parent Needs to Know.* 2nd ed. Rosenblatt AI, Carbone PS, eds. American Academy of Pediatrics; 2019

Autism Speaks is a national organization dedicated to promoting solutions across the spectrum and throughout the life span for the needs of individuals with autism spectrum disorder and families. Its website is constantly updated and is a rich resource for parents and educators. There are detailed descriptions of all the therapeutic modalities we address in this book.

https://www.autismspeaks.org

The New York Times. Understanding Autism: Research and Science; Family Matters; Help and Support. The New York Times; March 27, 2020

A comprehensive look at current understanding of autism spectrum disorder in all its forms, this publication is a collection of articles on research and science, family life, and help and support.

Gray C. *The New Social Story Book.* 15th anniversary ed. Future Horizons; 2015

Many parents and educators swear by the use of social stories to help kids anticipate challenging social situations. This is a workbook for adults and kids to use together.

Silberman S. *NeuroTribes: The Legacy of Autism and the Future of Neurodiversity.* Avery; 2016

Attention-Deficit/Hyperactivity Disorder

Wolraich ML, Hagan JF Jr. *ADHD: What Every Parent Needs to Know.* 3rd ed. American Academy of Pediatrics; 2019

ADDitude magazine is both a print subscription and a website with useful evidence-based articles for parents and individuals of any age with attention-deficit/hyperactivity disorder (ADHD). There is a wealth of information on remote learning strategies for learners with ADHD that is especially useful in 2020.

https://www.additudemag.com

CHADD (Children and Adults with Attention-Deficit/Hyperactivity Disorder) is a national nonprofit that holds in-person and virtual parent and patient support groups. Toolkits for parents about ADHD and other comorbidities can be found here. These are endorsed by the American Academy of Pediatrics.

https://chadd.org

HowToADHD is a YouTube channel run by a young woman with ADHD that adolescents and young adults enjoy.

https://www.howtoadhd.com

Rief SF. *The ADHD Book of Lists: A Practical Guide for Helping Children and Teens with Attention Deficit Disorders.* 2nd ed. Jossey-Bass; 2015

Bertin M. *The Family ADHD Solution: A Scientific Approach to Maximizing Your Child's Attention and Minimizing Parental Stress.* St. Martin's Press; 2011

Managing in School

We highly recommend the Mindset Kit for families and educators. The Mindset Kit supports the notion that intelligence can be developed, that's it not a fixed construct, and that when kids believe they belong in school, they will learn.

https://www.mindsetkit.org

For Adolescents and Young Adults

Nichols S, Moravcik GM, Tetenbaum SP. *Girls Growing Up on the Autism Spectrum: What Parents and Professionals Should Know About the Pre-Teen and Teenage Years.* Jessica Kingsley Publishers; 2009

Hartman D. *The Growing Up Book for Boys: What Boys on the Autism Spectrum Need to Know!* Jessica Kingsley Publishers; 2015

Attwood S. *Making Sense of Sex: A Forthright Guide to Puberty, Sex and Relationships for People with Asperger's Syndrome.* Jessica Kingsley Publishers; 2008

Bair-Merritt M, Broder-Fingert S, Rothman EF. *Safer Dating for Youth on the Autism Spectrum.* https://www.bmc.org/sites/default/files/Patient_Care/Specialty_Care/Pediatrics%20-%20Autism/resources/Safer-Dating-ASD.PDF. Published January 2020. Accessed September 21, 2020

This is a document created by 3 colleagues at Boston Medical Center, 2 pediatricians and a clinical psychologist. It's a terrific resource about safe dating for individuals on the autism spectrum. We highly recommend it.

Index